DA

# Mammography and Beyond: Developing Technologies for the Early Detection of Breast Cancer

Committee on Technologies for the Early Detection of Breast Cancer

Sharyl J. Nass, I. Craig Henderson, and Joyce C. Lashof, *Editors*

National Cancer Policy Board

INSTITUTE OF MEDICINE

and

Division of Earth and Life Studies
NATIONAL RESEARCH COUNCIL

NATIONAL ACADEMY PRESS
Washington, DC

NATONAL ACADEMY PRESS • 2101 Constitution Avenue, N.W. • Washington, DC 20418

NOTICE: The project that is the subject of this report was approved by the Institute of Medicine and the Governing Board of the National Research Council, whose members are drawn from the councils of the National Academy of Sciences, the National Academy of Engineering, and the Institute of Medicine. The members of the committee responsible for the report were chosen for their special competences and with regard for appropriate balance.

Support for this project was provided by the Breast Cancer Research Foundation, the Carl J. Herzog Foundation, Mr. John K. Castle, the Jewish Healthcare Foundation (Pittsburgh, PA), the Josiah Macy, Jr., Foundation, the Kansas Health Foundation, and the New York Community Trust. The views presented in this report are those of the Committee on Technologies for Early Detection of Breast Cancer and are not necessarily those of the sponsors.

**Library of Congress Cataloging-in-Publication Data**

Mammography and beyond : developing technologies for the early detection of breast cancer / Committee on the Early Detection of Breast Cancer ; Sharyl J. Nass, I. Craig Henderson, and Joyce C. Lashof, editors ; National Cancer Policy Board, Institute of Medicine and Commission on Life Sciences, National Research Council.
    p. ; cm.
    Includes bibliographical references and index.
    ISBN 0-309-07283-2
    1. Breast—Cancer—Diagnosis. 2. Breast—Imaging. 3. Medical screening.
I. Nass, Sharyl J. II. Henderson, I. Craig. III. Lashof, Joyce C. IV. Institute of Medicine (U.S.). Committee on the Early Detection of Breast Cancer. V. National Cancer Policy Board (U.S.).
    [DNLM: 1. Breast Neoplasms—diagnosis. 2. Mammography. 3. Mass Screening. WP 870 M2649 2001]
    RC280.B8 M29 2001
    616.99′449075—dc21
                                              2001030885

Additional copies of this report are available from the National Academy Press, 2101 Constitution Avenue, N.W., Box 285, Washington, DC 20055. The full text of this report is available on line at **www.nap.edu**.

For more information about the Institute of Medicine, visit the IOM home page at **www.iom.edu**.

COVER: Rosalie Ann Cassell, *Waiting for the Biopsy*, 1998. 18″ x 22″. Watercolor and ink. http://www.breastcancerfund.org/gallery_6.html. Art. Rage. Us. The Art and Outrage of Breast Cancer.

# THE NATIONAL ACADEMIES

National Academy of Sciences
National Academy of Engineering
Institute of Medicine
National Research Council

The **National Academy of Sciences** is a private, nonprofit, self-perpetuating society of distinguished scholars engaged in scientific and engineering research, dedicated to the furtherance of science and technology and to their use for the general welfare. Upon the authority of the charter granted to it by the Congress in 1863, the Academy has a mandate that requires it to advise the federal government on scientific and technical matters. Dr. Bruce M. Alberts is president of the National Academy of Sciences.

The **National Academy of Engineering** was established in 1964, under the charter of the National Academy of Sciences, as a parallel organization of outstanding engineers. It is autonomous in its administration and in the selection of its members, sharing with the National Academy of Sciences the responsibility for advising the federal government. The National Academy of Engineering also sponsors engineering programs aimed at meeting national needs, encourages education and research, and recognizes the superior achievements of engineers. Dr. William A. Wulf is president of the National Academy of Engineering.

The **Institute of Medicine** was established in 1970 by the National Academy of Sciences to secure the services of eminent members of appropriate professions in the examination of policy matters pertaining to the health of the public. The Institute acts under the responsibility given to the National Academy of Sciences by its congressional charter to be an adviser to the federal government and, upon its own initiative, to identify issues of medical care, research, and education. Dr. Kenneth I. Shine is president of the Institute of Medicine.

The **National Research Council** was organized by the National Academy of Sciences in 1916 to associate the broad community of science and technology with the Academy's purposes of furthering knowledge and advising the federal government. Functioning in accordance with general policies determined by the Academy, the Council has become the principal operating agency of both the National Academy of Sciences and the National Academy of Engineering in providing services to the government, the public, and the scientific and engineering communities. The Council is administered jointly by both Academies and the Institute of Medicine. Dr. Bruce M. Alberts and Dr. William A. Wulf are chairman and vice chairman, respectively, of the National Research Council.

MICHAEL W. VANNIER, M.D., Professor and Head, Department of Radiology, University of Iowa College of Medicine, Iowa City, Iowa

DEREK VAN AMERONGEN, M.D., M.S., FACOG, Chief Medical Officer, Humana/ Choice Care, Cincinnati, OH

### Liaison for the National Cancer Policy Board

ROBERT DAY, M.D., M.P.H., Ph.D., Emeritus President and Director, Fred Hutchinson Cancer Research Center, Seattle, WA

### Consultants

LARRY NORTON, M.D., Chief, Solid Tumors, Memorial Sloan-Kettering, New York, NY

BARRON LERNER, M.D., Ph.D, Assistant Professor of Medicine and Public Health (in the Center for the Study of Society and Medicine), Columbia University, New York, NY

### Staff

SHARYL J. NASS, Ph.D., Study Director

ROBERT COOK-DEEGAN, M.D., Director, National Cancer Policy Board (through August 2000)

ROGER HERDMAN, M.D., Director, National Cancer Policy Board (from September 2000)

CARMIE CHAN, Research Assistant (through August 2000)

MARYJOY BALLANTYNE, Research Assistant (from August 2000)

BIANCA TAYLOR, Project Assistant

JOHN KUCEWICZ, Intern

KEVIN COLLINS, Intern

ELLEN JOHNSON, Administrative Assistant (through June 2000)

NICCI DOWD, Administrative Assistant (from August 2000)

GARY WALKER, Financial Associate (through September 2000)

JENNIFER CANGCO, Financial Associate (from September 2000)

### Commissioned Writers

(for lay summaries of the report, workshop proceedings, and current practice in breast cancer diagnosis)

MARGIE PATLAK

(see http://www4.nationalacademies.org/IOM/IOMHome.nsf/Pages/ Breast+Cancer+Detection)

LAURA NEWMAN, M.A.

(see http://www.nap.edu/catalog/9893.html» and http:// www.nap.edu/catalog/10011.html)

# Reviewers

This report has been reviewed in draft form by individuals chosen for their diverse perspectives and technical expertise, in accordance with procedures approved by the NRC's Report Review Committee. The purpose of this independent review is to provide candid and critical comments that will assist the institution in making its published report as sound as possible and to ensure that the report meets institutional standards for objectivity, evidence, and responsiveness to the study charge. The review comments and draft manuscript remain confidential to protect the integrity of the deliberative process. We wish to thank the following individuals for their review of this report:

**Thomas F. Budinger, M.D., Ph.D.**, Head, Center for Functional Imaging, E.O. Lawrence Berkeley National Laboratory

**Webster K. Cavanee, Ph.D.,** Director, Laboratory of Tumor Biology, Ludwig Institute for Cancer Research, University of California-San Diego

**Joann G. Elmore, Ph.D.,** Assistant Professor, Department of Medicine, University of Washington

**Samuel Hellman, M.D.,** A.N. Pritzker Distinguished Service Professor, Center for Advanced Medicine, The University of Chicago

**Barbara J. McNeil, M.D., Ph.D.,** Professor and Head, Department of Health Care Policy, Harvard Medical School

**Susan Scherr,** Director, Survivorship Programs, National Coalition for Cancer Survivorship, Silver Spring, MD

Although the reviewers listed above have provided many constructive comments and suggestions, they were not asked to endorse the conclusions or recommendations nor did they see the final draft of the report before its release. The review of this report was overseen by **Barbara Hulka, M.D., M.P.H.,** Kenan Professor, Department of Epidemiology, University of North Carolina at Chapel Hill, appointed by the Institute of Medicine, and **Mary Jane Osborn, Ph.D.**, Department of Microbiology, University of Connecticut Health Center, appointed by the NRC's Report Review Committee, who were responsible for making certain that an independent examination of this report was carried out in accordance with institutional procedures and that all review comments were carefully considered. Responsibility for the final content of this report rests entirely with the authoring committee and the institution.

# Preface

Breast cancer remains a leading cause of cancer death among women in the United States. More than 180,000 new cases of invasive breast cancer are diagnosed each year, and more than 40,000 women die of the disease. Recent years, however, have seen improvements in survival attributed to better treatment and earlier diagnosis. Research efforts have been directed toward better treatment, preventive strategies, and early detection. Although mammography has been the mainstay of early detection, its limitations are well recognized and the search for more effective technologies for early detection has been receiving increased attention. As part of this increased attention, the Institute of Medicine (IOM) convened a committee to examine the current state of the art in early breast cancer detection, to identify promising new technologies, and to examine the many steps in medical technology development and the policies that influence their adoption and use. The IOM committee consisted of a 16-member interdisciplinary group with a wide range of views and expertise in breast cancer, medical imaging, cancer biology, epidemiology, economics, and technology assessment. The committee examined the peer-reviewed literature, met four times, held two workshops that dealt with new technologies as well as policies related to their adoption and dissemination, and consulted with experts in the field.

Early detection is widely believed to save lives by facilitating intervention early in the course of the disease, at a stage when cancer treatment is most likely to be effective. This concept, however, belies a number of complexities, not the least of which is the need to understand the basic biology of breast cancer. The committee recognized the need for research on the natural history of breast cancer to more clearly define the significance of early lesions, the need for the development of biomarkers, and the importance of assessing the effectiveness of new technologies in decreasing morbidity and mortality. This report describes many novel technologies that are being developed for the purpose of early breast cancer detection, as well as recent technological advances in detection modalities already in use. Because the many technologies that the committee examined were at different stages of development and thus the evidence of their accuracy and effectiveness varied, the committee found it difficult to predict which of the many new technologies were likely to play a role in the future of early breast cancer detection.

The committee also identified a number of barriers to both the development and the dissemination of new technologies and made recommendations for actions that can be taken to overcome them. Many new technologies are on the horizon and intriguing research in basic biology is under way, but much remains to be done. We are hopeful that this report will contribute in some small way to the efforts to improve our ability to detect breast cancer at an early stage. The committee was impressed with the dedication and commitment of the researchers in both the public and the private sectors and with the governmental personnel working to save the lives of women, and we are hopeful that their efforts will prove fruitful.

Joyce C. Lashof
*Chair*

# Acknowledgments

The committee wishes to thank all of the people who contributed to this report. First and foremost we wish to acknowledge the outstanding work of the study director, Sharyl Nass. Sharyl was responsible for the extensive literature search, for selecting an outstanding group of speakers for the two workshops, as well as preparing the initial drafts and revisions of the entire report. Her ability to identify the key issues as well as the key players was instrumental in carrying out the work of the committee. She was responsive to the committee members throughout, and we all found it a pleasure to work with her. We also thank Carmie Chan and MaryJoy Ballantyne who provided invaluable research assistance. We were further assisted by two interns, John Kucewicz and Kevin Collins, who made substantial contributions to the completion of Chapters 2 and 6, respectively. We also appreciate the efforts of Bianca Taylor, who took primary responsibility for organizing the logistics of all the committee meetings and workshops and who was very helpful in keeping the study on schedule. The senior staff of the National Cancer Policy Board (Roger Herdman, Robert Cook-Deegan, Maria Hewitt, and Hellen Gelband) all provided valuable feedback on drafts of the report.

We also wish to thank all of the workshop speakers and participants, as well as a host of others who contributed to the study by speaking at meetings or by providing data and other written materials. The names and affiliations of all the speakers and other contributors are listed in Appendix A.

All of the committee members gave generously of their time and were important collaborators throughout the deliberations and preparation of the report. Several members made primary contributions in drafting the report, and are noted for their efforts as follows: Chapter 1, Daniel Hayes; Chapter 2, Janet Baum and Michael Vannier; Chapter 3, Craig Allred, Jean Latimer, and Kenneth Offitt; Chapter 5, Suzanne Fletcher, Marthe Gold, Derek Van Amerongen, and Wade Aubry. In addition, Carolina Hinestrosa provided valuable and insightful comments that were incorporated into all the chapters of the report. We also thank Craig Henderson, vice-chair of the committee, for his thoughtful advice and insight throughout.

Finally, we owe a debt of gratitude to the seven independent foundations and individuals who provided the funds needed to undertake this study. This report could not have been produced were it not for the generosity of the Breast Cancer Research Foundation, the Carl J. Herzog Foundation, Mr. John K. Castle, the Jewish Healthcare Foundation, the Josiah Macy, Jr., Foundation, the Kansas Health Foundation, and the New York Community Trust.

# Acronyms

ABBI        advanced breast biopsy instrumentation
ABR         American Board on Radiology
ACRIN       American College of Radiology Imaging Network
ACS         American Cancer Society
AHRQ        Agency for Healthcare Research and Quality
ART         Advanced Research and Technology
AT          ataxia telangiectasia
ATP         Advanced Technology Program

BBE         Biofield Breast Examination
BCBSA       Blue Cross/Blue Shield Association
BC-PRG      Breast Cancer Progress Review Group
BCRP        Breast Cancer Research Program
BCSC        Breast Cancer Surveillance Consortium
BIRADS      Breast Imaging Reporting and Data System
BISTIC      Biomedical Information Science and Technology
                Implementation Consortium
BRCA        breast cancer-associated tumor suppressor gene
BSE         breast self-examination

CAD         computer-aided detection or diagnosis
CBE         clinical breast examination
CDC         Centers for Disease Control and Prevention
cDNA        complementary deoxyribonucleic acid
CEA         carcinoembryonic antigen
CGAP        Cancer Genome Anatomy Project

| CIA   | Central Intelligence Agency |
| CLIA  | Clinical Laboratory Improvement Amendments |
| CNB   | core-needle biopsy |
| CPTA  | Center for Practice and Technology Assessment |
|       | |
| DOD   | U.S. Department of Defense |
|       | |
| EITS  | electrical impedance tomography system |
| EPC   | evidence-based practice centers |
| ESS   | elastic scattering spectroscopy |
|       | |
| FDA   | Food and Drug Administration |
| FDAMA | Food and Drug Administration Modernization Act |
| FFDM  | Full-field digital mammography |
| FISH  | fluorescent in situ hybridization |
| FNA   | fine-needle aspiration |
| FNAB  | fine-needle aspiration biopsy |
| FSM   | film-screen mammography |
|       | |
| GAO   | General Accounting Office |
|       | |
| HCFA  | Health Care Financing Administration |
| HEI   | Hall effect imaging |
| HGRI  | National Human Genome Research Institute |
| HIP   | Health Insurance Plan of Greater New York |
| HMEC  | human mammary epithelial cells |
| HRSA  | Health Resources and Services Administration |
|       | |
| IBC   | invasive breast cancer |
| IDE   | investigational device exemption |
| IGF1  | insulin-like growth factor type 1 |
| IMDS  | Imaging Diagnostic System, Inc. |
| IOM   | Institute of Medicine |
| IRB   | institutional review board |
|       | |
| LCIS  | lobular carcinoma in situ |
| LOH   | loss of heterozygosity |
|       | |
| MCAC  | Medicare Coverage Advisory Committee |
| MIBI  | technetium-99m sestamibi |
| MMG   | magnetomammography |
| MQSA  | Mammography Quality Standards Act of 1976 |
| MRI   | magnetic resonance imaging |

| | |
|---|---|
| mRNA | messenger ribonucleic acid |
| MRS | magnetic resonance spectroscopy |
| | |
| NAF | nipple aspiration fluid |
| NCHCT | National Center for Health Care Technology |
| NCI | National Cancer Institute |
| NEMA | National Electrical Manufacturers' Association |
| NIH | National Institutes of Health |
| NIST | National Institute of Standards and Technology |
| NMD | National Mammography Database |
| | |
| OBBB | Office of Bioengineering, Bioimaging, and Bioinformatics |
| OTA | Office of Technology Assessment |
| OWH | Office on Women's Health |
| | |
| PCR | polymerase chain reaction |
| PET | positron emission tomography |
| PMA | premarketing approval |
| PPV | positive predictive value |
| PSA | Prostate specific antigen |
| PTEN | tumor suppressor gene |
| | |
| QALY | quality-adjusted life year |
| | |
| RCP | riboflavin carrier protein |
| RNA | ribonucleic acid |
| RO1 | a type of grant from the National Institutes of Health |
| RT | reverse transcription |
| RVU | relative value unit |
| | |
| SACGT | Secretary's Advisory Committee on Genetic Testing |
| SBI | Society of Breast Imaging |
| SBIR | Small Business Innovative Research |
| SNP | single nucleotide polymorphism |
| SPECT | Single-photon emission computed tomography |
| SQUID | superconducting quantum interference device |
| STTR | Small Business Technology Transfer Research |
| | |
| TACT | tuned aperture computed tomography |
| TCT | thermoacoustic computed tomography |
| TEC | Technology Evaluation Center |
| | |
| USAMRMC | U.S. Army Medical Research and Materiel Command |
| USPSTF | U.S. Preventive Services Task Force |

# Contents

# Mammography and Beyond:

# Executive Summary

Breast cancer takes a tremendous toll in the United States. After lung cancer, breast cancer is the second leading cause of death from cancer among women in the United States and is the most common non-skin-related malignancy among U.S. women. Each year, more than 180,000 new cases of invasive breast cancer are diagnosed and more than 40,000 women die from the disease. Until research uncovers a way to prevent breast cancer or to cure all women regardless of when their tumors are found, early detection will be looked upon as the best hope for reducing the burden of this disease. The hope is that early detection of breast cancer by screening could be as effective at saving lives as the Papanicolaou smear (Pap smear) used for cervical cancer screening.

Early detection is widely believed to reduce breast cancer mortality by allowing intervention at an earlier stage of cancer progression. Clinical data show that women diagnosed with early-stage breast cancers are less likely to die of the disease than those diagnosed with more advanced stages of breast cancer. A thorough annual physical breast examination and monthly breast self-examination can often detect tumors that are smaller than those found in the absence of such examinations, but data on the ability of physical examinations alone to reduce breast cancer mortality are limited. X-ray mammography, with or without a clinical examination, has been shown in randomized clinical trials both to detect cancer at an earlier stage and to reduce disease-specific mortality. As a result, screening mammography has secured a place as part of routine health maintenance procedures for women in the United States. The mortality rate from breast cancer has been decreasing in the United States by about 2 percent per year over the last decade, suggesting that early detection and improved therapy are both having an impact on the disease.

Mammography is not perfect, however. Routine screening in clinical trials resulted in a 25 to 30 percent decrease in breast cancer mortality among women between the ages of 50 and 70. A lesser benefit was seen among women ages 40 to 49. The benefit of screening mammography for women over age 70 is more difficult to assess because of a lack of data for this age group from randomized clinical trials. Screening mammography cannot eliminate all deaths from breast cancer because it does not detect all cancers, including some that are detected by physical examination. Some tumors may also develop too quickly to be identified at an early, "curable" stage using the standard screening intervals. Furthermore, it is technically difficult to consistently produce mammograms of high quality, and interpretation is subjective and can be variable among radiologists. Mammograms are particularly difficult to interpret for women with dense breast tissue, which is especially common in young women. The dense tissue interferes with the identification of abnormalities associated with tumors, leading to a higher rate of false-positive and false-negative test results among these women. These difficulties associated with dense tissue are especially problematic for young women with heritable mutations who wish to begin screening at a younger age than what is recommended for the general population.

Mammography can also have deleterious effects on some women, in the form of false-positive results and overdiagnosis and overtreatment. As many as three-quarters of all breast lesions that are biopsied as a result of suspicious findings on a mammogram, turn out to be benign; that is, the mammographic findings were falsely positive. (Many tissue biopsies performed on lumps found by physical examination are also benign, but the false-positive rate for physical examination has not been carefully studied.) "Overdiagnosis" is the labeling of small lesions as cancer or precancer when in fact the lesions may never have progressed to a life-threatening disease if they had been left undetected and untreated. In such cases, some of the "cures" that occur after early detection may not be real, and thus, such women are unnecessarily "overtreated." Technical improvements in breast imaging techniques have led to an increase in the rate of detection of these small abnormalities, such as carcinoma in situ, the biology of which is not well understood. Currently, the methods for classification of such lesions detected by mammography are based on the appearance of the tissue structure, and the ability to determine the lethal potential of breast abnormalities from this classification is crude at best.

The immense burden of breast cancer, combined with the inherent limitations of mammography and other detection modalities, have been the driving forces behind the enormous efforts that have been and that continue to be devoted to the development and refining of technologies for the early detection of breast cancer. The purpose of the study described in this report was to review the breast cancer detection technologies in development and to examine the many steps in medical technology development as they specifically apply to methods for the early detection of breast cancer. The study committee was charged with surveying existing technologies and identifying promising new technologies for early detection, and assessing the technical and scientific opportunities. The committee was further charged with examining the policies that influence the development, adoption, and use of technologies. Funding for the study was provided by seven independent foundations and individuals, including the Breast Cancer Research Foundation, the Carl J. Herzog Foundation, Mr. John K. Castle, the Jewish Healthcare Foundation, the Josiah Macy, Jr., Foundation, the Kansas Health Foundation, and the New York Community Trust.

## TECHNOLOGIES IN DEVELOPMENT

Most of the progress thus far in the field of breast cancer detection has resulted in incremental improvements in traditional imaging technologies. These technical advances have likely led to more consistent detection of early lesions, but clinical trials have not been undertaken to determine whether their use has also resulted in a greater reduction in breast cancer mortality compared with that of older technologies. Many technical improvements have been made to mammography since its initial introduction. One recent example is full-field digital mammography (FFDM). FFDM systems are identical to traditional film-screen mammography (FSM) systems except for the electronic detectors that capture and display the X-ray signals on a computer rather than directly on film. This digital process provides the opportunity to adjust the contrast, brightness, and magnification of the image without additional exposures. Many consider FFDM to be a major technical advance over traditional mammography, but studies to date have not demonstrated a meaningful improvement in screening accuracy. Although one could argue that studies thus far have not directly tested the full potential of FFDM through the use of "soft-copy" image analysis (on a computer screen as opposed to film), difficulties remain with regard to the limited resolution and brightness of the soft-copy display. The technology could potentially improve the practice of screening mammography in other ways, for example, by facilitating electronic storage, retrieval, and transmission of mammograms. Computer-aided detection, through the use of sophisticated computer programs designed to recognize patterns in images, has also shown potential for improving the accuracy of screening mammography, at least among less experienced readers. However, questions remain as to how this technology will ultimately be used and whether it will have a beneficial effect on current screening practices.

Other breast imaging technologies approved by the Food and Drug Administration (FDA) include ultrasound, magnetic resonance imaging (MRI), scintimammography, thermography, and electrical impedance imaging (Table 1). Ideal detection performance may ultimately depend on

**TABLE 1**  Current Status of Imaging and Related Technologies Under Development for Breast Cancer Detection

| Technology | Current Status | | |
|---|---|---|---|
| | Screening | Diagnosis | FDA approved for breast imaging/ detection |
| Film-screen mammography (FSM) | +++ | +++ | Yes |
| Full-field digital mammography (FFDM) | ++ | ++ | Yes |
| Computer-assisted detection (CAD) | ++ | o | Yes |
| Ultrasound (US) | + | +++ | Yes |
| Novel US methods (compound, three-dimensional, Doppler, harmonic) | o | o | No |
| Elastography (MR and US) | o | o | No |
| Magnetic resonance imaging (MRI) | + | ++ | Yes |
| Magnetic resonance spectroscopy (MRS) | -/o[a] | +/o[a] | No |
| Scintimammography | o | + | Yes |
| Positron emission tomography (PET) | o | o | Yes |
| Optical imaging | o | + | No |
| Optical spectroscopy | - | o | No |
| Thermography | o | + | Yes |
| Electrical potential measurements | o | + | No |
| Electrical impedance imaging | o | + | Yes |
| Electronic palpation | o | NA | No |
| Thermoacoustic computed tomography, microwave imaging, Hall effect imaging, magnetomammography | NA | NA | No |

NOTE:  This table is an attempt to classify a very diverse set of technologies in a rapidly changing field and thus is subject to change in the near future.

[a]Ex vivo analysis of biopsy material/in vivo MRS.

Current Status Explanation of Scale
- -    Technology is not useful for the given application
- NA  Data are not available regarding use of the technology for  given application
- o    Preclinical data are suggestive that the technology might be useful for breast cancer detection, but clinical data are absent or very sparse for the given application.
- +    Clinical data suggest the technology could play a role in breast cancer detection, but more study is needed to define a role in relation to existing technologies
- ++   Data suggest that technology could be useful in selected situations because it adds (or is equivalent) to existing technologies, but not currently recommended for routine use
- +++  Technology is routinely used to make clinical decisions for the given application

multimodality imaging, as no single imaging technology to date can accurately detect all significant lesions. Ultrasound and MRI in particular have shown potential as adjuncts to mammography for diagnostic and screening purposes, especially for women in whom the accuracy of mammography is not optimal, such as those with dense breasts. MRI and ultrasound imaging may also facilitate new minimally invasive methods for the treatment of early lesions that are under investigation, but clinical trials are needed to assess the value of the procedures.

Many additional technologies are at earlier stages of development, but to date, it appears that no quantum steps forward have been taken in this area. Furthermore, improved imaging technologies that allow detection of more lesions at an earlier, precancer stage may or may not lead to reduced breast cancer mortality and may lead to more overtreatment of women. The dilemma of overtreatment could potentially be overcome by coupling imaging technologies with biologically based technologies, such as functional imaging, that can determine which lesions are likely to become lethal. The benefit of discovering early lesions could also be enhanced by developing new and effective preventive and therapeutic interventions that are minimally invasive and more acceptable to women. Thus, a great deal of work remains to be done to optimize the benefits and minimize the risks of breast cancer screening.

A number of technologies that may help to define the biological nature of breast lesions are being developed, including culture of breast cancer cells in the laboratory, measurement of protein expression in cancer cells, identification of markers of cancer cells or the proteins that they secrete in blood or breast fluid, or identification of genetic changes in tumors (Table 2). Further progress in this field will depend on the establishment, maintenance, and accessibility of tissue specimen banks, as well as access to new high-throughput technologies and bioinformatics. Technologies based on biology could potentially contribute to improved patient outcomes in several ways. For example, they could distinguish between early lesions that require treatment because they are highly likely to become lethal and those that are not. In many instances, these technologies could also potentially identify fundamental changes in the breast that appear before a lesion can be detected by current imaging methods. Thus, they may identify women at high risk of developing breast cancer or, more importantly, women at high risk of dying from breast cancer. Such women could then undergo more frequent screening or would perhaps benefit from newer imaging technologies. Some women might also choose to explore a "risk reduction strategy" that would affect all breast cells (e.g., bilateral prophylactic mastectomy), although current strategies for risk reduction are less than ideal. Improved understanding of the biology and etiology of breast cancer could also lead to better prevention strategies, which would further increase the benefits of early detection.

**TABLE 2** Technologies Under Development for Biological Characterization and Detection of Breast Cancer

| Detection Objective | Techniques | Stage of Development | Current Limitations |
| --- | --- | --- | --- |
| Identify germ-line mutations associated with cancer risk | Various genetic tests for BRCA1, BRCA2, p53, and AT | In clinical use | ≤10% of women with breast cancer affected<br>Survival benefit not proven |
| | DNA arrays | Preclinical stage | |
| Identify polymorphisms associated with cancer risk | Various sequencing techniques | Used as research tools | Value for predicting cancer risk poorly defined |
| Identify and characterize somatic mutations and epigenetic changes | Fluorescent In Situ Hybridization (FISH), Comparative Genomic Hybridization, Polymerase Chain Reaction (PCR) for loss of heterozygosity (LOH), DNA arrays, DNA methylation assays | Used as research tools | Diagnostic and prognostic values of mutations are poorly defined; tumors are heterogeneous |
| Measure changes in RNA expression in cancer cells[a] | Northern analysis Reverse transcription-PCR, cDNA array | Used as research tools | Same as directly above; difficult to assess small samples;<br>Need computer algorithms for array data |

| | | | |
|---|---|---|---|
| Measure changes in levels of protein expression in cancer cells[a] | Immunohistochemistry (IHC) | Some IHC in clinical use | |
| | Two-dimensional gel electro-phoresis, Mass spectroscopy | All used as research tools | Same as directly above |
| Identify markers of cancer in breast fluids | Nipple aspiration Breast lavage | Used as research tools, early stage of clinical testing | Sensitivity and specificity are low; appropriate markers to be examined are not clear |
| Identify markers of cancer or risk in serum or blood | Various tests for protein markers | Some in clinical use for monitoring disease Others are research tools | Same as directly above |
| | Isolation and analysis of cancer cells in circulation | Early stage of development | |
| Culture of breast cells | Various tissue culture methods | Used as research tools | Primary cultures have been difficult to grow Prognostic value of newer methods unproven |

[a]Potential targets of functional imaging.

## TECHNOLOGY DEVELOPMENT PROCESS

The pathway from technical innovation to accepted clinical practice is long, arduous, and costly. Although the activity and investment in research aimed at developing new technologies for early breast cancer detection have increased substantially over the last decade, biomedical research has also become more complex and capital intensive. Moreover, in addition to the developers of new technologies, many groups participate in the process, including FDA, health care insurers and managed care organizations, and other technology assessment institutions. These public and private organizations and policy makers play a role in evaluating medical technologies at various points along the way, making decisions about FDA approval, insurance coverage, and reimbursement that ultimately determine whether new technologies will be adopted and disseminated. Those who evaluate the potential of new technologies consider many factors, including clinical need, technical performance, clinical performance, economic issues, and patient and societal perspectives.

Government funding of research in the health care sector has traditionally focused primarily on basic scientific discovery, but recently, a new emphasis on the translation of science into practice through the development of technology has received considerable attention, including the creation of joint public- and private-sector initiatives. The private sector has made considerable investment in this area as well, although private investment in breast imaging technologies appears to be less attractive than investment in other areas of the health care industry. A variety of factors may contribute to this phenomenon, but it is likely due to the perception that there is a high degree of economic risk in this field, including considerations of the time and resources needed to develop technologies, the size of the potential market, and the remuneration possible. The end results of research are always unpredictable, but for medical devices, the requirements for FDA approval and insurance coverage have been variable and unpredictable, adding additional levels of risk to the development process. Furthermore, because technical innovations are often first introduced into the system in rather crude form, it can be difficult and problematic to judge them solely on the basis of their early versions.

## ASSESSMENT OF NEW TECHNOLOGIES

The dominant framework for medical technology regulation and evaluation has historically been based on therapeutics, whereas early detection relies on screening and diagnostic methods. The evaluation of therapeutic and detection technologies, however, may be intrinsically different. The stages of development for drugs are more standardized, and therapeutic interventions generate direct outcomes that can be observed in patients. In contrast, most patient-level effects of screening and diagnostic tests are mediated by subsequent therapeutic decisions. Screening and diagnostic tests also generate information that is subject to interpretation. Furthermore, this information is only one of the inputs into the decision-making process. Hence, the evaluation of detection technologies is fundamentally an assessment of the value of information. The development process for devices also tends to be iterative, and thus, assessment at early stages of development may not recognize the full potential of a new medical device. That is, most technologies that ultimately achieve widespread use go through successive stages of development, variation, and appraisal of the actual experience in the market.

With the exception of mammography, new breast cancer detection technologies have been evaluated by diagnostic studies that primarily measure sensitivity (the proportion of people with the disease who test positive) and specificity (the proportion of people without the disease who test negative). Even if the technologies ultimately are intended to be used for screening, they are generally not evaluated through screening studies that measure health outcomes. Adoption of new detection technologies for screening purposes before assessment of their effects on clinical outcome has been common and quite problematic for technologies used to screen for other diseases because data on detection accuracy are not adequate to assess the potential value of new technologies for screening. The ideal end points for assessment of screening technologies are reductions in disease-specific mortality or morbidity, or both, but the clinical trials needed to measure those end points are quite large, lengthy, and costly. Surrogate end points for morbidity and mortality are difficult to define because the net effect of new detection technologies could be either positive (more accurate detection, leading to lower breast cancer mortality) or negative (capable of identifying more lesions but not changing disease-specific mortality and thus leading to greater morbidity and higher screening costs).

## TECHNOLOGY DISSEMINATION

After the hurdles of FDA approval, insurance coverage, and reimbursement have been cleared, the adoption and dissemination of new breast cancer detection technologies will ultimately depend on whether women and their health care providers find them acceptable. Much is already known about the adoption and dissemination of screening mammography, and this knowledge may prove instructive for other developing technologies. Experience from current mammography programs suggests that outreach to women, education of women and providers, and access to facilities and services are all essential components of successful dissemination.

The use of screening mammography has increased greatly in the last decade, but a significant number of women still do not get screened, and many others do not undergo screening at the recommended intervals. Women often express concerns about discomfort from the procedure, the inconvenience of scheduling an annual test, lack of access to screening facilities, and fear of what could be found (including false-positive results). Studies indicate that physician recommendation is the single most influential factor in determining whether women are screened.

Access to screening facilities may be particularly difficult for women who lack health insurance. The National Breast and Cervical Cancer Early Detection Program was established through the Centers for Disease Control and Prevention with the goal of providing screening examinations for uninsured women. The program has grown considerably since it was launched 10 years ago, but it still only reaches about 12 to 15 percent of eligible women nationwide. New federal legislation that would allow Medicaid coverage for treatment of breast cancer detected through the program was recently passed, but adoption of this program by the states is pending.

As more women adopt the practice of routine screening and the number of women eligible for screening mammography increases (because of the aging U.S. population), there will be increased demands for trained mammographers and certified screening facilities. There are anecdotal reports that inadequate numbers of mammographers and mammography technologists are being trained to fulfill current and future needs, but quantitative data to support these assertions are not available. Concerns have also been expressed among radiologists and health care administrators that the reimbursement rate for mammography is too low to cover the procedure's actual costs (including the costs of complying with federally mandated quality standards, which are unique to mammography) and that this situation could lead to a reduction in the availability of screening services. Quantitative data are unavailable to confirm or refute these concerns. If the rate of reimbursement for mammography truly is artificially low, then cost comparisons with new technologies may also unfairly favor mammography.

When mammography was introduced, it was a "void-filling" technology and thus had no competition during the dissemination process. New technologies face a much different scenario. Evaluation will likely include comparison with mammography, and adoption of a new technology will require competition with other detection technologies that are currently available. A goal of new technologies is to provide additional choices for women and their physicians, allowing an individualized approach to screening and diagnosis depending on a woman's specific needs and characteristics. At the same time, new technologies may add layers of complexity to the decision-making processes associated with screening and diagnosis, making it more challenging to establish practice guidelines and to define a standard of care.

## RECOMMENDATIONS

The committee's recommendations fall into two general categories: those that aim to improve the development and adoption processes for new technologies (Recommendations 1 to 5) and those that aim to make the most of the technologies currently available for breast cancer detection (Recommendations 6 to 10).

**1. Government support for the development of new breast cancer detection technologies should continue to emphasize research on the basic biology and etiology of breast cancer and on the creation of classification schemes for breast lesions based on molecular biology.** A major goal of this research should be to determine which lesions identified by screening are likely to become lethal and thus require treatment. This approach would increase the potential benefits of screening while reducing the potential risk of screening programs.

- Funding should focus on the development of biological markers and translational research to determine the appropriate uses and applications of the markers, including functional imaging.
- Research on cancer markers should focus on screening as well as on downstream decisions associated with diagnosis and treatment.
- Funding priorities should include specimen banks (including specimens of early lesions), purchase and operation of high-throughput technologies for the study and assessment of genetic and protein markers, and new bioinformatics approaches to the analysis of biological data.

**2. Breast cancer specimen banks should be expanded and researcher access to patient samples should be enhanced.**

- Health care professionals and breast cancer advocacy groups should educate women about the importance of building tumor banks and encourage women to provide consent for research on patient samples.
- Stronger protective legislation should be enacted at the national level to prevent genetic discrimination and ensure the confidentiality of genetic test results.
- The National Cancer Institute (NCI) should devise and enforce strategies to facilitate researcher access to the patient samples in specimen banks. For example, the costs associated with the sharing of samples with

collaborators should be included in the funding for the establishment and maintenance of the specimen banks, and specimen banks supported by government funds should not place excessive restrictions on the use of the specimens with regard to intellectual property issues.

**3. Consistent criteria should be developed and applied by the Food and Drug Administration (FDA) for the approval of screening and diagnostic devices and tests.**

• Guidance documents for determination of "safety and effectiveness," especially with regard to clinical data, should be articulated more clearly and applied more uniformly.
• Given the complexity of assessing new technologies, the FDA advisory panels could be improved by including more experts in biostatistics, technology assessment, and epidemiology.

**4. For new screening technologies, approval by the Food and Drug Administration (FDA) and coverage decisions by the Health Care Financing Administration (HCFA) and private insurers should depend on evidence of improved clinical outcome. This pursuit should be streamlined by coordinating oversight and support from all relevant participants (FDA, NCI, HCFA, private insurers, and breast cancer advocacy organizations) at a very early stage in the process.** Such an approach should prevent technologies that have been approved for diagnostic use from being used prematurely for screening in the absence of evidence of benefit. Technology sponsors generally lack the resources and incentive to undertake large, long-lasting, and expensive screening studies, but a coordinated approach would make it easier to conduct clinical trials to gather the necessary outcome data. The proposed process should provide for the following:

• FDA should approve new cancer detection technologies for diagnostic use in the traditional fashion, based on evidence of the accuracy (sensitivity and specificity) of new devices or tests in the diagnostic setting. In the case of "next-generation" devices (in which technical improvements have been made to a predicate device already on the market), technical advantages such as patient comfort or ease of data acquisition and storage could be considered in the determination of approval.
• If a new device that has been approved for diagnostic use shows potential for use as a screening tool (based on evidence of accuracy) and the developers wish to pursue a screening use, an investigational device exemption should be granted for this use and conditional coverage should be provided for the purpose of conducting large-scale screening trials to assess clinical outcomes.

• Trials should be designed and conducted with input from FDA, NCI, HCFA, the Agency for Healthcare Research and Quality, and breast cancer advocacy organizations. Informed consent acknowledging the specific risks of participating in a screening trial would be necessary.

• HCFA and other payers should agree to conditionally cover the cost of performing the test in the approved clinical trials, whereas NCI and the technology's sponsors should take responsibility for other trial expenses. Participation by private insurers would be particularly important for the assessment of new technologies intended for use in younger women who are not yet eligible for Medicare coverage. Although this expense may initially seem burdensome to private insurers, the cost of providing tests within a clinical trial would be much less than the costs associated with broad adoption by the public (and the associated pressure to provide coverage) in the absence of experimental evidence for improved clinical outcome.

• Trial data should be reviewed at appropriate intervals, and the results should determine whether FDA approval should be granted (for those deemed sufficiently effective) and coverage should be extended to use outside of the trials. (A prior approval for diagnosis would remain in place regardless of the decision for screening applications.)

• The ideal end point for clinical outcome is decreased disease-specific mortality. However, given the length of time required to assess that end point and the fact that early detection by screening mammography has already been proven to reduce breast cancer mortality, a surrogate end point for breast cancer detection is appropriate in some cases. As a general rule, a screening technology that consistently detects early invasive breast cancer could be presumed efficacious for the purposes of FDA approval. Detection of premalignant or preinvasive breast lesions, however, cannot be assumed to reduce breast cancer mortality or increase benefits to women, and it is not an appropriate surrogate end point for FDA approval, given the current lack of understanding of the biology of these lesions.

**5. The National Cancer Institute should create a permanent infrastructure for testing the efficacy and clinical effectiveness of new technologies for early cancer detection as they emerge.** The NCI Breast Cancer Surveillance Consortium and the American College of Radiology Imaging Network may provide novel platforms for this purpose through the creation of databases and archives of clinical samples from thousands of study participants.

**6. The Health Care Financing Administration should analyze the current Medicare and Medicaid reimbursement rates for mammography, including a comparison with other radiological techniques, to de-**

termine whether they adequately cover the total costs of providing the procedure. The cost analysis of mammography should include the costs associated with meeting the requirements of the Mammography Quality Standards Act. A panel of external and independent experts should be involved in the analysis.

7. **The Health Resources and Services Administration (HRSA) should undertake or fund a study that analyzes trends in specialty training for breast cancer screening among radiologists and radiologic technologists and that examines the factors that affect practitioners' decisions to enter or remain in the field.** If the trend suggests an impending shortage of trained experts, HRSA should seek input from professional societies such as the American College of Radiology and the Society of Breast Imaging in making recommendations to reverse the trend.

8. **Until health insurance becomes more universally available, the U.S. Congress should expand the Centers for Disease Control and Prevention screening program to reach a much larger fraction of eligible women, and state legislatures should participate in the federal Breast and Cervical Treatment Act by providing funds for cancer treatment for eligible women.** The Centers for Disease Control and Prevention should be expected to reach 70 percent of eligible women (as opposed to the current 15 percent). This objective is based on the stated goals of the U.S. Department of Health and Human Services' *Healthy People 2010* report, which by the year 2010 expects 70 percent of women over age 40 to have had a recent (within the last 2 years) screening mammogram.

9. **The National Cancer Institute should sponsor large randomized trials every 10 to 15 years to reassess the effects of accepted screening modalities on clinical outcome.** These trials would compare two currently used technologies that are known to have different sensitivities. Breast cancer-specific mortality would be the principal outcome under evaluation. Such studies are needed because detection technologies and treatments are both continually evolving. Hence, the benefit of a screening method may change over time.

10. **The National Cancer Institute, through the American College of Radiology Imaging Network or the Breast Cancer Surveillance Consortium, should sponsor further studies to define more accurately the benefits and risks of screening mammography in women over age 70.** As the age distribution of the U.S. population continues to shift toward older ages, the question of whether these women benefit from screening mammography will become increasingly important.

# I
# Introduction

Breast cancer is the most common non-skin-related malignancy and the second leading cause of cancer death among women in the United States[1]. Each year, more than 180,000 new cases of invasive breast cancer are diagnosed and more than 40,000 women die from the disease. Until research uncovers a way to prevent breast cancer or to cure all women regardless of when their tumor is found, early detection will be looked upon as the best hope for reducing the heavy toll of this disease. The early detection of cervical cancer by screening with the Papanicolaou smear (the Pap smear) dramatically reduced mortality from that cancer, and the rationale for the early detection of breast cancer is similar.

Fifty years ago, there was no established method for the detection of breast cancer at an early stage or for screening of the general population, but advances in technology, policy recommendations by various organizations, and legal mandates have thoroughly changed that situation (Figure 1-1). Although the use of X-ray imaging for the detection of breast cancer was first suggested in the early 1900s, mammography did not begin to emerge as an accepted technology until the 1960s, after a number of technical innovations that produced higher-quality images that were more reproducible and easier to interpret were introduced. Subsequently, some physicians began ordering mammograms to help with the diagnosis of complicated cases, and the technology was also tested as a screening

---

[1]Lung cancer is the leading cause of cancer deaths among U.S. women, with more than 65,000 deaths annually (American Cancer Society, 2000; http://www3.cancer.org/cancerinfo/).

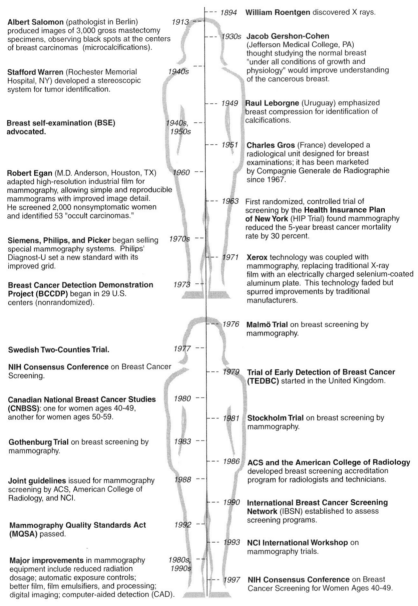

**Albert Salomon** (pathologist in Berlin) *1913* produced images of 3,000 gross mastectomy specimens, observing black spots at the centers of breast carcinomas (microcalcifications).

*1894* **William Roentgen** discovered X rays.

*1930s* **Jacob Gershon-Cohen** (Jefferson Medical College, PA) thought studying the normal breast "under all conditions of growth and physiology" would improve understanding of the cancerous breast.

**Stafford Warren** (Rochester Memorial *1940s* Hospital, NY) developed a stereoscopic system for tumor identification.

*1949* **Raul Leborgne** (Uruguay) emphasized breast compression for identification of calcifications.

**Breast self-examination (BSE)** *1940s,* **advocated.** *1950s*

*1951* **Charles Gros** (France) developed a radiological unit designed for breast examinations; it has been marketed by Compagnie Generale de Radiographie since 1967.

**Robert Egan** (M.D. Anderson, Houston, TX) *1960* adapted high-resolution industrial film for mammography, allowing simple and reproducible mammograms with improved image detail. He screened 2,000 nonsymptomatic women and identified 53 "occult carcinomas."

*1963* First randomized, controlled trial of screening by the **Health Insurance Plan of New York** (HIP Trial) found mammography reduced the 5-year breast cancer mortality rate by 30 percent.

**Siemens, Philips, and Picker** began selling *1970s* special mammography systems. Philips' Diagnost-U set a new standard with its improved grid.

*1971* **Xerox** technology was coupled with mammography, replacing traditional X-ray film with an electrically charged selenium-coated aluminum plate. This technology faded but spurred improvements by traditional manufacturers.

**Breast Cancer Detection Demonstration** *1973* **Project (BCCDP)** began in 29 U.S. centers (nonrandomized).

*1976* **Malmö Trial** on breast screening by mammography.

**Swedish Two-Counties Trial.** *1977*

**NIH Consensus Conference** on Breast Cancer Screening.

*1979* **Trial of Early Detection of Breast Cancer (TEDBC)** started in the United Kingdom.

**Canadian National Breast Cancer Studies** *1980* **(CNBSS):** one for women ages 40-49, another for women ages 50-59.

*1981* **Stockholm Trial** on breast screening by mammography.

**Gothenburg Trial** on breast screening by *1983* mammography.

*1986* **ACS and the American College of Radiology** developed breast screening accreditation program for radiologists and technicians.

**Joint guidelines** issued for mammography *1988* screening by ACS, American College of Radiology, and NCI.

*1990* **International Breast Cancer Screening Network** (IBSN) established to assess screening programs.

**Mammography Quality Standards Act** *1992* **(MQSA)** passed.

*1993* **NCI International Workshop** on mammography trials.

**Major improvements** in mammography *1980s,* equipment include reduced radiation *1990s* dosage; automatic exposure controls; better film, film emulsifiers, and processing; digital imaging; computer-aided detection (CAD).

*1997* **NIH Consensus Conference** on Breast Cancer Screening for Women Ages 40-49.

Currently, screening mammography is advocated in 22 countries.

**FIGURE 1-1**   A History of Breast Cancer Screening.
SOURCES: Gold et al. (1990), Kevles (1997); Jatoi (1999), Moss (1999), and Lerner (2001).

tool (reviewed by Lerner, 2001). X-ray film mammography and physical examination of the breast are now the mainstays for early detection of breast cancer. Screening for early cancer detection has been credited for part of the recent reduction in breast cancer mortality, which had been stagnant for 40 years (Blanks et al., 2000; Hakama et al., 1997; Mettlin, 1999; Peto et al., 2000) (Figure 1-2). (Adjuvant therapy is also credited with reducing breast cancer mortality). New or improved technologies are also rapidly emerging and providing new hope of early detection.

Over the past decade, the investment in breast cancer research, including early detection, has increased substantially. Research has intensified with federal funding, and private firms have turned more attention to breast cancer detection. Programs within the U.S. Department of Health and Human Services and the U.S. Department of Defense support large numbers of investigators working on breast cancer, and recently, the National Aeronautics and Space Administration and several intelligence services have agreed to apply their imaging expertise to mammography (Table 1-1). Biotechnology and device companies have proliferated, with many developing technologies that might improve the ability to detect breast cancer early, and established firms have also turned their attention to breast cancer, in part as the result of findings derived from the rising federal research investment.

Advances in imaging (see Chapter 2) include reducing the dose of X rays needed, enhancement of digital images, computer-assisted analysis of images, and use of alternatives to X rays such as ultrasound, magnetic resonance imaging (MRI), and optical imaging. Techniques for high-resolution imaging and image processing, many of which were developed for other applications such as space science, are now being applied to breast imaging, with hopes of improved accuracy, speed, ease of use, and perhaps lower cost. Advances in genetics and increased knowledge of the basic biology and etiology of breast cancer may also lead to novel, biologically based early detection and diagnostic methods. Use of molecular markers (see Chapter 3) may increase the accuracy of diagnostic techniques and offer new opportunities for the characterization of early disease as well as for the refinement and improvement of treatments.

However, early detection depends on more than just the development of technologies and the advance of new science. Technological advances must be thoroughly evaluated before they can become widely used by women. This evaluation takes place in many stages, including Food and Drug Administration (FDA) approval (when it is a device), adoption by health plans and providers, approval of payment for screening and detection, acceptance by women, and marketing by private firms. A wide range of factors must be considered at the various stages, including safety, accuracy, cost-effectiveness, and negative side effects. The level of evidence needed to establish efficacy, how effectiveness should be es-

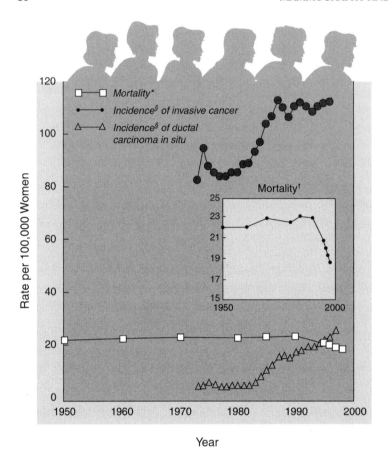

Year

**FIGURE 1.2**   Breast cancer incidence and mortality rates in the United States, 1950-1998.

*Age-adjusted to the 1940 U.S. standard population. SOURCE: *Health, United States 2000*, National Center for Health Statistics, National Vital Statistics System, Centers for Disease Control and Prevention.

§Age-adjusted to the 1970 U.S. standard population. SOURCE: *SEER Cancer Statistics Review, 1973-1996* (Ries et al., 1999). Numbers are calculated using cancer incidence rates from the regions of the U.S. included in the National Cancer Institute's Surveillance, Epidemiology, and End Results (SEER) program and population data collected by the U.S. Bureau of the Census.

†Inset: Mortality data on a compressed scale to demonstrate the recent decrease. Between 1990 and 1998, mortality decreased by ~2%/year on average.

tablished, how costs should be measured, and how much evidence is needed before decisions about coverage are made—including offering and paying for screening—are all critical questions that need to be addressed. According to Edward Golub at the Pacific Center for Ethics and Applied Biology: "We are on the verge of an era of technological change in which the ability to do tests can determine whether we do them, which ones we do, and on whom they are done; it is crucial to understand the value and limits of [screening] tests, and how they fit into the goals of medicine. We are in danger of behaving as if all technological change is progress, and of confusing being swept along on the wave of changes with responsible exercise of the authority that society has given to the clinician in that which matters most to people, their health" (Golub, 1999, p. 14).

The purpose of the study presented in this report was to review breast cancer detection technologies in development and to examine the many steps in medical technology development as they specifically apply to methods for the early detection of breast cancer. The study committee was charged with 'surveying existing technologies and identifying promising new technologies for early detection, assessing the technical and scientific opportunities.' The committee was further charged with examining the 'policies that influence the development, adoption, and use of technologies.'

## THEORY AND PRINCIPLES OF CANCER SCREENING

The practice of screening for cancer is based on the premise that early detection will have a positive effect on the outcome of the disease through medical intervention. The goal of screening is to reduce disease-specific morbidity and mortality through early treatment by identifying clinically occult (asymptomatic) tumors that are likely to become lethal. It is widely believed that early detection of such tumors will allow surgical removal of the cancer before the cells have begun to metastasize.

Policy decisions regarding the use of screening in large populations depends on data from clinical studies (R. Harris, 1999). In 1968, the World Health Organization proposed guidelines for clinical trials of tests used to screen for diseases (Wilson and Jungren, 1968):

1. The disorder screened for should be an important cause of morbidity, disability, or mortality.

2. The tests must have acceptable performance characteristics (for example, high levels of sensitivity and specificity, see Box 1-1 for definitions of screening test performance).

3. The tests must be available and acceptable to the target population and that population's physicians.

**TABLE 1.1** Examples of Funding Sources for Research in Early Detection of Breast Cancer

| Funder or Program | Amount ($) | Type of Projects Supported |
|---|---|---|
| *Government Funders*<br>Early Detection Research Network, NCI, NIH; established 1999 (edrn.nci.nih.gov) | $8 million awarded 10/99 to fund 18 biomarker development laboratories. $18 million awarded 5/00 to fund nine clinical/epidemiological centers, three biomarker validation labs, and a data center.<br>Additional $2 million for Steering Committee. | Development of biomarkers for earlier detection of cancer and risk assessment. Four components of the multi-institutional consortium: biomarker developmental laboratories, biomarker validation laboratories, Clinical/epidemiological centers, data management, and a coordination center.<br>Breast cancer is one focus activity. |
| Unconventional Innovations Program, NCI, NIH, OTIR; announced 1999 (amb.nci.nih.gov/UIP.HTM) | Initial estimate of $48 million over next 5 years. | Development of noninvasive methods of detecting defined signatures of cancerous and precancerous cell types and developing directed interventions toward detected cells. Promotes multidisciplinary collaboration among researchers with expertise in diverse scientific fields. |
| Phased Innovation Award NCI, NIH, OTIR; announced 1999 (otir.nci.nih.gov/funding/phasein.html) | 6 months, $100,000. | Fosters the translation of emerging technologies from pilot research to research development, speeding the adoption of near-term technological opportunities. Example of an award includes Innovative Technologies for the Molecular Analysis of Cancer, encompassing methods and tools that enable research, such as instrumentation, techniques, devices, and analysis tools. |

Continued on next page

| | | |
|---|---|---|
| Phased Technology Application Award, NCI, NIH, OTIR announced 1999 (otir.nci.nih.gov/funding/phasetech.html) | 2 years, $750,000. | Developed to complement the Phased Innovation Award. Fosters the translation of emerging technologies from evaluation to pilot application, speeding the adoption of near-term technological opportunities. |
| Cooperative Trials in Diagnostic Imaging (ACRIN), NCI, NIH; March 1999 (www.acrin.org) | $3 million in FY 1999, $23 million through FY 2003. | Network established to facilitate multi-institutional clinical trials in diagnostic imaging related to cancer, with breast cancer as one focus area. |
| Director's Challenge: Toward a Molecular Classification of Tumors, NCI, NIH; announced 1999 (grants.nih.gov/grants/guide/rfa-files/RFA-CA-98-027.html) | Ten 5-year grants awarded, totaling $4.1 million for first 6 months. Anticipated total cost of $50 million for 5 years. | Discovery of molecular profiles toward goal of precise molecular diagnosis of cancer. Breast cancer is one of eight cancers targeted. |
| Development and Testing of Digital Mammography Displays and Workstations (PA), NCI, NIH; announced April 1999 | Open application; no set-aside. | Development of displays and workstation design for improved image interpretation. |
| Early Clinical Advanced Technology Program, NIST, U.S. Department of Commerce; began in 1990 (www.atp.nist.gov) | $22 million over 5 years, starting in FY 2001, to support a total of 56 trials. | Will support phase I and II clinical trials to rapidly evaluate new technologies in molecular level targeted imaging such as imaging probes, ligands, radiopharmaceuticals, and contrast agents. |
| Trials of Imaging Agents, NCI, NIH; announced March 2000 | | |

**TABLE 1.1**  Continued

| Funder or Program | Amount ($) | Type of Projects Supported |
|---|---|---|
| Advanced Technology Program, NIST U.S. Department of Commerce; Began in 1990 (www.atp.nist.gov) | NA (breast cancer portion unknown) | Encourages innovation by bridging the gap between research laboratory and marketplace through partnerships with the private sector. Accelerates development of promising novel technologies through early-stage investment. |
| Breast Cancer Research Program (BCRP), U.S. Department of Defense began in 1992 (cdmrp.army.mil/) | $135 million in FY 1999. | Supports the spectrum of breast cancer research, from basic research to clinical science. Examples of award mechanisms include special mammography awards and computer-aided diagnosis support. Has also funded research in telemammography, ultrasound, MRI, PET, and molecular targets. |
| U.S. Department of Energy (www. doe.gov) | $72 million in FY1999 for the Life Sciences Division (breast cancer portion unknown) | Life Sciences Division supports research in the molecular basis of breast cancer, as well as technologies for detection (Center for Functional Imaging). |
| National Science Foundation (www.nsf.gov) | In 1999, more than $2.8 billion for research (unknown how much to breast cancer research) | Research grants include projects related to early detection of breast cancer (e.g., digital mammography). Photonics Partnership Initiative will investigate possibilities for early breast cancer detection. |

*Private Foundations*

| | | |
|---|---|---|
| California Breast Cancer Research Program; established in 1993 (www.ucop.edu/srphome/bcrp) | $75 million since 1994.; $16 million in 1999. | Earlier detection is one priority area of the program and encompasses the development of new technologies, biomarkers, and improved access for all women. |
| Susan G. Komen Breast Cancer Foundation; established in 1982 (www.komen.org) | In 1998, $14.1 million distributed in research grants. Current funding for imaging technology projects has maximum amount of $250,000 for 2-year period. | Grant program supports research in imaging technology to improve screening and diagnosis, in addition to basic, clinical, and translational research in breast cancer. Program in imaging technology dedicated to research and development for early detection and diagnosis of breast cancer. |
| Breast Cancer Research Foundation; established in 1993 (www.bcrfcure.org) | In 1999, gave out $6 million in grants. Minimum annual grant of $100,000 per institution. | Funds clinical and genetic research in the causes and treatments of breast cancer, including technologies for early detection. |
| Breast Cancer Fund; established in 1992 (breastcancerfund.org) | Grants range from $15,000 to $50,000. | One objective of the Innovative Research Grant category is to replace mammography with a safer, more accurate screening method. |
| Whitaker Foundation; established in 1975 (www.whitaker.org) | In 1998, $52 million for awards and programs. Maximum award is $240,000 over 3 years. | Supports the field of biomedical research. Past grants have been awarded to research in technologies for breast cancer detection, including digital mammography, microwave imaging, optical tomography, etc. |

*Continued on next page*

**TABLE 1.1** Continued

| Funder or Program | Amount ($) | Type of Projects Supported |
|---|---|---|
| Friends…You Can Count On; established in 1995 (www.earlier.org) | Small Grants in Cancer Detection/ Screening; awards up to $40,000 offered, may be used over 3-year period. | Funds research on new methods to improve detection of early breast cancer, especially in the areas of biological or immunological methods for the detection of early-stage breast cancer. |
| *New Initiatives and Collaborations* | | |
| NASA/NCI collaboration: Workshop on Sensors for Bio-Molecular Signatures, June 1999 | | Development of sensory and imaging systems that will help NASA detect life on other planets and NCI to detect cancer cells in humans. These technologies would have sensitivities and detection capabilities at the molecular level and the ability to transmit information to external systems. |
| NCI-Industry Forum & Workshop on Biomedical Imaging in Oncology, NCI, industry, HCFA, FDA September 1999 | | Discussed importance of coordination between various agencies and industries to improve the present system of technology development. |

NOTE: NIH, National Institutes of Health; OTIR, Office of Technology and Industrial Relations; FY, fiscal year; NIST, National Institute of Standards and Technology; PET, positron emission tomography; NASA, National Aeronautics and Space Administration; HCFA, Health Care Financing Administration.

## BOX 1-1
## Definitions of Screening Test Performance

The performance of a screening test is often defined by three related measurements: sensitivity, specificity, and positive predictive value. The sensitivity of a screening test is the proportion of people with the disease who test positive. Specificity is the proportion of people without the disease who test negative. There is often a trade-off between sensitivity and specificity, with an increase in one leading to a decrease in the other. The positive predictive value is the portion of individuals with a positive screening test result who actually have the disease. If screened individuals are assigned a position in a two-by-two classification scheme on the basis of their disease status and test result, values for the three measurements can be calculated as follows:

Actual Disease Status

|  |  | + | − |
|---|---|---|---|
| Test | + | True Positive (TP) | False Positive (FP) |
| Result | − | False Negative (FN) | True Negative (TN) |

| *Measurement* | *Question Answered* |
|---|---|
| Sensitivity (se) = $\dfrac{TP}{TP + FN}$ | How often does the test correctly identify women with breast cancer? |
| Specificity (sp) = $\dfrac{TN}{TN + FP}$ | How often does the test correctly identify women without the disease? |
| Positive predictive value $= \dfrac{TP}{TP + FP}$ | Among women with an abnormal test result, what proportion actually have the disease? |

The positive predictive value (PPV) is a function of sensitivity, specificity, and disease prevalence (P), with the following mathematical relationship:

$$PPV = \frac{(P)(se)}{[(P)(se) + (1 - P)(1 - sp)]}$$

4. Appropriate follow-up of individuals with positive findings must be ensured.

5. Screening should provide a net benefit to the target population, and the resources required to administer the tests under screening conditions must be justified in terms of the net benefits.

In other words, the natural history of the disease should be sufficiently well known, treatments should be sufficiently effective, risks resulting from screening should be acceptably low, and efficacy in reducing disease-specific morbidity and mortality should be high enough to conclude that early detection of the disease will be beneficial. Clearly, these standards are subject to value judgments in determining the relative importance of each condition and whether the conditions are adequately met. However, it is quite useful to refer to these recommendations when evaluating potential screening technologies.

The methods used to assess the efficacy of a screening method are quite different from the approach used to assess new treatments. For instance, treatment outcome is often measured by using short-term surrogate end points that have previously been correlated with long-term outcome, but such surrogate end points generally do not exist for screening methods.

There are many difficulties in accurately determining the real benefit of any cancer screening technology or program. Two inherent biases[2] must be taken in account: lead-time bias and length bias (Figure 1-3). These biases can be minimized (but not completely eliminated) only by evaluating a screening modality through a randomized, controlled trial in which mortality is the end point. Lead-time bias is due to the assumption that the identification and treatment of tumors at an earlier point in the progression of the disease will necessarily alter the rate of progression. Thus, a woman who survives 4 years after the diagnosis of a cancer identified during screening may be thought to have an increased survival time compared with that for an unscreened woman who finds a lump and dies 2 years after the diagnosis. However, once a cancer is identified by screening and is treated, it is impossible to know how long the woman would have survived if the cancer would have gone undetected until it became palpable. Likewise, it is impossible to know whether earlier detection and treatment of the woman with a 2-year postdiagnosis survival time would have resulted in a longer life for the woman if her cancer had been detected and treated sooner.

---

[2]Here, "bias" is defined as a process at any stage of inference that tends to produce results that depart systematically from the true values.

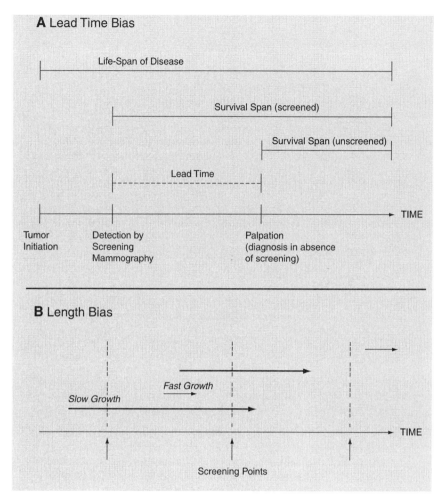

**FIGURE 1-3**   Lead-time (A) and length (B) biases. In panel B, the length of the arrows represents the time required for the tumor to reach a palpable size. For a more detailed description of lead-time and length biases, see the accompanying text in Chapter 1.

Length bias reflects the fact that screening tests detect a disproportionate number of women with slowly progressing tumors. A cancer that takes several years to reach a palpable size will be detected as a smaller tumor by regular screening than one that grows to the same size in a much shorter time period. If an aggressive, fast-growing tumor is more likely to become life-threatening than a slow-growing tumor, then many women whose tumors were identified through a screening program will inherently have a more favorable outcome following treatment.

**BOX 1.2**
**Cancer Risk**

The term "risk" refers to the quantitative measure of the probability of developing or dying from a particular disease such as cancer. Several basic measures of risk may be used to make decisions for cancer screening, including estimates of absolute risk or relative risk, as defined below.

*Absolute risk* is a measure of risk over time in a group of individuals and may be used to measure lifetime risk or risk over a narrower time period. For example, the absolute risk of developing breast cancer during any given decade of life will be lower than the absolute risk of developing breast cancer over a lifetime, which is essentially a cumulative risk over successive decades of life. It is a function of two factors that vary at different ages: the incidence rate of disease and the rate of death from other causes, both of which increase with age but which have opposite effects on the absolute risk of developing breast cancer. Thus, the lifetime risk of developing breast cancer is 14.4 percent, whereas the absolute risk of developing breast cancer over the decade between the ages of 40 and 50 is 1.8 percent, that over the decade between the ages of 50 and 60 is 3.2 percent, and that over the decade between the ages of 60 and 70 is 4 percent (Wun et al., 1998).

*Relative risk* is a comparative measure and is based on a comparison of disease incidence in two populations. It compares the risk of developing cancer in people with a certain exposure or genetic trait (i.e., environmental or genetic risk factors) with that in people without this exposure or trait. A relative risk greater than 1 implies elevated risk for the disease, whereas a value less than 1 implies a protective effect for the given factor. For example, smokers are 10 times more likely to develop lung cancer than nonsmokers and are thus said to have a 10-fold relative risk of developing lung cancer compared to nonsmokers (American Cancer Society, 2000). However, most relative risks for cancer are not this large. In the case of breast cancer, the relative risk associated with most defined risk factors is 2 or less. For example, women with a first-degree (mother, sister, or daughter) family history of breast cancer have about a two-fold relative risk of developing breast cancer compared with that for women without such a family history.

Relative risks may seem large while the corresponding absolute risk may be relatively small. For example, the relative risk for thyroid cancer following therapeutic radiation therapy is increased 16-fold compared with the risk for the general population; however, this translates to an absolute risk of 1.7 percent over the 20-year period following radiation exposure (Hancock et al., 1991). Absolute risks may be directly compared with one another, whereas relative risks may vary depending on the reference (control) population being studied.

Additional difficulties encountered in the assessment of screening programs include selection bias and overdiagnosis. Selection bias assumes that women who are at higher risk (see Box 1-2 for a definition of "risk") for breast cancer will be more likely to participate in screening trials and will be more compliant with the recommended guidelines for screening mammography. Since cancer screening may be more beneficial and cost-effective for high-risk populations than for the general population, a selection bias may result in overestimation of the value of implementing a screening program for the general population.

"Overdiagnosis" is the result of labeling small lesions as cancer or precancer when in fact the lesions may never have progressed to a life-threatening disease if left undetected and untreated. In such cases, some of the "cures" following early detection may not be real. This issue will be revisited in the next sections.

## CURRENT PRACTICE OF BREAST CANCER DETECTION

Breast cancer detection currently entails three distinct stages. The first stage is identification of an abnormality in the breast tissue either by physical examination or by an imaging technique (most commonly, mammography). Once identified, the abnormality must be diagnosed as benign or malignant by using additional imaging modalities or by biopsy and microscopic examination of the tissue morphology (Figure 1-4). In the third stage, abnormalities labeled as malignant must be further characterized biochemically and staged according to tumor size and extent of invasion and metastasis to determine a prognosis and an appropriate course of treatment.

Monthly breast self-examination (BSE) is a common method of identifying lumps and other abnormalities in the breast. BSE in conjunction with screening mammography is currently advocated by many organizations,[3] but it is also recommended for younger women who are not yet being screened by mammography. BSE was first advocated in the 1940s and 1950s, before the advent of screening mammography. Breast surgeons saw many patients whose tumors were too large for surgical removal, and they believed that regular self-examination of the breasts would result in earlier detection when surgery was still an option. Although the goal of finding smaller tumors at an earlier stage may be attained by BSE (Coleman, 1991), to date the evidence is not definitive that BSE improves the survival rate for women with breast cancer. Furthermore, BSE can lead to an increase in unnecessary biopsies, especially in younger women (Semiglazov et al., 1992, 1999; Thomas et al., 1997). Two large, randomized trials are ongoing in Russia and China[4] and may help to answer some of these questions more definitively.

---

[3]The U.S. Preventive Services Task Force does not currently recommend routine BSE. See Table 6.1 for more information.

[4]Preliminary results from the first 5 years of the study in China showed no significant difference in the breast cancer mortality or tumor size at the time of diagnosis among women trained in BSE compared to the control group. However, women trained in BSE did find more benign breast lesions. Longer follow-up of participants in this trial is required before a final assessment of BSE can be made (Thomas et al., 1997).

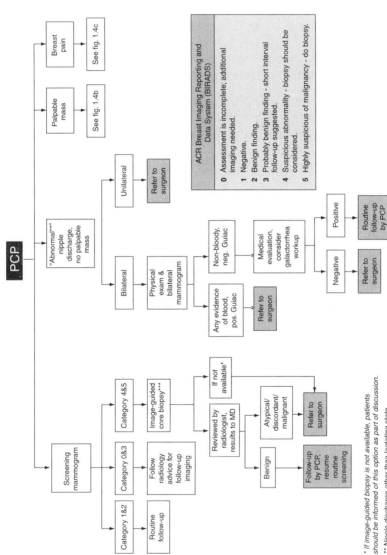

PCP

Screening mammogram

- Category 1&2 → Routine follow-up
- Category 0&3 → Follow radiology advice for follow-up imaging
- Category 4&5 → Image-guided core biopsy***

Image-guided core biopsy*** →
- If not available*
- Reviewed by radiologist, results to MD
  - Atypical/ discordant/ malignant → Refer to surgeon
  - Benign → Follow-up by PCP, resume routine screening

If not available* → Refer to surgeon

"Abnormal"*** nipple discharge, no palpable mass

- Bilateral → Physical exam & bilateral mammogram
  - Any evidence of blood, pos. Guiac → Refer to surgeon
  - Non-bloody, neg. Guiac → Medical evaluation, consider galactorrhea workup
    - Positive → Routine follow-up by PCP
    - Negative → Refer to surgeon
- Unilateral → Refer to surgeon

Palpable mass → See fig. 1.4b

Breast pain → See fig. 1.4c

**ACR Breast Imaging Reporting and Data System (BIRADS)**

0  Assessment is incomplete; additional imaging needed.
1  Negative.
2  Benign finding.
3  Probably benign finding - short interval follow-up suggested.
4  Suspicious abnormality - biopsy should be considered.
5  Highly suspicious of malignancy - do biopsy.

* If image-guided biopsy is not available, patients should be informed of this option as part of discussion.

** Nipple discharge other than lactating state.

*** If palpable mass present and/or core needle biopsy not available, consider FNA.

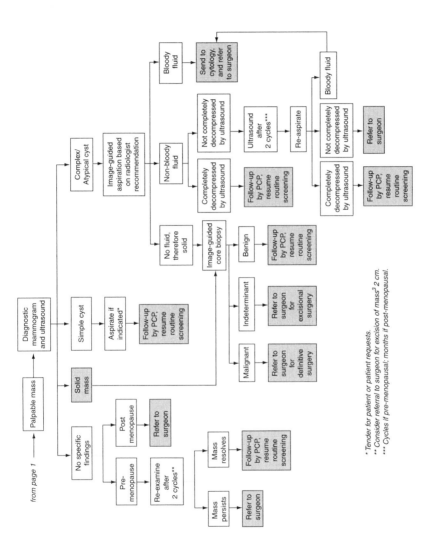

**FIGURE 1-4** Breast cancer management algorithm. SOURCE: Risk Management Foundation, Boston Massachusetts (May 23, 2000).

32

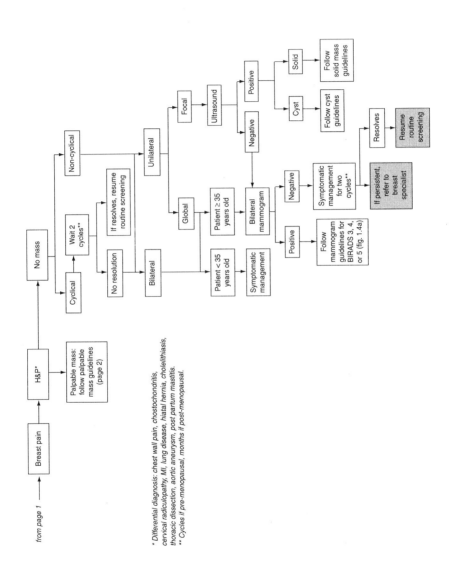

from page 1 → Breast pain → H&P* → Palpable mass: follow palpable mass guidelines (page 2)

No mass

Cyclical / Non-cyclical

Cyclical → Wait 2 cycles** → If resolves, resume routine screening / No resolution

Non-cyclical → Unilateral / Bilateral

Bilateral → Patient < 35 years old → Symptomatic management

Patient ≥ 35 years old → Bilateral mammogram

Unilateral → Focal / Global

Focal → Ultrasound → Positive / Negative

Positive → Solid → Follow solid mass guidelines

Cyst → Follow cyst guidelines

Bilateral mammogram → Positive → Follow mammogram guidelines for BIRADS 3, 4, or 5 (fig. 1.4a)

Negative → Symptomatic management for two cycles**

Resolves → Resume routine screening

If persistent, refer to breast specialist

\* Differential diagnosis: chest wall pain, chostochondritis, cervical radiculopathy, MI, lung disease, hiatal hernia, cholelithiasis, thoracic dissection, aortic aneurysm, post partum mastitis.
\*\* Cycles if pre-menopausal, months if post-menopausal.

Breast physical examination by physicians is also widely practiced and advocated for women of all ages. Although clinical breast examination (CBE) has been studied in conjunction with mammography and one study has shown it to be beneficial in that context (the Health Insurance Plan of New York [HIP] trial), its use as a stand-alone screening tool has not yet been fully assessed. A large trial is being undertaken in India to determine the impact of screening by physical examination alone on breast cancer mortality (Jatoi, 1999). In Canada, a large randomized clinical trial has directly compared CBE alone with screening mammography plus CBE.[5] The results showed no significant difference in breast cancer mortality rates between the two study arms at 7 and 13 years after the initiation of screening (Miller et al., 1993, 2000)[6], although mammography identified smaller tumors than physical examination did. The study does not question the assertion that mammography lowers breast cancer mortality, but the results suggest that a very careful standardized physical examination (lasting an average of 10 minutes) can achieve the same reduction in mortality as screening mammography. The investigators in that study did not address the question of whether mammography led to reduced morbidity as a result of less aggressive treatment for the smaller tumors found by that screening approach. This is the only study to date to directly compare CBE to screening mammography, so there are no data to confirm or refute the findings, although the undertaking of such a confirmatory study has recently been suggested (Mittra et al., 2000). However, even if the data are sound, it might be more difficult in practice to recapitulate the benefits of CBE observed in this clinical trial (that is, more difficult than it would be for mammography) because mammography is highly standardized and regulated in the United States (see the discussion of the Mammography Quality Standards Act below), whereas CBE is not. A number of recommendations for improving the practice and standardization of CBE have been made based on a review of the literature (Barton et al., 1999).

Nevertheless, physical examination will always be important, but it is not sensitive enough to identify very small tumors. Although a pad to help women perform BSE was recently approved by the FDA[7] and some electronic palpation devices are under development (see Chapter 2), pros-

---

[5]In contrast, the other five randomized clinical trials compared screening mammography (or mammography plus clinical examination) to no screening. When the Canadian National Breast Screening Study was launched, the organizers believed that it was unethical to randomize women to forego screening entirely.

[6]The conclusions drawn from this study are controversial because many radiologists have criticized the study for a variety of reasons. For an overview, refer to Baines (1994).

[7]B-D Sensability Breast Self-Examination Aid (Becton Dickinson, Franklin Lakes, New Jersey) (Primary Care and Cancer, 1999).

pects for improving physical detection methods may depend more on increasing the number of people who do it carefully and thoroughly after training and education than on technological advances.

Screening mammography is promoted as the key to the continued reduction in breast cancer mortality through early detection. A number of organizations, including the National Cancer Institute (NCI), the American Cancer Society (ACS), and the American College of Radiology , currently recommend routine screening every 1 to 2 years for women over age 40 (U.S. Preventive Services Task Force, 1996). Several randomized controlled studies have been undertaken in four countries to assess the value of screening mammography (reviewed by Moss [1999] and Jatoi [1999]) (Table 1-2). Most of them demonstrated a substantial reduction in rates of death from breast cancer (about 25 to 30 percent) among women screened by mammography, and meta-analysis has confirmed a clear benefit of screening mammography for women over age 50 (Kerlikowske et al., 1995; Kerlikowske, 1997). (A recent review published in *The Lancet* criticized six of the eight trials for methodological inadequacies in randomization procedures that led to baseline imbalances and for determining the cause of death without blinding [Gotzsche and Olsen, 2000]. The authors concluded that because the two studies without these problems showed no reduction in mortality rates for the screened groups, screening for breast cancer by mammography is unjustified. An accompanying editorial and several letters to the editor rebutted the review, pointing out that the baseline differences were very small, that many other criteria are important for the assessment of screening trials, and that one trial did not assess screening but, rather, compared two different methods of screening.) The reported reduction in breast cancer mortality among women aged 40-49 appears to be less than that of older women, with a longer time period between initiation of routine screening and observation of reduced mortality. As a result, the value of screening women younger than age 50 is still controversial, as will be discussed later in this chapter.

There are now a variety of venues for mammography breast cancer screening, including doctors' offices, private radiology practices, hospital radiology departments, imaging centers, breast clinics, and mobile mammography vans. Because the effectiveness of screening mammography is dependent on the quality of the facilities and personnel, a federal law requires all mammography facilities to be certified by FDA. The intent of the Mammography Quality Standards Act (MQSA)[8] was to ensure that

---

[8]MQSA was passed in 1992 and enacted in 1994, with FDA inspections starting in 1995. On October 1, 1998, an extension of MQSA, called MQSRA (R = reauthorization), was enacted, with an extension given until 2002. MQSRA has more stringent regulations for facilities and personnel. These final regulations became effective in April 1999, with inspections under these changes beginning in 2000.

**TABLE 1-2**  Results of Randomized Clinical Trials of Screening Mammography

| Trial | Entry Years | Age at Entry(years) | Number of Women | Follow-up Period (years) | RR (95% CI) |
|---|---|---|---|---|---|
| HIP Trial[a] | 1963-69 | 40-64 | 60,696 | 18 | 0.77 (0.61-0.97) |
| Malmö | 1976-86 | 45-69 | 41,478 | 12 | 0.81 (0.62-1.07) |
| Two-County | 1977-85 | 40-74 | 133,065 | 11 | 0.70 (0.58-0.85) |
| Stockholm | 1981-85 | 40-64 | 59,176 | 7.4 | 0.71 (0.4-1.2) |
| Gothenburg | 1982-88 | 40-59 | 49,553 | 10 | 0.86 (0.54- 1.37) |
| Edinburgh | 1978-85 | 45-64 | 54,671 | 10 | 0.82 (0.61- 1.11) |
| Canada NBSS I[a] | 1980-87 | 40-49 | 50,430 | 10 | 1.10 (0.78- 1.54) |
| Canada NBSS II[b] | 1980-87 | 50-59 | 39,405 | 8.3 | 0.97 (0.62- 1.52) |

NOTE:  RR, relative risk (a value less than 1 indicates fewer breast cancer deaths among screened women); CI, confidence interval, NBSS, national breast screening study.

[a]Compared mammography plus CBE with no screening.
[b]Compared mammography plus CBE with CBE alone (all others compared mammography with no screening).

SOURCES: adapted from Jatoi (1999), Kerlikowske et al. (1995), and Moss (1999).

**TABLE 1-3** Mammographic Diagnostic Assessment Categories (Breast Imaging Reporting and Data System) – BIRADS

| BIRADS Category | Assessment | Recommendations |
| --- | --- | --- |
| 0 | Incomplete | Other mammographic views and techniques or ultrasound needed |
| 1 | Negative, no findings | Routine screening |
| 2 | Benign finding | Routine screening |
| 3 | Probably benign | Short-term follow-up to establish stability |
| 4 | Suspicious abnormality | Biopsy should be considered |
| 5 | Highly suggestive of malignancy | Appropriate action should be taken |

SOURCE: American College of Radiology: Breast Imaging Reporting and Data System (BIRADS). Reston, Virginia, American College of Radiology, 1998.

all facilities meet federal standards for equipment, personnel, and practices.[9] Since its inception, the quality of mammograms has improved (Suleiman et al., 1999; U.S. General Accounting Office, 1998a,b; Wagner, 1999). However, mammography is the only medical examination that is federally regulated in this way, and the regulations substantially increase the cost of performing mammography (Inman, 1998; Wagner, 1999).

A screening mammogram actually consists of two X-ray films, taken from the side (referred to as the "mediolateral oblique view") and from above (referred to as the "craniocaudal view"), for each breast. A diagnostic mammogram, which may include additional views or magnifications, is usually performed following a suspicious finding on a screening mammogram or when a woman has a new symptom such as a breast lump. To create a uniform system of assessing mammography results, the American College of Radiology developed the Breast Imaging Reporting and Data System (BIRADS)[10] (Table 1-3). This system includes five categories

---

[9]It is noteworthy that mammography performed in the randomized clinical trials with an older technology would not meet today's MQSA standards.

[10] The American College of Radiology has also recently established the National Mammography Database (NMD) with the goal of improving mammography quality. NMD is a national comparative database of mammography reporting information for breast imaging facilities, regions, and states to allow a national mammography audit of practices by use of the BIRADS lexicon.

of assessment with increasing suspicion of malignancy, along with standard follow-up recommendations for each category.

Ultimately, mammograms do not detect cancer per se. Rather, they provide a means for the identification of tissue abnormalities, which are subject to interpretation by human observers who introduce variability into the process on the basis of their prior experience, training, perceptual capabilities, vigilance, and so on. Radiologists look for microcalcifications (tiny calcium deposits), architectural distortions, asymmetrical densities, masses, and densities that have developed since the previous mammogram. In some cases, breast ultrasound may be ordered as a follow-up to mammography to rule out cysts (fluid-filled lesions) or to better characterize the lesion and its solid components. For women with a BIRADS score of 4 or 5, biopsy and histological examination are generally necessary to determine whether the abnormality identified by imaging methods is benign and harmless or malignant and life threatening.

Traditionally, a diagnostic biopsy entails an open surgical incision to remove a lump or tissue sample. In the case of nonpalpable lesions, the surgeon may be guided to the position of the abnormal tissue by "wire localization," in which a fine wire is inserted into the suspicious area and placement of the tip is confirmed by mammography. More recently, two minimally invasive biopsy methods have been developed for breast cancer diagnosis: fine-needle aspiration (FNA) for cytology and core-needle biopsy (CNB) for pathological assessment of breast tissue (Fajardo and DeAngelis, 1997; Morrow, 1995; Scott and Morrow, 1999; Sneige, 1991). A very thin needle and syringe can be used to remove either fluid from a cyst (standard FNA) or clusters of cells from a palpable mass (fine-needle aspiration biopsy [FNAB]). It is most frequently used to confirm a cyst by removing the cyst fluid. If the mass proves to be solid or only partially filled with fluid, the needle is quickly pushed back and forth through the solid tissue while suction is applied to free some cells, which are aspirated and analyzed by a cytopathologist. The sensitivity of FNAB cytology depends on the quality of the sample obtained and the experience of the cytologist, but it generally falls in the range of 65 to 98 percent (Scott and Morrow, 1999). Unfortunately, the ability to obtain samples of sufficient size from nonpalpable lesions is limited, and the retrieval of such samples can be done only with imaging guidance (ultrasound or mammography). Thus, FNA is not as useful in such instances (Pisano et al., 1998b). Other limitations of this procedure are that it cannot distinguish between invasive cancer and in situ lesions, and it may produce inconclusive findings that require an additional core or open biopsy procedure.

CNB, although more traumatic for the patient, affords a higher rate of sensitivity. CNB uses a larger needle with a special cutting edge. The needle is inserted, under local anesthesia, through a tiny incision in the skin, and 5 to 10 small cores of tissue are removed. Tissue cores obtained by CNB are usually sufficiently large to allow pathologists to distinguish between invasive and noninvasive types of breast cancer. For nonpalpable lesions, CNB must be combined with an imaging modality (X ray, ultrasound, or less frequently, MRI) to target the suspicious tissue. The choice of guidance method depends on the experience of the radiologist or surgeon, the equipment available, and the type of lesion.

Novel CNB systems are also being developed with the goal of improving accuracy (Velanovich et al., 1999; Wong et al., 2000). One example is a vacuum-assisted biopsy instrument, also known as a Mammotome, in which suction is applied to the tissue while CNB is performed. This results in more tissue being drawn into the needle. In one study that compared standard stereotactic CNB with vacuum-assisted biopsy in patients with microcalcifications, CNB missed calcifications in nearly 10 percent of the patients, but vacuum-assisted biopsy did not miss calcifications in any of the 106 patients (Meyer et al., 1997). The Advanced Breast Biopsy Instrument (ABBI) is an example of a new system for removal of a larger core biopsy specimen than is possible with a Mammotome or by traditional CNB. The ABBI method uses a rotating circular knife and a thin wire heated with an electrical current to remove a large cylinder of tissue containing the abnormality.

## LIMITATIONS OF CURRENT TECHNOLOGIES

Despite its demonstrated ability to detect breast cancer early and reduce disease-specific mortality rates to some degree, mammography has inherent limitations and risks like any cancer screening technology (including physical examination). Because the sensitivity and specificity are not 100 percent, screening programs will necessarily produce some false findings, both false-positive and false-negative findings, which can have detrimental effects on the screened population. Furthermore, identification of breast cancer by screening mammography does not guarantee that a woman will not die of breast cancer. Even small tumors may develop the ability to metastasize, and in these cases, early detection and treatment will not necessarily produce a cure. Some cancers will also rapidly develop during the period between screenings (termed interval cancers), and such aggressive tumors may not be amenable to treatment.

### False-Positive Results

One limitation with the current technology for mammography is the high rate of false-positive results, which are abnormal findings in patients who are subsequently found to be free of breast cancer. To avoid large numbers of false-positive results, the specificity of a test must reach 99 percent or more, but most screening tests for cancer have much lower specificities. For published reports on mammography, specificities generally fall in the range of 90 to 98 percent (Mushlin et al., 1998). The risk of having a false-positive result by mammography during routine yearly screening may be as high as 10 percent (Brown et al., 1995). One study suggests that among women who receive annual mammograms for 10 years, half will have at least one false-positive result that leads to additional tests such as diagnostic mammography, ultrasound, or biopsy (Christiansen et al., 2000; Elmore et al., 1998a). Currently, as many as three-fourths of all biopsy specimens turn out to be benign lesions. As acceptance and use of mammographic screening become more widespread, the increasing number of false-positive results becomes a cause for concern.

Short-term studies have shown that abnormal mammograms negatively affect a woman's psychological and emotional state (Lowe et al., 1999). Even when further evaluation rules out cancer, some women report impaired moods and daily functioning for up to 3 months after a suspicious finding on a mammogram (Lerman et al., 1991). A study in Norway examined perceptions of quality of life 18 months following a false-positive mammogram. Most women in that study regard their experience with a false-positive mammogram as one of the many minor stressful life incidences, with only a temporary decrease in quality of life (Gram et al., 1990). However, women with false-positive mammograms also experience heightened levels of concern about breast cancer (Lowe et al., 1999; Gram et al., 1990). Previously, it was commonly believed that fear could prevent women from returning for a second screening following a false-positive result. However, a recent study showed that women with false-positive mammograms, especially those who had no previous mammograms, were actually more likely to come in for their next scheduled visit (Burman et al., 1999; Pisano et al., 1998a).

The medical procedures that are necessary after a suspicious mammogram have additional consequences, both physical and financial. Follow-up work to an initial screening test can include diagnostic mammograms, ultrasound examinations, and needle or surgical biopsies. Pain and reduced sexual sensitivity due to surgical biopsy are possible side effects (Gram et al., 1990). Lost productivity as a result of time off for surgery and recuperation is an additional cost. Retrospective studies show that the additional costs of evaluating false-positive results can add up to one-third of the total cost of screening for all women (Elmore et al., 1998a; Lidbrink et al., 1996). Furthermore, scarring of the tissue following surgical biopsy may result in cosmetic concerns and could potentially interfere with subsequent cancer detection. However, improvements in biopsy techniques have led to smaller and less invasive procedures and have thus reduced some of these concerns.

## False-Negative Results

No screening or diagnostic technology is perfect, and thus, some false-negative results are inevitable. A normal mammogram does not guarantee that a woman is free of breast cancer because some tumors are not detected by mammography. The sensitivity of screening mammography (ability to detect occult cancer) ranges from 83 to 95 percent in published studies (Mushlin et al., 1998). Failure to detect breast cancer can generally be attributed to one of four main reasons: inherent limitations of mammography, inadequate radiographic technique, subtle or unusual lesion characteristics, and errors of interpretation. A number of studies have shown that a significant portion of breast cancers detected at follow-up mammography are visible in retrospect on the previous mammogram that was interpreted as normal (Harvey et al., 1993; van Dijck et al., 1993; Warren Burhenne et al., 2000). Regardless of the cause, a false-negative finding on a mammogram can be quite harmful to the woman whose cancer has been missed. Normal findings on a mammogram may produce a false sense of security that could prevent women from seeking appropriate medical attention, even for symptomatic lesions. A delay in diagnosis will delay treatment, perhaps in some cases to the point where treatment will no longer be effective because the tumor has had sufficient time to progress and metastasize. Because of these potential dire consequences associated with false-negative findings, the number of medical malpractice lawsuits stemming from missed cancer diagnoses has increased considerably since screening programs were widely introduced. In fact, a recent report suggests that lawsuits alleging a missed or delayed breast cancer diagnosis are now the most prevalent of all medical malpractice suits filed against radiologists and physicians in general (Berlin, 1999; Physicians Insurers Association of America, 1995, 1997) (see Chapter 6).

## Lack of Data for Older Women

The risk of breast cancer increases with age throughout a woman's lifetime, and the sensitivity and positive predictive value of screening mammography also improve as women age (Kerlikowske et al., 1993; Mushlin et al., 1998) (Table 1-4). However, few data are available on the benefits of screening mammography in women age 70 and older, and thus, uniform recommendations do not exist for women in this age group. The efficacy of mammography in older women is unknown because only two randomized controlled trials included women over age 65, and the numbers were too small too provide meaningful results (Table 1-2). Furthermore, screening of some older women may be less beneficial and cost-effective because of their shortened life expectancies compared with those

**TABLE 1-4**   The Probability of Developing
Breast Cancer is Age Dependent

| Age | Probability |
| --- | --- |
| by age 30 | 1 out of 2,525 |
| by age 40 | 1 out of 217 |
| by age 50 | 1 out of 50 |
| by age 60 | 1 out of 24 |
| by age 70 | 1 out of 14 |
| by age 80 | 1 out of 10 |

SOURCE: National Cancer Institute, Surveillance, Epidemiology, and End Results (SEER) Program, Publication
97-3536, 1997.

for women in younger age groups. When a woman has serious comorbid
conditions that are life limiting and would deter intervention if a tumor
were discovered, screening mammography would not be helpful and is
generally not recommended. However, because of the lack of data, it is
difficult to determine who is likely to benefit from screening, and thus,
the decision is often made on an individual basis. Recently, a retrospective cohort study among women ages 66 to 79 years suggested that some
women in this age group might benefit from the continuation of screening
mammography. Results indicated an increased probability for detecting
localized breast cancer in conjunction with a significantly reduced risk for
detecting metastatic breast cancer among screened women (Smith-
Bindman et al., 2000). A case-control study from Holland found that regular screening mammography for women ages 65 to 75 was associated
with a 55 percent reduction in mortality from breast cancer, although
there was no reduction in breast cancer mortality associated with screening of women over age 75 (Van Dijck et al., 1996). Another recent study
suggests that for women over age 70, screening mammography may be
most beneficial and cost-effective for individuals with higher bone min-
eral density, a characteristic associated with a higher risk for breast cancer
(Kerlikowske et al., 1999).

### Challenges in Younger Women

Breast cancer screening for women under age 50 remains controversial (Lerner, 2001). Some studies have reported a survival benefit of mammography, and many organizations advocate regular screening in this
age group, but questions have been raised as to whether the benefits
outweigh the risks and costs of screening younger women (Table 1-5). As
a result of the controversy, some effort has been made to develop guidelines based on risk to help women make individual decisions about when

**TABLE 1-5** Results of Randomized Controlled Trials for Women Ages 40 to 49 years

| Trial | Start Date | Age at Entry (years) | Follow-up Period (years) | RR (95% CI) |
|---|---|---|---|---|
| HIP | 1963 | 40-49 | 10 | 0.77 (0.50-1.16) |
| Malmö I | 1976 | 45-49 | 14 | 0.67 (0.35-1.27) |
| Malmö II | 1978 | 45-48 | 12 | 0.69 (0.44-1.09) |
| Two-County: | | | | |
| Östergötland | 1977 | 40-49 | 13 | 1.02 (0.52-1.99) |
| Kopparberg | 1977 | 40-49 | 13 | 0.73 (0.37-1.41) |
| Stockholm | 1981 | 40-49 | 11.4 | 1.08 (0.54-2.17) |
| Gothenburg | 1983 | 39-49 | 12 | 0.56 (0.32-0.98) |
| Edinburgh | 1978-82[a] | 45-49 | 10-14 | 0.73 (0.43-1.25) |
| Canada NBSS I | 1980 | 40-49 | 10.5 | 1.14 (0.83-1.56) |

NOTE: RR, relative risk; CI, confidence interval.

[a]Initial randomization was 1978; additional women ages 45-49 years were randomized starting in 1982.
SOURCE: adapted from Kerlikowske (1997).

to begin screening (Gail and Rimer, 1998). It was beyond the charge of the present committee to revisit the issue of whether women under age 50 should undergo routine screening mammography, so the discussion in this report will simply review some of the issues behind the controversy, with an emphasis on how technology development may overcome some of the difficulties associated with the screening of women in this age group.

Statistical analysis of pooled data from seven randomized clinical trials indicated that screening mammography reduced breast cancer mortality by about 16 to 18 percent in women under age 50 (Berry, 1998; Kerlikowske 1997; National Institutes of Health, 1997). However, the lag time between initiation of screening and clear demonstration of a reduced mortality was more than 10 years, whereas it was about 5 years for women over age 50. The lower absolute risk of cancer among women under age 50 implies that even if relative mortality benefits were equal for women under and over age 50, absolute risk reduction would remain considerably lower for younger women. This disparity would not be corrected by improved screening technology or adjustment of screening intervals (Sirovich and Sox, 1999). Furthermore, because breast cancer is less common among women under age 50 than among older women, more individuals need to be screened to identify a case of occult breast cancer or to prevent a death from breast cancer.

One of the difficulties with screening women in their 40s is that most such women are premenopausal and are therefore likely to have greater breast density than postmenopausal women, whose breast tissue often (but by no means always) contains a higher percentage of fatty tissue. (However, postmenopausal women on estrogen replacement therapy may have similar difficulties [Laya et al., 1996], and the number of women on such therapy has been increasing.) This tissue density can make mammograms more difficult to interpret and can thus lead to missed diagnoses, as well as increased rates of false-positive findings (resulting in unnecessary biopsies). One study found that the accuracy of screening mammography in premenopausal women varies with the phase of a woman's cycle at the time of screening (White et al., 1998), suggesting that accuracy might be improved by scheduling the mammogram during a particular phase (the follicular phase during the first 2 weeks of the cycle), but this is not standard practice at present. Physical examination (CBE and BSE) may also be impeded by dense breast tissue (Heimann et al., 1998).

Other screening modalities that are not affected by breast density might be helpful for the screening of women with dense tissue at any age, especially since there may actually be a correlation between breast density and cancer risk (Byng et al., 1998). A number of studies have been undertaken to test other technologies in this population, as discussed in more detail in Chapter 2.

Younger women also tend to have a faster average cell growth rate, meaning that interval cancers may be more common and, thus, that screening may need to be conducted more frequently (e.g., annually or, among high-risk women, perhaps even semiannually) to be effective for women in this age group (Kerlikowske et al., 1996; Tabar et al., 1999).

These concerns associated with the screening of younger women are especially relevant to women at high risk. For example, women with inherited mutations in breast cancer susceptibility genes such as BRCA1 and BRCA2 are faced with the decision of choosing between prophylactic bilateral mastectomy or screening, often beginning at an earlier age than the general population (Burke et al., 1997). Women may also opt to participate in chemoprevention trials. Thus far, there are no definitive data to guide the decision-making process. Because of the limitations of mammography, especially for younger women, improved screening methods are seriously needed for this high-risk group. Several institutions are now studying whether alternate screening modalities, such as MRI or ultrasound, may be more effective and cost-effective for this relatively small, specific group.

### Radiation Sensitivity and Breast Cancer Screening

Since mammography was first introduced, some concerns have been raised about the potential risks associated with repeated exposure of the breast to ionizing radiation (i.e., X rays). There is no direct evidence of carcinogenic risk from mammography, but there is a hypothetical risk from screening because higher than normal rates of breast cancer have been noted in women with high-level radiation exposures to the breast that occurred from the 1930s to the 1950s as a result of exposure to atomic bomb radiation, multiple chest X rays, and radiation therapy treatments for benign disease or Hodgkin's lymphoma (Clemons et al., 2000; Feig and Hendrick, 1997). However, extrapolation of cancer risk from these very high radiation doses, which are unlike any dose a woman might receive from mammography, is difficult, if not impossible (Land, 1980), and most experts agree that the potential benefits of mammography outweigh the risks from radiation (Feig and Hendrick, 1997). Furthermore, technical improvements to mammographic methods over the years have greatly reduced the dose of radiation necessary to obtain quality mammograms.

Nonetheless, the risk of cancer following radiation exposure may not be uniform among all women. For example, a number of rare hereditary syndromes, usually diagnosed in children, are associated with cancer predisposition as well as sensitivity to ionizing radiation. Among these is ataxia telangiectasia (AT), a rare autosomal recessive disorder. It was observed by Swift and coworkers that mothers of children with AT devel-

**TABLE 1-6** Prevalence of AT Mutations in Women with Early Onset or Bilateral Breast Cancer

| Study | No. of Women | Type of Breast cancer | No. (%) of Women with *AT* mutations |
|---|---|---|---|
| FitzGerald et al., 1997 | 202 | Early (<40) onset | 2 (1) |
| Broeks et al., 2000 | 82 | Early (<45) onset | 7 (8.5)[a] |
| Izatt et al., 1999 | 100 | Early (<40) onset no FH | 0 |
| Shafman et al., 2000 | 57 | Contralateral | 0 |
| Chen et al., 1998 | 88 | FH | 3 (3.4) |
| Chen et al., 1998 | 100 | FH | 1 (1) |

NOTE: FH, family history; AT, ataxia telangiectasia gene.
[a]Significantly increased from population frequency.

oped breast cancer more frequently than predicted for the general population and that the breast cancers in these individuals were often associated with exposure to diagnostic radiation (Swift et al., 1991). Because 1 percent of the general population was predicted to be carriers of mutations of the *AT* gene, there was a concern that a large subset of women would be more susceptible to diagnostic radiographic procedures. Since the identification and cloning of the *AT* gene, a number of studies have been designed to address this important public health question. Of five studies conducted to date, only one reveals an increased risk for breast cancer in *AT* heterozygotes (Table 1-6).

In addition to these studies of early-onset or contralateral breast cancers occurring after radiation therapy, other study designs have thus far failed to reveal a significant role of *AT* heterozygosity as a risk factor for radiation-associated breast cancer. One of these studies included 52 patients with a second malignancy after receiving therapeutic radiation for Hodgkin's disease (Nichols et al., 1999). In addition, the adverse effects of radiation were not associated with *AT* mutations in 57 patients in two studies (Appelby et al., 1997; Shayeghi et al., 1998). Thus, the current literature does not support the theory that mutation of the *AT* gene is a major risk factor for radiation-induced breast cancer, although additional studies are needed.

Recent studies have also raised concerns regarding the radiation sensitivity of carriers of *BRCA* mutations. Initial reports showed that mice lacking the protein products of the *BRCA1* and *BRCA2* genes were extremely sensitive to ionizing radiation (Connor et al., 1997; Sharan et al., 1997). Recently, human tumor cell lines containing one normal copy and one mutated copy of the *BRCA1* gene also showed many classical signs of radiation sensitivity (Foray et al., 1999). These results raise the possibility that *BRCA* mutations in humans may result in deleterious effects (due to the accumulation of radiation-induced mutations) in women exposed to ionizing radiation. However, the doses of gamma radiation used in these cell line experiments (in the range of 1 to 2 grays [Gy]) were far in excess of the doses that normal tissues receive during diagnostic irradiation (in the range of 1 rad, or 0.01 Gy). Further study is needed to address this issue.

## Overtreatment of Early Lesions

New technologies do not merely detect breast cancer earlier, but they can also complicate the screening and treatment processes. Improvements in the sensitivity of breast imaging techniques have led to an increase in the identification of small abnormalities whose biology is not well understood. For example, many consider ductal carcinoma in situ (DCIS) to be a premalignancy because it appears cancerous but has not invaded surrounding tissues or metastasized (Figure 1-5).

The number of women diagnosed with DCIS has greatly increased since screening mammography was widely adopted. Between 1973 and 1983, DCIS accounted for only 0.3 to 5.2 percent of all cases of breast cancer diagnosed, depending on the age group. In contrast, between 1983 and 1992, DCIS constituted 12 to 18 percent of all newly diagnosed cases of breast cancer and may account for as much as 30 percent of breast cancer cases identified by screening mammography (Ernster et al., 1996). Among women ages 40 to 49, as many as 40 percent of all cases of breast cancer detected by mammography are DCIS (Ernster and Barclay, 1997). Although some DCIS lesions will develop into invasive cancers, there is no method for determination of whether a particular DCIS will develop into a life-threatening metastatic cancer. In fact, one study reported finding occult DCIS at autopsy in 40 percent of women between 40 and 50 years of age who died from other causes (Nielsen et al., 1987), although the incidence in other similar studies (6 to 18 percent) has not been quite so high (see Welch and Black [1997] and references therein).

Initially, DCIS was often treated by mastectomy, but more recently, lumpectomy (removal of tissue surrounding the lesion) followed by radiation has become more common, as it has with invasive breast cancer. However, the pattern of treatment varies greatly, and because the rate of DCIS detection has increased, thousands of mastectomies for DCIS are still performed each year (Ernster et al., 1996). In some cases, the treatment decision may be due to a patient's inaccessibility to facilities that provide radiation therapy (e.g., because of where a woman lives or because she lacks medical insurance).

Another type of noninvasive high-risk breast lesion, referred to as "lobular carcinoma in situ" (LCIS), is as perplexing or even more so than

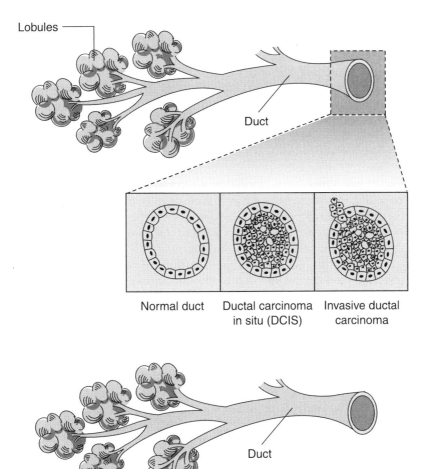

Lobules

Duct

Normal duct

Ductal carcinoma
in situ (DCIS)

Invasive ductal
carcinoma

Duct

Lobules

Normal lobule

Lobular carcinoma
in situ (LCIS)

Invasive
lobular
carcinoma

**FIGURE 1-5** Schematic representation of ductal (a) and lobular (b) carcinoma of the breast. SOURCE: adapted from Love (1995, p. 220).

DCIS in terms of biological understanding and clinical management. Epidemiological studies have shown that patients with a history of LCIS are as likely as those diagnosed with DCIS to eventually develop invasive breast cancer (relative risk, ~10 times that for age-matched controls) (Rosen et al., 1980; Rosen, 1981). Unlike DCIS, the risk associated with LCIS is bilateral, suggesting that LCIS may be a marker for rather than a precursor of invasive breast cancer. Furthermore, LCIS is often multifocal and bilateral, suggesting that it may arise in response to a carcinogenic "field defect." Recent studies have unequivocally demonstrated that LCIS shares identical genetic defects with invasive cancer in the same breast (Lu et al., 1998; Nayar et al., 1997), consistent with the notion that LCIS may be both a marker for and a direct precursor to invasive tumors. LCIS is present in about 5 percent of breast biopsy specimens. It is almost always clinically occult and is encountered as an incidental finding in breasts biopsied for some other reason. Surgery is not considered an option for patients with LCIS because of its multifocal nature, and there is no universally agreed upon approach to the management of LCIS because it is not a true malignancy. In the recent chemoprevention trial conducted by the National Surgical Adjuvant Breast and Bowel Project, a history of LCIS was one of the enrollment criteria. There was a 50 percent reduction in the incidence of invasive breast cancer in the LCIS group receiving tamoxifen compared with the incidence in the group receiving a placebo, suggesting that tamoxifen may be reasonable therapy for patients with LCIS (Fisher et al., 1998a).

Increasing the ability to identify DCIS and LCIS raises important questions in regard to breast cancer screening. What are clinicians looking for, and what should they do when they find it? The biology of these small lesions and how to treat them are not as well studied, and research has been possible only since it became possible to detect them, so clarity about optimal treatment will take many years to develop.

## DILEMMA OF "EARLIER" DETECTION

The efforts to develop technologies capable of pushing back the detection timeline to a stage that is even earlier than what is currently possible could provide new opportunities for early intervention, but such opportunities could also increase the difficulties associated with "overdiagnosis." The underlying assumption in promoting early detection held by many investigators, most physicians, and almost all members of the lay population is that early detection provides an opportunity to reverse the malignancy process more effectively and perhaps with less toxicity than if the condition were identified later. The notion that earlier detection is better requires the following three assumptions: (1) that development of carcinoma of the breast proceeds through a relatively orderly

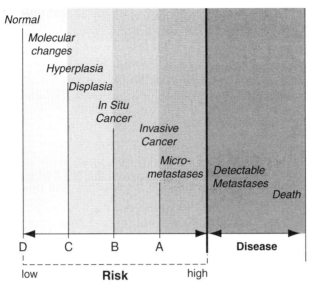

**FIGURE 1-6** Hypothetical illustration of breast cancer initiation and progression. Although most patients and physicians would consider a histological diagnosis of breast cancer, even when it is totally in situ, a "disease," a more precise definition of disease is "a condition that causes morbidity and mortality." In this sense, breast cancer is only a disease when one of these two conditions exists. Morbidity and mortality occur almost exclusively in the setting of clinically detectable metastases. Thus, all other stages of breast abnormalities are shown here as having variable levels of risk for the development of morbidity and mortality (i.e., disease). For more detail, refer to the section Dilemma of "Earlier" Detection in the text.

series of steps (Figure 1-6); (2) that this process includes an irreversible checkpoint (which may vary for different patients) and that once an individual is past this checkpoint the process steadily progresses so that only some sort of external intervention can prevent the ultimate inevitability of morbidity and mortality; and (3) that detection of this process before establishment of metastatic deposits will permit external intervention to prevent disease-specific morbidity and mortality more efficiently than after metastases are established. These points of detection are illustrated as A, B, C, and D, respectively by the vertical lines on Figure 1-6.

The fundamental support for these assumptions comes from the randomized clinical trials described earlier in this chapter, which showed that mammography screening of asymptomatic women results in early treatment of breast cancers that are detected and reduces disease-specific mortality by approximately 20 to 30 percent compared with that for women who have not been screened.[11] Why is the decrease in mortality not greater? There are several possible answers to this question. Simply put, screening mammography is insufficiently sensitive in two ways: (1) it does not detect all cancers at point B, and (2) it does not detect any cancers at point C. One might argue that improvements in imaging technologies might allow clinicians to increase the number of tumors detected at point B or even move detection to point C. However, a second reason that reductions in breast cancer mortality rates due to screening mammography are limited might be embedded in the biology of the cancer itself. Some cancers may metastasize at a time well before point B on the breast cancer continuum, whereas others may do so much later. Thus, the question of whether detection is early enough to allow effective intervention may vary from one woman to the next.

The assumptions presented above raise several considerations. A distinction should be made between screening for an asymptomatic but precise condition that is considered undesirable and establishing that the individual is at risk for such a condition but does not yet and may never have it. Indeed, taken to its extreme, this distinction is blurred and perhaps even abolished in the definition of "disease." For example, most patients and physicians would consider a histological diagnosis of breast cancer, even when it is totally in situ, a "disease." However, a more precise definition of disease is "a condition that causes morbidity and mortality." In this sense, breast cancer is only a disease when one of these two conditions exists. Morbidity and mortality occur almost exclusively in the setting of clinically detectable metastases.

Before the increased awareness of breast cancer and adoption of screening mammography, almost all patients who presented with breast cancer did so because the condition was at a stage at which it was truly a disease: it caused symptoms or even death. However, in more modern times, most patients are diagnosed with asymptomatic breast cancer. In this setting, almost all treatment for breast cancer (surgical removal of the primary tumor, local-regional radiation to sterilize the area, and adjuvant systemic therapy) could be considered prophylactic or preventive. Such treatments are applied to reduce the chances that the patient will develop morbidity or mortality (or "disease"). A substantial body of literature describing the results of randomized clinical trials demonstrates that each of these strategies does, in fact, reduce to some extent the individual's chances of developing morbidity or mortality from breast cancer.

Why are these distinctions important? No single condition, other than actually having symptomatic disease, carries a 100 percent chance (or risk) of developing what is designated, in this discussion, disease. How-

---

[11]As noted earlier, a single study compared screening mammography to CBE and found that although mammography could detect tumors at a smaller size than CBE can, this "earlier" detection did not translate to improved survival (Miller et al., 2000). These findings remain controversial (see footnote 6, this chapter).

ever, as one moves from left to right on the theoretical breast cancer continuum illustrated in Figure 1-6, an individual's chances of ultimately developing morbidity and mortality increase. Estimating this risk is quite difficult because, at least in the last century, few patients were left untreated once they had a diagnosis of "breast cancer," and therefore, it is impossible to determine what percentage of patients, if any, might never have progressed to experience morbidity or mortality from breast cancer if they were left untreated.

However, one might extrapolate from certain experiences to suggest that among women at a given point in the continuum, not all will progress to the next or subsequent steps. For example, a number of pathological features such as the presence of axillary lymph nodal micrometastases are known to identify women more likely to develop morbidity and mortality after local-regional therapy. However, 20 to 30 percent of node-negative patients subsequently develop symptomatic, incurable metastases, and up to 25 percent of node-positive patients do not (Cocconi, 1995; Weidner, 1995). More recently, clinical investigators have reported that detection of distant micrometastatic breast cancer cells in circulation or even bone marrow is associated with a poorer prognosis (Braun et al., 2000; Pantel et al., 1999). However, a substantial fraction of these "positive" patients also survive without systemic therapy. Other molecular features, such as hormone receptor content, measures of proliferation, and *HER-2* gene amplification, may help to fine-tune prognostic estimates, but they are far from absolute in dividing a population into those who are destined to develop "disease" and those who are not.

DCIS presents an even greater dilemma than early invasive cancers. DCIS hypothetically lies to the left of invasive cancer on the theoretical continuum illustrated in Figure 1-6. Since DCIS does not contain cells that have invaded the surrounding tissue layer, it should not be associated with metastatic cells or a very high, if any, risk of developing morbidity and mortality. Therefore, in theory, DCIS would be the preferred lesion to detect by screening (rather than invasive cancer). However, it is not known what percentage of breast cancers pass through the DCIS phase. In other words, do some breast cancers progress from left to right in Figure 1-6 with only a brief sojourn as DCIS, or do some perhaps skip it completely? Moreover, few patients who have been diagnosed with this condition have ever been studied or followed without excising of the lesion. Therefore, it is not known whether some or many in situ breast cancers would never progress beyond this phase. Indeed, it is likely that a certain proportion of these lesions might remain as in situ cancer or even regress to a less worrisome histologic state. Nonetheless, recent randomized clinical trials have suggested that women with excised DCIS who do not receive further local (surgery, radiation) or systemic (hormonal) therapy are more likely to suffer a recurrence of cancer in the breast with either the same diagnosis or a more advanced diagnosis (further to the right on the continuum illustrated in Figure 1-6), such as invasive breast cancer (Fisher et al., 1998; Hetelekidis et al., 1999; Silverstein and Lagios, 1997).

In summary, current definitions of breast cancer, as determined by histopathology of biopsy specimens taken from the breast, are only imperfect surrogates of whether patients will develop true disease, as defined here. A diagnosis of anything other than "normal" or "benign" breast tissue places the patient into a higher risk category, whereas treatment with surgery or with radiation or systemic therapy places the patient in a lower risk category. Treatment in this setting is always applied inefficiently because there is no effective way of determining who will benefit from it. Thus, many women receive "preventive" therapy, even though they would never develop metastatic disease, in order to reduce the risk of morbidity and mortality for those who would. Preventive therapy is less efficient the further to the left on the breast cancer continuum in Figure 1-6 one goes. As a woman's condition moves farther to the right on the continuum, women are more willing to accept previously unacceptable preventive therapies because they perceive their risk of death from breast cancer to be higher.

## SUMMARY

X-ray mammography is now the mainstay for the detection, diagnosis, and localization of breast cancers. It is currently the only medical imaging procedure used as a screening tool. Screening mammography has definitively been shown to reduce, but not eliminate mortality from breast cancer when it is performed at regular intervals and followed by appropriate interventions. In randomized clinical trials, screening mammography reduced breast cancer mortality by about 25 to 30 percent among women ages 50 to 70 and by about 18 percent among women between the ages of 40 and 50. Although the incidence of breast cancer increases with age, data on the benefits of screening for older women are lacking because most randomized trials excluded women over age 70. Recent observational studies suggest that mammography is also beneficial for women over age 70, but further documentation of benefit is important. There is also some indirect evidence that screening mammography has been effective in reducing the number of deaths from breast cancer in the general population. Mortality from breast cancer in the United States, as well as some European countries, has been decreasing in recent years, and some of this reduction is consistent with the effect of screening.

However, there is clearly room for improvement in the screening and diagnosis of breast cancer because of both the technical and the biological limitations of the current methods. Although the clinical practice of mammography is federally regulated for quality assurance (the only clinical procedure regulated in this way), it is still technically difficult to consistently produce mammograms of high quality, and interpretation is subjective and can be variable among radiologists. Furthermore, mammography does not detect all breast cancers, including some that are palpable, and as many as three-quarters of all breast lesions biopsied because of a suspicious finding on a mammogram turn out to be benign. Mammograms are particularly difficult to interpret for women with dense breast tissue, who are at increased risk of breast cancer. The dense tissue interferes with the identification of abnormalities associated with tumors. This leads to higher rates of false-negative and false-positive findings in these women. In addition, optimal screening intervals are poorly defined because some tumors develop too quickly to be identified at the current screening intervals, especially in younger women.

The current limitations of mammography and other existing technologies (as described in this chapter) have been driving forces behind the efforts to improve mammography and other diagnostic techniques and to develop additional novel methods for the early detection of breast cancer. The purpose of the study presented in this report is to examine some of the many technologies under development (Chapters 2 and 3) and to identify potential impediments to the development of new breast cancer screening and diagnostic procedures (Chapters 4, 5, and 6). Many factors can influence the development, adoption, and use of medical technologies, including the availability of research funds, the regulatory approval process, coverage and reimbursement decisions, acceptability to the target population, and difficulties in ensuring broad access. Although many technologies described in this report are at a relatively early stage of development and it is difficult to predict their ultimate value or use, they all must clear many hurdles if they are to become part of the standard of care for women and thus play a role in reducing the toll of breast cancer.

In assessing new technologies, three distinct goals regarding early detection, listed below, need to be considered and addressed. These are revisited frequently throughout the remaining chapters.

1. Identification of a higher percentage of women with an early stage of breast cancer. This aim could be achieved by improving the accuracy (sensitivity and specificity) and accessibility of mammography and also by developing other technologies that can identify cancers that are often missed by mammography. This is the goal of many of the technologies described in Chapter 2.

2. Development of technologies that can detect early changes before the appearance of a true malignancy that increase a woman's risk of de-

veloping invasive or metastatic breast cancer. A number of potential technologies could accomplish this aim, as described in Chapters 2 and 3.
However, as these develop, the specificity (that is, the magnitude to which
a woman's risk is increased as a result of having a positive test) must be
considered. Women may or may not consider a given magnitude sufficient to accept a given preventive strategy. Thus, it is important that
investigators and physicians not assume that if a new technology identifies a breast abnormality, even one that appears, histologically, to represent cancer, it must move a patient to the right on the cancer continuum
(as illustrated in Figure 1-6). In the absence of data, such an assumption
would unfairly lead a patient to accept therapies that she previously believed were unacceptable.

3. Discover more acceptable and effective means of risk reduction for
women at early points along the continuum of breast cancer initiation and
progression. Research on the biological processes that increase a woman's
risk may also lead to new intervention strategies directed toward those
processes.[12] An underlying context of this discussion of early detection is
that new, more acceptable preventive strategies could be applied more
widely and efficiently. That is, a therapy with little or no toxicity or adverse consequences would be much more acceptable to women with only
a low or a moderate risk.

In the meantime, enthusiasm for new technologies should be tem-
pered by consideration of the ultimate goal: to reduce the morbidity and
mortality from breast cancer among women. It is important to keep in
mind that the ability to move toward detection at an earlier point in the
continuum of abnormalities does not necessarily mean that further
progress toward decreasing disease-specific morbidity and mortality will
occur. It is also essential to understand what is being detected and how to
appropriately intervene. Decisions about the use of new technologies
should be firmly grounded in scientific evidence if investigators are to optimize the benefits and minimize the risks of early breast cancer detection.

---

[12]Like screening trials, prevention trials are large, long, and costly when the incidence of
cancer is used as an end point. Recently, an alternative approach to the streamlining of
investigations in this field has been proposed by a task force of the American Association
for Cancer Research. The group recommends using the incidence of breast intraepithelial
neoplasia (IEN) as a surrogate end point for prevention studies (Fabian et al., 2000). IEN is
defined as a condition associated with a change in morphology, molecular expression, genetic makeup, and relative risk of breast cancer. IEN includes proliferative breast disease,
atypical hyperplasia, and carcinoma in situ.

# 2
# Breast Imaging and Related Technologies

Medical imaging is central to breast cancer screening, diagnosis, and staging. Mammography is the most sensitive technique available for the detection of nonpalpable breast lesions, and thus, screening mammography has secured a routine place in health maintenance for women in the United States. Although it is less than perfect, screening mammography can reduce breast cancer mortality when combined with appropriate interventions (see Chapter 1).

Conventional X-ray mammography is a mature technology that provides high-quality images at low radiation doses in the majority of patients. However, conventional film-based mammography may not provide adequate diagnostic information for some women with radiodense breast tissue. It has been estimated that this technology misses about 15 percent of breast cancer lesions (Mushlin et al., 1998). In addition, studies have reported that the positive predictive value[1] of conventional mammography ranges only from 15 to 40 percent (Kerlikowske et al., 1993; Kopans, 1992; Kopans et al., 1996). Consequently, 60 to 85 percent of lesions detected by mammography are benign, and thus, many biopsies could potentially be avoided. This situation creates an important incentive for the development of novel technologies to improve detection, diagnosis, and staging and monitoring of treatment for breast cancer.

Accordingly, other imaging technologies, particularly nonionizing

---

[1]The positive predictive value is the number of cancers diagnosed per number of biopsies recommended (see Box 1-1).

modalities such as magnetic resonance imaging and ultrasound, are being tested for application to breast cancer, with promising results. At present, these methods may provide additional diagnostic specificity over X-ray mammography alone. Additional tools such as scintimammography, positron emission tomography, magnetic resonance spectroscopy, and optical imaging are under investigation as well. To date, no single imaging method appears to offer both high sensitivity and high specificity for the detection and diagnosis of breast cancer.

The previous chapter summarized the main technologies in current use for breast cancer detection, whereas this chapter looks more closely at imaging modalities under development (Tables 2-1 and 2-2). The various technologies can roughly be divided into three categories: (1) those that are currently in use, such as X-ray mammography and ultrasound, but that are being further refined; (2) those that are commonly used for medical imaging, such as magnetic resonance imaging (MRI), but that are still experimental with regard to breast cancer detection; and (3) and novel imaging modalities that may be used in the future. A 1996 report, *The Mathematics and Physics of Emerging Biomedical Imaging*, explains the technical background of many of these promising new technologies in greater detail than is possible here (Institute of Medicine, 1996).

The chapter describes the current state of the art as well as technological roadblocks associated with promising near-term imaging technologies. Potential longer-term solutions using alternative modalities, such as optical or microwave imaging, are also briefly addressed. In addition, this chapter describes how novel technologies may affect breast cancer detection in ways beyond image acquisition, including image processing, display, management, storage, and transmission. Common to all imaging systems is the increasing use of digital methods for signal processing, which also offers the possibility of computer-aided detection by texture analysis and pattern recognition.

## FUNDAMENTALS OF IMAGING ANALYSIS

Breast imaging technologies are being developed with three distinct goals in mind: (1) to identify abnormal tissues, (2) to localize the abnormalities within the breast to facilitate further examination or treatment, and (3) to characterize the abnormalities and aid the decision-making process following identification. An ideal imaging modality would accomplish all three goals in a single use, but in reality, most current technologies cannot achieve this, so developers tend to focus on optimizing one goal at a time. In addition to these technical goals, developers hope to generate detection methods that are more practical, inexpensive, harmless, and appealing to the patient than current methods.

Many of the current medical imaging methods are used to map struc-

**TABLE 2-1** Current Status of Imaging and Related Technologies Under Development for Breast Cancer Detection

| Technology | Current Status | | FDA approved for breast imaging/ detection |
| --- | --- | --- | --- |
| | Screening | Diagnosis | |
| Film-screen mammography (FSM) | +++ | +++ | Yes |
| Full-field digital mammography (FFDM) | ++ | ++ | Yes |
| Computer-assisted detection (CAD) | ++ | o | Yes |
| Ultrasound (US) | + | +++ | Yes |
| Novel US methods (compound, three-dimensional, Doppler, harmonic) | o | o | No |
| Elastography (MR and US) | o | o | No |
| Magnetic resonance imaging (MRI) | + | ++ | Yes |
| Magnetic resonance spectroscopy (MRS) | -/o[a] | +/o[a] | No |
| Scintimammography | o | + | Yes |
| Positron emission tomography (PET) | o | o | Yes |
| Optical imaging | o | + | No |
| Optical spectroscopy | - | o | No |
| Thermography | o | + | Yes |
| Electrical potential measurements | o | + | No |
| Electrical impedance imaging | o | + | Yes |
| Electronic palpation | o | NA | No |
| Thermoacoustic computed tomography, microwave imaging, Hall effect imaging, magnetomammography | NA | NA | No |

NOTE: This table is an attempt to classify a very diverse set of technologies in a rapidly changing field and thus is subject to change in the near future.

[a]Ex vivo analysis of biopsy material/in vivo MRS.

Current Status Explanation of Scale
-    Technology is not useful for the given application
NA   Data are not available regarding use of the technology for given application
o    Preclinical data are suggestive that the technology might be useful for breast cancer detection, but clinical data are absent or very sparse for the given application.
+    Clinical data suggest the technology could play a role in breast cancer detection, but more study is needed to define a role in relation to existing technologies
++   Data suggest that technology could be useful in selected situations because it adds (or is equivalent) to existing technologies, but not currently recommended for routine use
+++  Technology is routinely used to make clinical decisions for the given application

tural or morphological differences in tumors, such as microcalcifications, tissue masses, angiogenesis, asymmetry, and architectural distortion. Some of the more recently developed techniques can provide information about the biological or functional differences between tumors and normal tissues (Glasspool and Evans, 2000; Hoffman and Menkens, 2000). Such information is critical for making the "quantum leap" in fully achieving

**TABLE 2-2**  Imaging Technologies Being Developed for Detection of Breast Cancer

| Technology | Description, Mechanism |
| --- | --- |
| Full Field Digital Mammography (FFDM) | Detector responds to X-ray exposure, sends electronic signal to computer to be digitized and processed. Separates detector and image display. |
| Computer-Aided Detection and Diagnosis (CAD) | Computer programs to aid in identification of suspicious mammograms and classification as benign or malignant. Serves as a second opinion to radiologists. |
| Ultrasound | Use of high-frequency sound waves to generate an image. |

[New ultrasound technologies, in early stages of development]

Compound imaging: uses several ultrasound beams that strike the tissue from different angles. Significantly reduces speckle and improves contrast and definition of small masses and microcalcifications. May cause reduction in display of some masses.

Three-dimensional ultrasound imaging: permits display of a volume of tissue rather than a single slice. Examination of tumor volume and changes in tumor size over time.

| Stage of Development | Potential Strengths | Current Limitations |
|---|---|---|
| General Electric's Senographe 2000 D has FDA approval for use as both hard-copy and soft-copy displays. Studies are under way to compare FFDM with FSM. | Ability to manipulate contrast and magnification with one exposure. Ease of image storage and retrieval. Facilitates CAD, digital tomo-synthesis, and tele-mammography. | Spatial resolution and luminance of digital display are lower than those for FSM. Old film screens difficult to digitize for comparisons. Cost may be prohibitive. |
| R2 Technology, Inc. has a program on the market. General Electric has agree-ment with R2 Technologies to use GE FFDM machine with R2's CAD system. | Retrospective studies show that CAD can improve radiologists' readings and improve rate of false-negative results. | CAD used alone has very low specificity. Sensitivity and specificity are undetermined for general screening population. |
| Currently used as follow-up to mammography, to determine if lesion is a cyst or solid mass, or to characterize or localize a mass. | Studies suggest potential for increased use in diagnosis and perhaps even screening, especially for women with dense breasts. | Poor ability to detect microcalcifications due to speckle. Compound imaging may help reduce speckle. |

Three-dimensional and power Doppler imaging: use of Doppler technology may allow assessment of tumor vascularity; it is potentially useful for predicting biological activity and predicting responses to treatment. Can be coupled with contrast agents.

Ultrasound elastography: uses information from ultrasound signal to generate images showing elastic properties of tissue. Detects differences in tissue stiffness and may detect features not visible with mammography or conventional ultrasound.

*continued on next page*

**TABLE 2-2**  Continued

| Technology | Description, Mechanism |
|---|---|
| Magnetic Resonance Imaging (MRI) | Image generated by signals from excitation of nuclear particles in a magnetic field. Breast tumors show increased uptake of contrast agent. |

[Other MRI technologies under development.]
Minimally invasive prognosis and therapy monitoring: different cancer types that
 display distinct MRI enhancement characteristics may be important as prognostic
indicators.

| | |
|---|---|
| MR Spectroscopy (MRS) | Use of magnetic resonance spectra and "functional" molecular markers to measure biochemical components of cells and tissues. |
| Scintimammography | Image created with radioactive tracers, which concentrate more in cancer tissues than in normal tissues. Measures spatial concentration of radio-pharmaceuticals to generate planar or three-dimensional images by SPECT. |

| Stage of Development | Potential Strengths | Current Limitations |
|---|---|---|
| National Cancer Institute trials are under way to study three-dimensional high-resolution and dynamic contrast MRI in conjunction with mammography. Completion by 2001. | Benefits in detection:<br>• detection of multiple malignancies<br>• detection of invasive lobular carcinoma<br>• screening for high-risk women with dense breasts<br>• detection of recurrent cancers | Lack of uniform interpretation criteria. Cannot reliably detect microcalcifications and small tumors, especially if they do not pick up the contrast agent.<br>Overlap in uptake time course of benign and malignant tumors. |

"Smart" MRI contrast agents: agents "activated" by biochemical processes are then detected by MRI; can correlate cell functions with disease state, and can track cell growth and behavior. Limited by identification of appropriate markers and lack of clinical data. Pursued commercially by Metaprobe in Pasadena, CA.
MR Elastography: image elastic properties of tissue.

| | | |
|---|---|---|
| Studied as potential adjunct to mammography, fine needle aspirates, and assessment of lesions in vivo. | MRS spectra of samples mayincrease accuracy of FNA analysis. Potential noninvasive method of characterizing lesions. | High cost and low sensitivity and specificity for detection of small lesions. |
| MIBI approved by FDA. Other radioactive compounds being studied. Used as adjunct to mammography to localize tumors, distinguish malignancies versus benign lesions, and identify meta-static cells in distal regions of the body. | MIBI scans unaffected by dense tissue, implants, or scarring. Used when mammograms are indeterminate; can avoid the need for follow-up mammograms. High-resolution scinti-mammography uses a gamma camera and may improve resolution. Potential for SPECT monitoring of multidrug resistance. | Radiation health risks similar to those from X rays, although small doses generally considered safe except for pregnant women. MIBI more expensive than ultrasound or mammography, but less expensive than MRI. MIBI unable to detect cancers smaller than 1 cm and less accurate for nonpalpable masses. |

*continued on next page*

**TABLE 2-2**   Continued

| Technology | Description, Mechanism |
| --- | --- |
| Positron emission tomography (PET) | Uses tracers such as labeled glucose to identify regions in the body with altered metabolic activity, which is common in malignant tumors. |
| Radioactive antibodies | Target antigens specific to breast cancer, include carcinoembryonic antigen and certain growth factor receptors. |
| Optical imaging<br>Elastic scattering spectroscopy (ESS), "Optical Biopsy" | Use of fiber-optic probes to obtain spectral measurements of elastically scattered light from tissue. Generates spectral signatures that reflect architectural changes at cellular and subcellular levels. |
| Optical tomography | Use of light to image the breast. |
| Infrared thermography | Measures heat emitted by the body. Tumors can raise skin surface temperature by 2 to 3 degrees C, with heat detected by infrared cameras. Dynamic Area Telethermometry detects changes in blood flow. |
| Electrical potential measurements | Measurement of electrical potential at the skin surface. Proliferation of epithelial tissue disrupts normal polarization. |

| Stage of Development | Potential Strengths | Current Limitations |
| --- | --- | --- |
| More studies needed to determine clinical utility. | In theory, could be useful in women with dense breasts, implants, or scars. | Currently no technique to target biopsy specimens that are identified by PET but not visible on mammograms. PET scanners expensive and not readily available. |
| Only small studies to date; need more clinical studies to determine role in breast cancer diagnosis. | Some agents show promising sensitivity and specificity for breast cancer. | Scans can be difficult to interpret. Need to identify optimal markers for imaging. |
| Early clinical studies on transdermal needle diagnostic. | Portable, designed for convenient clinical use. Instant diagnosis would reduce patient anxiety and allow immediate treatment. | Currently depends on endoscopic approach, which may not be relevant to breast tissue. |
| Systems being developed by Imaging Diagnostic Systems Inc., Dynamics Optical Breast Imaging Medical Systems, and Advanced Research Technologies, Inc. | Low cost, speed, comfort, and noninvasiveness. Optical scans can be digitized for image manipulation and serial studies. | Must optimize accuracy and resolution and improve target-to-background ratios. Variations in breast tissues due to age, hormone status, and genetic makeup. |
| FDA approval in December 1999 to OmniCorder for its BioScan System, based on Dynamic Area Tele-thermometry. Computerized Thermal Imaging, Inc., is testing its system in clinical trials. | Noninvasive, does not require compression or radiation exposure. New cameras offer improved spatial and thermal resolutions. | Results of numerous studies have been inconsistent. Old technology, especially infrared cameras, has hindered development. |
| Biofield Breast Exam (BBE) has received CE Mark Certification that allows the company to sell in Europe. FDA approval pending. | BBE gives a single, numerical result that objectively determines malignancy. Inexpensive, does not require an expert reader, no discomfort, and speedy procedure. | Two large clinical studies demonstrated specificity of 55 to 60%. |

*continued on next page*

**TABLE 2-2**  Continued

| Technology | Description, Mechanism |
|---|---|
| Electrical impedance imaging | Measures voltage at skin surface while passing small current through breast. Cytological and histological changes in cancerous tissue decrease impedance of tissue. |
| Electronic palpation | Quantitative palpation of breast using pressure sensors. |
| Thermoacoustic Computed Tomography (TCT) | Breast is irradiated with radio waves, causing different thermal expansion of tissue and generating sound waves, from which a three-dimensional image is constructed. |
| Microwave imaging | Transmits low-power microwaves into tissue and collects backscattered energy to create three-dimensional image. Higher water content in malignant tissues causes more scatter. |
| Hall Effect Imaging (HEI) | Induces vibrations by passing electric pulse through tissue while exposed to a magnetic field. |
| Magnetomammography (MMG) | Tags cancerous tissue with magnetic agents that are imaged with SQUID magnetometers. |

| Stage of Development | Potential Strengths | Current Limitations |
| --- | --- | --- |
| FDA approval in 1999 to TransScan Medical (Ramsey, NJ) for use of T-Scan 2000 device as an adjunct to mammography for women with lesions in BIRADS[a] 3/4. | Potential as adjunct to mammography for women with certain indeterminate lesions. Painless, no breast compression or ionizing radiation. | Not to be used for women with clear indications for biopsy. Currently conducting more trials to validate technology. |
| Assurance Medical (Hopkinton, MA) is seeking FDA approval and is testing 400 women with suspicious lesions. Ultratouch (Paoli, PA) is developing robotic device (Palpagraph) and starting clinical studies for FDA approval. | Potential to standardize performance and documentation and serially monitor physical breast exams. Preliminary studies suggest use for general screening. | Limited sensitivity for small lesions. Clinical utility unproven. |
| Development in early stages. To date, no large published clinical trials. Optosonics plans to initiate a study of 80 women this year. | Does not use ionizing radiation and does not compress the breast. Retains three-dimensional structural information and images are highly consistent. | Three-dimensional images difficult to display or analyze; more time-consuming and costly than mammography. |
| To date, research focused on theoretical validation through computer modeling and studies with excised breast tissue. | Does not require compression or use ionizing radiation. In theory, should produce high-contrast image, regardless of tissue density. | Technology has been constrained by poor resolution, poor depth penetration, excessive power requirements, unsafe microwave levels, and intensive image reconstruction programs. |
| Early stages of development; first published account of HEI in 1998. To date, HEI tested only with excised and simulated tissue. | May be useful for a limited population of women. | Prohibitive cost; requires an expensive, super-conducting magnet. |
| Still untested; looking for an agent that is both magnetic and specific to cancerous tissue. | Would not require compression or ionizing radiation. Should be equally effective with dense breasts. | Poor spatial resolution, expensive to fabricate and operate. |

*continued on next page*

**TABLE 2-2** Continued

| Technology | Description, Mechanism |
| --- | --- |
| Three-dimensional interactive visualization | Includes technologies such as virtual reality. |

the third goal of diagnostic imaging described above: tumor characterization. Again, an ideal imaging tool would provide useful data on both structure and function, but this goal is quite challenging to achieve at present.

Imaging technologies for the breast are based on physical, mechanical, electrical, chemical, and biological properties of tissue (Figure 2-1). Although the technical applications of imaging tools vary, they all have a common theme. In each case, image assembly and analysis involve identification of a signal and separation of the signal from the background. A machine or a person may do the separation step, which depends on image contrast.

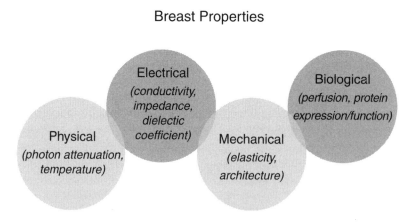

**Breast Properties**

**FIGURE 2-1** Properties of breast tissue exploited by different modes of imaging. Examples of these categories are listed.

| Stage of Development | Potential Strengths | Current Limitations |
| --- | --- | --- |
| Primarily developed for non-medical applications. Some early clinical research (e.g., breast MRI) | Could potentially be used for image visualization, training, and procedure planning and support. | Significant advances required in virtual reality technologies, including novel algorithms for breast imaging. |

## DIGITAL MAMMOGRAPHY

Full-field digital mammography (FFDM) systems are identical to traditional film-screen mammography (FSM) systems except for the electronic detectors that capture and facilitate display of the X-ray signals on a computer or laser-printed film (Figures 2-2 and 2-3). Proper positioning and compression of the breast are still critical for producing quality digital mammograms. The digital detector array responds to X-ray exposure and then sends an electronic signal for each detector location to a computer, where it is digitized, processed, and stored as a specific signal and location (pixel). The goal of digital mammography—to identify and localize breast abnormalities—is similar to that of traditional mammography. The primary motivation behind the development of digital X-ray mammography is the belief that it has the potential to improve image quality and therefore lesion detection (especially for dense breasts) with a lower

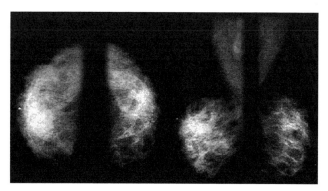

**FIGURE 2-2** Examples of Film Screen Mammography images of the breast. Source: Miraluma Educational CD-ROM, DuPont Radiopharmaceutical Division, The DuPont Merck Pharmaceutical Company.

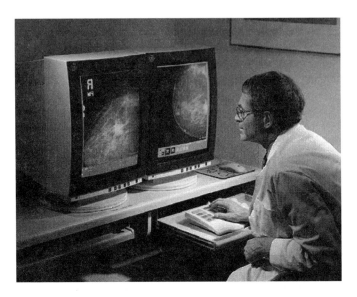

**FIGURE 2-3**   Example of Full-Field Digital Mammography images of the breast, and current technology.  Source:  General Electric Medical Systems.

dose of radiation compared with that required for conventional film-based mammography.

Digital mammography separates image acquisition from image display, offering an infinite ability to manipulate contrast, brightness, and magnification with one exposure, a feat that is not possible with traditional FSM (Pisano et al., 2000). The ability to fine-tune the digital image can enable a more detailed examination of questionable areas without requiring a new X-ray exposure. Digital processing can also enable dynamic or real-time imaging (e.g., to assist with biopsy and localization procedures) and can enable direct use of computer-aided detection and diagnosis (CAD; see below). In addition, the technology may facilitate digital tomosynthesis—reconstruction of a three-dimensional image or hologram of the breast by combining information from different detection angles. Ease of digital image archiving, retrieval, and transmission is another advantage. For example, studies on the feasibility of satellite or long-distance transmission of digital mammograms for consultation, a process known as telemammography, are under way.

When an image is displayed on a cathode ray tube (CRT) monitor (or "soft-copy" display), digital image processing can potentially improve the lesion-to-background contrast and enhance subtle details that might be missed in a standard mammogram film. Fine-tuning of the image has not yet been proved to be beneficial for breast cancer detection, but in theory, image processing could improve detection of lesions in dense breast tissue, which can obscure precancerous and cancerous lesions. Manipulation of the image, however, could theoretically reduce the visibility of the lesions as well as enhance them. Thus, optimal use of digital processing may depend on image processing algorithms similar to those used with computed tomography (CT) scans.

Digital mammography currently faces some fundamental technological problems that may impede its implementation. One current limitation of digital mammography is that the spatial resolution and luminance range of images displayed on a CRT—even with the most advanced CRT technology—are significantly lower for digital mammography than for conventional FSM. Film-screen mammograms have spatial resolutions up to 20 line-pairs per millimeter (mm). The current digital display systems have, at best, 12.5 line-pairs per mm (40 micrometers [mm] per pixel) of spatial resolution. The increased contrast resolution possible in digital mammography (the ability to display subtle differences in the number of photons absorbed in adjacent areas of the breast) may or may not compensate for its lower spatial resolution. Digital mammograms can also be printed on film with a laser printer. Such a hard-copy display increases the spatial resolution and the gray-scale range so that they are comparable to those for standard FSM. However, film for use in a laser printer is costly, and often, more than one version of the mammogram must be printed to obtain optimal readability. Thus, there is a great need for the development and testing of cost-effective digital displays for high-resolution, high-contrast, large-field-of-view visualization combined with a practical rate of display and light output.

Also key to enhancing interpretation of digital mammograms is determining how to display the most important information in the image in the best (and fastest) possible way for the clinician. This requires development of computer workstations with practical user interfaces for clinical radiologists (e.g., multi-resolution, "region-of-interest" displays and "bright-light" display equivalents). Another initial limitation of FFDM is that prior films taken by standard FSM cannot be imported easily into digitized formats for serial comparisons, posing a problem for the comparison of images over time, but this will be a dilemma for any new imaging modality. Communication hardware and software also need to be developed or improved to achieve workable collaborative efforts between specialists at different locations.

Current efforts to further develop digital mammography include photostimulatable phosphors, scanning detectors, optically coupled two-dimensional arrays, large-area detectors, and new detector materials. Ideally, the detector system should be compatible with existing mammography system geometries. Specifically, the detector must image all breast tissue up to the chest wall.

Currently, at least four manufacturers have digital mammography systems with different spatial resolutions: both the Fuji and the General Electric systems have resolutions of 100 μm, that of Fischer's system is 54 μm, and Hologic's[2] digital mammography system can obtain a 41-μm resolution. (For a more detailed description of the technology associated with each of these digital detectors, see Pisano et al. [2000]). In January 2000 the Food and Drug Administration (FDA) approved the first digital mammography machine, General Electric's Senographe 2000 D digital mammography system. However, it was approved for use only with hard-copy displays, which eliminates the opportunity for enhanced soft-copy manipulation and makes computer-aided detection more difficult. In November 2000, General Electric was granted FDA approval to use the Senographe 2000 D system for soft-copy mammogram reading.[3]

Most clinical testing of FFDM systems has been conducted by manufacturers to obtain FDA approval, and results have not been published in many cases. However, a multicenter trial supported by the U.S. Army Breast Cancer Research and Materiel Command is comparing FFDM with FSM in a general screening population of nearly 7,000 women over age 40. Results thus far suggest that digital mammography performs no better than standard FSM in detecting malignant lesions but so far has led to fewer recalls of women for further examination than conventional mammography in a screening population (Lewin et al., 2000).

The sensitivity was 53 percent for FFDM, whereas it was 67 percent for FSM (the difference was not statistically significant) (Lewin et al., 2000). These sensitivities were lower than the typically cited values for mammography (83 to 95 percent [Mushlin et al., 1998]) because each technique detected tumors that were not detected by the other one. The use of both technologies also resulted in a higher cancer detection rate (6.4 cancers per 1,000 women screened) than would normally be expected. Among a general population of women being screened for the first time, about four to six cancers are found per 1,000 women screened. In subsequent screening rounds, about three to four cancers will be identified per 1,000 women screened.

One potential advantage of FFDM was noted in the study results (Lewin et al., 2000). The rate of calling women back for further evaluation after FFDM (11.3 percent) was lower compared with that after FSM (15 percent). This difference was statistically significant ($p < 0.001$). If this difference is in fact real, projection of these data to all U.S. women receiv-

---

[2]The system was originally developed by Trex Medical (Danbury Connecticut), which was recently acquired by Hologic Corp. (Bedford, Massachusetts).

[3]See http://www.fda.gov/cdrh/mammography/mmweb/mmweb74/rws.html.

ing screening mammograms (about 25 million) could result in half a million fewer women being called back for follow-up procedures.

Both FSM and FFDM missed a significant number of cancers in this study (Figure 2-4). In fact, more than 800 of the first 5,000 screening examinations by FFMD and FSM had discordant interpretations (Lewin, 1999). The cause of the discrepancy in most cases was due to small differences in breast positioning and compression, even though the same technologist took the two mammograms sequentially on nearly identical machines. For the remaining one-third of the individuals with discrepant results, the difference between readings was primarily due to interpretation, which is known to vary considerably from double-reading studies (Beam et al., 1996; Thurfjell et al., 1994). Contrary to conventional wisdom, only a few of the cancers detected in individuals with discrepant results were in areas of dense tissue (Lewin, 1999).

Given the information currently available, FFDM does not appear to offer significant improvements over FSM with regard to breast cancer detection. However, the study described above is not yet complete, and the preliminary data may have insufficient statistical power to reveal important differences between FFDM and FSM. The U.S. Department of Defense will not be supporting further patient accrual to this trial, but further studies are under way. The American College of Radiology Imaging Network trial of digital mammography may be especially important in answering unresolved issues (see Chapter 4). FFDM is also at a relatively early stage of development compared with FSM and so may have more room for improvement. Furthermore, novel applications and analysis of the digital information, including tomosynthesis, telemammography, and CAD may offer additional value over FSM even if FFDM cannot detect more cancers, but the clinical utility of these applications is not yet certain.

## OTHER TECHNICAL ADVANCES IN X-RAY IMAGING WITH POTENTIAL APPLICATION TO BREAST CANCER

A number of technical innovations have been suggested as ways to further improve X-ray mammography. A few examples are listed below, but relatively few data are available to assess the potential value of these techniques.

Capillary optic arrays are bundles of hollow glass capillaries that guide X rays in a manner similar to the way in which fiber optics guide light. Focused postpatient capillary optic arrays have the potential to significantly improve both contrast and resolution of mammographic images compared with those of conventional antiscatter grids (Kruger et al., 1996).

Phase-contrast X-ray imaging with coherent (or monoenergetic) X

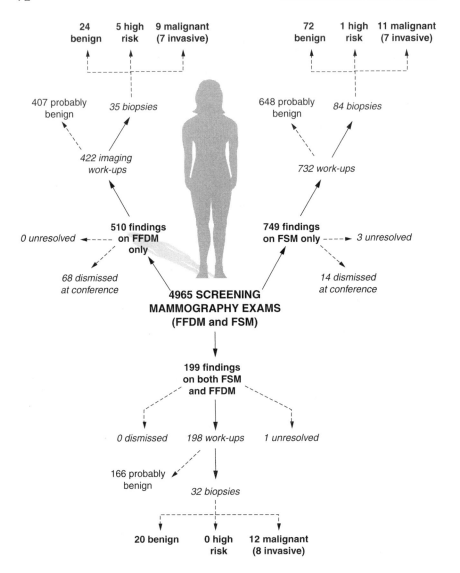

**FIGURE 2-4** Results from the Department of Defense study for the clinical evaluation of full field digital mammography for breast cancer screening. Note: updated results from this study were presented at the annual meeting of the Radiological Society of North America in November, 2000. After screening 6,768 women, 51 confirmed cancers were found; 18 were detected by both FFDM and FSM, 9 by FFDM only, and 16 by FSM only. 8 additional interval cancers were found within a year of screening. Statistically, there was still no difference between the sensitivity of the two methods. SOURCE: Lewin et al., 2001.

rays can be a powerful technique for the detection of low-contrast details in weakly absorbing objects. Synchroton accelerators can generate near-monoenergetic X rays as an alternative to the X rays emitted by the X-ray tubes used in conventional mammography. Another potential source of near monoenergetic X-ray radiation is the free electron laser. Phase-contrast X-ray imaging may be useful in diagnostic radiology applications such as mammography when imaging of low-contrast details within soft tissue by conventional x-ray imaging does not give satisfactory results. By using radiation doses smaller than or comparable to the doses needed for standard mammographic examinations, details that have low levels of X-ray absorption and that are invisible by conventional techniques may be detected by phase-contrast X-ray imaging (Arfelli et al., 1998a,b; 2000; Burattini et al., 1995). However, the interpretation of images through tissues with complex geometries and heterogeneous tissue types will require substantially more research.

X-ray CT has been used for more than 20 years to generate three-dimensional images of the body. X-ray computed tomographic mammography (CT/M) was first reported in 1977 to detect both benign and malignant breast disease in fatty and dense breasts. CT may also be capable of diagnosing early cancer in women who have had radiation therapy or surgery (Chang et al., 1977). CT/M imaging of the breast may facilitate diagnosis when mammography fails to detect a lesion or is unable to provide a definitive diagnosis, particularly when one is using a contrast medium (Chang et al., 1979). Although CT/M will not replace conventional mammography for routine breast examinations, it may provide an option for overcoming some limitations of mammography (Chang et al., 1980). These early development efforts resulted in a prototype product that was never brought to market, but other forms of digital CT applied to the breast are being investigated, although they have not yet been clinically evaluated in prospective trials (Nicklason et al., 1997; Pisano and Parham, 2000).

For example, tuned-aperture computed tomography (TACT) is a simpler method for tomographic viewing of individual breast tissue layers or retrieval of a true three-dimensional image. A reference system is used to reconstruct the projection geometry that produced the image. Once the projection geometry is known, it is possible to digitally reconstruct the three-dimensional image of the breast on the basis of optical aperture theory. The procedure is tailored for the breast so three-dimensional mammograms can be produced with increased patient comfort through less stringent requirements for breast compression. Multiple TACT images can be reconstructed with the same dose of radiation to the patient needed to obtain a single two-dimensional conventional digital mammogram (Webber et al., 1997).

## COMPUTER-AIDED DETECTION AND DIAGNOSIS

CAD systems consist of sophisticated computer programs that are designed to recognize patterns in images. They are intended for two different purposes: to help radiologists identify suspicious areas that may otherwise be overlooked on screening mammograms (detection schemes) and to classify breast lesions as benign or malignant (diagnosis schemes). CAD systems can be used directly on digital mammograms or on standard film-screen mammograms that have been digitized. Although CAD has a very low specificity when it is used alone without the judgment of a radiologist (Thurfjell et al., 1998), several studies now suggest that CAD can improve a radiologist's ability to detect and classify breast lesions in simulated clinical reading situations (reviewed by Nishikawa [1999]). However, further clinical studies are needed to more clearly define the value and appropriate use of the technology.

Image interpretation for screening mammograms is challenging for many reasons. Among the general screening population, about 1.5 to 6 cancers are identified for every 1,000 women screened, so radiologists must examine many films to detect a few cancers. Rapid interpretation of many images is necessary for mammography to be practical at a reasonable cost. As a result, some cancers are missed. Studies show that a significant number of cancers (as many as 30 to 65 percent) can be visualized on prior mammograms in retrospective reviews (Harvey et al., 1993; van Dijck et al., 1993; Warren-Burhenne et al., 2000). Double reading of mammograms by two radiologists can improve the cancer detection rate (by 4 to 15 percent) (Beam et al., 1996; Thurfjell et al., 1994), but such a practice is expensive and time-consuming. CAD is intended to improve detection rates in a more efficient and cost-effective manner. However, CAD use also increases the amount of time that a reader spends on each film.

Detection schemes generally use the following approach: (1) preprocessing of the image to increase the signal-to-noise ratio of the lesions being detected, (2) identification of all potential lesions, and (3) elimination of false-positive findings (using artificial neural networks and other analyses). Currently, detection schemes have a sensitivity of approximately 90 percent, with a rate of false-positive results of one to two per image (Nishikawa, 1999). It is critical to reduce the rate of false-positive results without decreasing sensitivity to increase the clinical acceptance of CAD. This is because the radiologist must scrutinize each false-positive finding which will reduce his or her productivity, decrease confidence in the computer-aided diagnosis, and, potentially, increase the number of unnecessary biopsies. Although different techniques have been developed, only two have been tested and shown to improve radiologists' performance.

A recent study of retrospective prior film review for about 500 women diagnosed with breast cancer found that CAD could potentially reduce the rate of false-negative results of radiologists by more than 70 percent (Warren-Burhenne et al., 2000). A common concern is that CAD might result in higher rates of callback and biopsies, only to eventually yield negative findings. However, recent data from five institutions that used conventional mammography showed no significant increase in callback rates before and after they started using CAD (~24,000 films interpreted before CAD installation and ~14,000 films read after CAD installation). In a concomitant study of more than 1,000 films for women previously diagnosed with breast cancer by screening mammography, CAD correctly labeled microcalcifications in 98 percent of the cases and masses in 75 percent of cases (Warren-Burhenne et al., 2000). However, the sensitivity and specificity of CAD in a general screening population have not yet been defined (although a study is under way[4]). Furthermore, detection of changes in a woman's mammograms over time is still technically challenging, and thus, new tools and techniques will be necessary to accomplish this goal. Comparison of serial images is confounded by variations in breast compression, patient positioning, and X-ray exposure parameters.

Further studies of CAD with digital mammography also are under way. In the United States, General Electric has an agreement with R2 Technologies, Inc. (Los Altos, California), to use R2 Technologies' detection algorithms with the FDA-approved General Electric digital mammography machine. To date, only the CAD software package produced by R2 Technologies has FDA approval and is being marketed in the United States. Several CAD detection systems are also being developed by other companies, such as Qualia Computing, Inc. (Beavercreek, Ohio), Scannis Inc. (Foster Creek, California), and CADx Medical Systems (Laval, Quebec, Canada), and these systems are being tested with populations around the world.

The commercially available CAD systems do not classify breast lesions as benign or malignant. Classification schemes work by merging features extracted from the radiograph (either automatically by the computer or manually by the radiologist) along with clinical and demographic information to give the likelihood that a lesion is cancerous. The typical techniques used are the same as those used with detection schemes. Current experimental systems used to distinguish benign and malignant lesions suggest that the positive predictive value of a radiologist's reading can be significantly increased by using CAD (Chan et al., 1999; Doi et al., 1997). The performance of CAD applied to mammography could potentially improve when direct digital image data become available.

---

[4]Qualia Computing, Inc. (Beavercreek, Ohio), is nearing completion on a study of their mammographic CAD system with 5,000 screening patients.

Similar computer algorithms could also be developed to assess digital breast images generated by other imaging modalities. Analysis of images from multiple three-dimensional breast imaging modalities could potentially enhance diagnosis and staging by combining anatomic, physiological, and biological tumor information in a single three-dimensional image. However, such technology does not currently exist.

## ULTRASOUND

Ultrasound waves are high-frequency sound waves that reflect at boundaries between tissues with different acoustic properties. The depth of these boundaries is proportional to the time intervals of reflection arrivals. Thus, ultrasound can map an image of tissue boundaries. Traditionally used as an adjunct to mammography in the identification of cysts and in guiding aspiration and biopsy, improvements in ultrasound technology have begun to expand the role of ultrasound in the differentiation of benign and malignant breast lesions and selection of patients for biopsy (Figure 2-5).

X-ray mammograms are frequently followed up with ultrasound imaging to determine whether a lesion that appeared on a mammogram is a cyst or a solid mass. Because a fluid-filled cyst has a different "sound

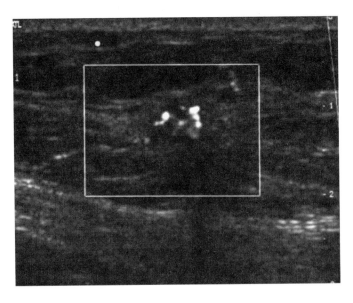

FIGURE 2-5  Example of an ultrasound image of the breast. Source: Janet Baum, Director, Breast Imaging, Beth Israel Deaconess Medical Center, Boston, MA.

signature" than a solid mass, radiologists can reliably use ultrasound to identify cysts, which are commonly found in breasts (Feig, 1999a,c). If ultrasound cannot make a distinction between a cyst and solid mass, ultrasound imaging may also be used to guide a needle into the abnormal tissue, from which fluid or cells may be taken (Feig, 1999a,c).

Ultrasound imaging of the breast may also help radiologists evaluate some lumps that can be felt but that are difficult to see on a mammogram, especially in dense breasts. Researchers have therefore begun to evaluate ultrasound in distinguishing malignant tumors from benign lesions (Ziewacz et al., 1999). In one study of 750 breast lesions that were subsequently biopsied, ultrasound accurately diagnosed benign conditions 99.5 percent of the time. If the ultrasound findings had been used to determine who should have a biopsy and who should be monitored, more than half of the biopsies would have been avoided (Stavros, 1995). Another study of 3,000 women who primarily had palpable lesions found that when ultrasound was used with standard mammography, 92 percent of breast cancers were detected. The specificity was 98 percent. In addition, when both imaging modalities indicated the lack of a malignancy, that diagnosis was correct more than 99 percent of the time (i.e., the rate of false-negative results was 1 percent) (Duijm et al., 1997).

This combined imaging is likely to be less accurate for nonpalpable tumors, but one 1998 screening study of more than 3,500 women with dense breasts found that ultrasound could detect some early-stage, clinically occult tumors that were missed by screening mammography (Kolb et al., 1998). Thus, there may be a future role for ultrasound in the screening of younger women with dense breasts and high risk factors. However, current ultrasound technology has a field of view limited to several centimeters at maximum resolution, making full breast examination difficult and time-consuming. This is in part a result of the traditional use of ultrasound for examination of masses that are already suspected. At present, larger arrays that would increase the field of view are technologically feasible at modest extra cost.

Conventional ultrasound has been limited in its ability to detect microcalcifications, which are frequently linked to breast cancer (Merritt, 1999). This difficulty is due in part to a phenomenon called "speckle," which arises from the interaction of the ultrasound field with the tissue. In the breast, speckle may produce small bright echoes within tissues, making them look like calcifications, so distinguishing artifacts from true calcifications can be difficult. Speckle and other noise also degrade the characterization of very small cysts and solid masses.

A new technique, called "compound imaging," significantly reduces speckle in breast images and improves the contrast and definition of small masses and even allows visualization of microcalcifications (Merritt, 1999). Conventional ultrasound generates images by using a beam that strikes tissues from a single direction. New ultrasound methods use several beams that strike the tissue from different angles. This reduces speckle and other artifacts, but it may also reduce resolution.

Three-dimensional ultrasound imaging of the breast is also under investigation. Three-dimensional ultrasound displays a volume of tissue rather than a single slice. Such three-dimensional images make it possible to simultaneously view multiple planes of observations and see through and around structures without the superimposition of overlying structures. Three-dimensional images may also permit more accurate measurement of tumor volume and comparison of changes in the sizes of masses over time. In contrast to fetal and gynecological ultrasound, for which three-dimensional methods have received considerable attention, three-dimensional breast sonography is early in its development.

Ultrasound can also provide information about blood flow by mapping the amount of acoustic frequency shift as a function of blood cell motion at a particular position in tissue, the Doppler effect. The detection of increased tumor blood flow could potentially play a role in the differentiation of benign and malignant masses (Carson et al., 1998; Mehta et al., 2000), but whether this will prove to be a reliable indicator for malignancy remains to be shown in controlled clinical studies. Power Doppler is a method that shows the amount of blood cells in motion and thus in effect shows vasculature. Its sensitivity may be limited because increased vascularity may not be seen in some cancers. Ultrasound contrast agents might improve the ability of Doppler ultrasound to evaluate tumor blood supply, particularly when coupled with new signal processing methods such as harmonic and pulse inversion contrast imaging. Several contrast agents are being tested in clinical trials. Assessment of tumor vascularity could also be useful to predict the biological activities of tumors and in monitoring responses to treatment.

Elastography is another novel use of ultrasound in the breast (Ophir et al., 1999). Like palpation, elastography detects differences in tissue stiffness and other mechanical properties. Physical breast examination by inspection and palpation enables detection of breast cancer by observing differences in mechanical properties, especially stiffness, since cancerous tissue is usually much more rigid and less easily deformable than normal breast tissue. However, cysts and certain benign lesions may have mechanical properties that can mimic malignant tumors, so finding a rigid mass within the breast does not confirm malignancy.

In elastography, the mechanical properties of breast tissue are measured from point to point within the breast by ultrasound or MRI (described in the next section). These measurements are mapped into images, often called "elastograms." There are many elastic properties of solids, including tissues, that can be determined by ultrasound or MRI measurements obtained before and after application of small deformations or by monitoring the propagation of mechanical (infrasonic) waves. Ultrasonic and magnetic resonance elastography have the potential to distinguish breast abnormalities, such as malignant tumors, from normal tissue, benign processes, and scars. Since, in general, elastography can be done noninvasively to form images for subjective and quantitative evaluations, these methods are under active investigation. Elastic properties are not directly measured, however, and must be inferred (mathematically) by one of numerous technical strategies used to model and display the images. No clinical trials of elastography in breast cancer have yet been reported, but some feasibility demonstrations have been completed, so human clinical trials are anticipated (Muthupillai et al., 1995; Plewes et al., 2000; Sinkus et al., 2000). However, assessment of elastography could be hampered by a lack of standardization with regard to which elastic parameters should be measured and by a lack of a published characterization of normal tissue.

In summary, ultrasound imaging is well established as an adjunct to mammography for distinguishing cysts from solid lesions and as a method for localizing tumors before biopsy. Several studies suggest that it could be more widely used to characterize tumors as benign or malignant and perhaps even as a screening adjunct for specific populations. More study is needed to assess these possibilities. Ongoing technological advances in ultrasound imaging have the potential to increase the use of ultrasound in breast cancer detection even more, but their stage of development is too early to predict their ultimate utility.

## MAGNETIC RESONANCE IMAGING

Magnetic resonance images are created by recording the signals generated after radiofrequency excitation of hydrogen nuclei (or other elements) in tissue exposed to a strong static magnetic field. The signals have characteristics that vary according to tissue type (e.g., fat, muscle, fibrotic tissue, and edema[5]). The method has minimal hazards from magnetic field effects and does not use ionizing radiation. The goal of breast MRI is similar to that of mammography: to identify structural abnormalities in the tissue. Some newer applications of MRI technology also aim to gather functional information about breast lesions. It is being developed primarily as a diagnostic tool to avoid unnecessary biopsies among women with dense breasts, but screening applications are also being studied among high-risk populations.

MRI has been used for a wide variety of medical applications since FDA approved the procedure in 1985. MRI of the human breast was first

---

[5]Women may experience some tissue edema in the first few months after surgery.

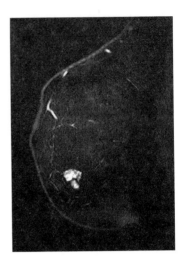

**FIGURE 2-6**  Example of a magnetic resonance image of the breast. Source: Drs. D. Plewes and R Shumak of Sunnybrook and Women's College Health Centre, University of Toronto.

attempted in the 1980s, but early results were disappointing. Subsequently, intravenous contrast agents were used with a dedicated breast MRI coil, offering a clear advance. In general, malignant tumors showed intense uptake of contrast agents, whereas the surrounding normal tissue did not (Figure 2-6). Following this discovery, MRI has been studied as an emerging but as yet unproven technology for breast cancer detection. Recently, a number of investigators in this field have demonstrated the potential of breast MRI, but it is currently confined to experimental protocols.

Two different MRI techniques are being evaluated to detect breast tumors: dynamic contrast imaging and three-dimensional high-resolution imaging. Dynamic imaging aims to pinpoint tumors on the basis of how quickly they take up the contrast agent. Because malignant tumors tend to have enhanced and leaky blood vessels compared with normal tissue, they generally take up more contrast agent faster. However, studies show that there is an overlap in contrast agent uptake between benign and malignant breast tumors (Farria et al., 1999). Dynamic contrast imaging typically images only a cross section of the breast. Three-dimensional high-resolution imaging, on the other hand, generates whole-breast images, which allow radiologists to detect additional breast lesions that may be missed by dynamic contrast imaging. In the future, faster imaging technology may allow dynamic imaging information to be obtained simultaneously with three-dimensional, high-resolution, whole-breast imaging.

Studies suggest that MRI may, in some cases, be useful for the diagnosis of breast lesions identified through screening mammography or clinical breast examination (Tan et al., 1999; Farria et al., 1999). The sensitivity of MRI for the detection of suspicious breast lesions ranges between 88 and 100 percent (10 studies reviewed by Farria et al., 1999). One study of 225 women found the combined sensitivity of MRI and standard mammography to be 99 percent (Bone et al., 1997). The reported specificity of MRI is more variable, ranging from 28 to 100 percent (Farria et al., 1999), depending on the patient population and the interpretation technique used. The relatively low degree of specificity of MRI in some studies was mainly due to its frequent inability to distinguish between malignant tumors and benign noncystic abnormalities, such as nonmalignant solid tumors (fibroadenomas) and ductal hyperplasia. The disparity between the very high degree of sensitivity and the relatively low degree of specificity of the technology can be problematic in that "serendipitous lesions"—unexpected lesions found incidentally in the breast during the MRI workup of a lump or breast abnormality detected by mammography—are often observed (Lawrence et al., 1998). This raises the question as to whether such lesions should also be monitored or biopsied. The likelihood that these lesions are in fact cancerous seems to be low, but further study is needed to improve the decision-making process following MRI (Lawrence et al., 1998). To increase confidence in the nature of the lesions detected by MRI (e.g., benign versus malignant lesions), follow-up studies or confirmation of diagnosis by tissue biopsy may be required. Moreover, biopsy of lesions seen on MRI images but not on images obtained by other imaging methods can be difficult because MRI localization for biopsy is not a standard practice. Accessible and easy-to-use guidance systems are required to perform localization or biopsy of lesions detected by MRI alone. For MRI-guided biopsy, magnet-compatible needles and other equipment using materials that do not cause image distortions in a magnetic field need further development.

MRI shows particular promise in defining the local extent (size, number, distribution) of cancer foci in women with known breast cancer who are candidates for breast-conserving therapy. Studies show that MRI may be particularly useful in defining the extent of a specific type of breast cancer, invasive lobular carcinoma. Although this type of cancer makes up only about 10 percent of all breast malignancies, it is frequently missed in mammograms and the extent of the cancer is difficult to determine by other methods. In one very small study of 20 women, MRI accurately predicted the extent of invasive lobular carcinoma in 85 percent of patients, whereas mammography accurately predicted the extent of invasive lobular carcinoma in only 31 percent of patients (Rodenko et al., 1996).

Unfortunately, MRI cannot reliably reveal microcalcifications, and MRI can miss small tumors, particularly if they do not selectively take up the contrast agent. However, despite these limitations, a negative MRI result could potentially rule out the presence of breast cancer in a patient whose mammogram, sonogram, and physical examination are not definitive. MRI is much more expensive than ultrasound or X-ray mammography, and MRI systems capable of imaging the human breast are not available at every institution. Nevertheless, a recent meta-analysis suggests that if the diagnostic performance of MRI is equal to or better than those reported recently, it could potentially be a cost-effective alternative to excisional biopsy in the follow-up of suspicious lesions identified by mammography (Hrung et al., 1999a).

To assess the usefulness of MRI for the diagnosis of breast cancer, the National Cancer Institute is conducting a large, multicenter study of three-dimensional high-resolution MRI and dynamic contrast MRI performed in conjunction with mammography (Farria et al., 1999). One of the goals of the study, which is expected to be completed in 2001, is to establish uniform interpretation criteria for MRI of the breast. A lack of standards has hampered the clinical usefulness of MRI in the diagnosis of breast cancer. Similar studies in the United Kingdom and Europe are also under way or are being planned.

Another potential use for MRI is detection of recurrent breast cancer in breasts previously subjected to lumpectomies, because MRI scans are usually not limited by scarring and edema, unlike mammography and ultrasound, which are sometimes limited by scarring. MRI scans can also reliably detect tumors in women with breast implants or dense breasts, both of which can interfere with interpretation of X-ray mammograms. Consequently, MRI is being tested as a screening technology for high-risk women, who may begin screening at a younger age and thus are more likely to have dense breast tissue. A recent prospective trial compared MRI, ultrasound, and mammography in 192 women at high risk for breast cancer on the basis of personal or family history (Kuhl et al., 2000). The sensitivities of mammography, ultrasound, and MRI, were 33, 33 (ultrasound and mammography combined), and 100 percent, respectively. MRI identified three breast cancers that were not detected by mammography. The specificity of MRI was 95 percent based on the experience of this group in interpreting patterns of contrast enhancement and through the use of short-term follow-up MRI studies performed with 10 percent of the women. Several studies at other institutions involving more than 5,000 high-risk patients worldwide are in progress. These studies should allow a more accurate assessment of the sensitivity and specificity of MRI for high-risk populations.

Other novel applications of MRI technology are also under investigation but are generally in the early stages of development. One example is MRI elastography, which measures the mechanical properties of tissue, as described in the previous section along with ultrasound elastography.

MRI could also potentially provide a noninvasive method for assessment of prognosis, in addition to its possible role in screening and diagnosis. In this role, functional imaging of molecular markers is required. Functional MRI differs from traditional MRI by combining anatomic examination with information about biological function. For example, different histological types of breast cancer display distinct differences in MRI enhancement characteristics (Knopp et al., 1999). These differences correlate with the density and permeability of tumor vasculature, which independently predict the outcomes of breast cancer (Craft and Harris, 1994; Weidner et al., 1992).

Newer "smart" magnetic resonance contrast agents may reveal additional biochemical and physiological information, such as gene expression and other physiological processes in the form of a three-dimensional magnetic resonance image (Louie et al., 2000). The technology uses gadolinium contrast agents within a molecular shell that are activated by specific biochemical processes inside the cell and that are then detected by conventional MRI. If the gadolinium agents were activated selectively in breast cancer cells, it could be detected in the images obtained by MRI. Imaging of cell functions like gene expression that can be correlated to disease states is in the very early stages of development, but it is being pursued commercially.[6] One ultimate goal of this novel imaging technique is to track cell growth and behavior in breast and other cancers (Straus, 2000), including imaging of intracellular protein communication, apoptosis (or programmed cell death), and angiogenesis (growth of new blood vessels, a hallmark of many cancers). However, so far, all research has been conducted with animals, and testing in clinical trials with humans is still likely years away. In addition, more studies must be done to identify the appropriate markers to be imaged, as discussed in more detail in the next chapter.

In addition to its potential role in screening and diagnosis, MRI may also be helpful in the development of novel minimally invasive therapies. Interactive monitoring of localized "thermotherapy" by MRI is being studied as a possible alternative to lumpectomy. The tumor cells are heated by lasers, radiofrequency ultrasound, or high-intensity focused ultrasound, and the resultant tumor cell destruction can be monitored by MRI. This method is in a very early stage of development, and its true clinical utility and potential have not been assessed in clinical trials (Farria et al., 1999). New interventions for early lesions that are simple, effective, and acceptable to women could enhance the net benefits of screening by reducing some of the problems associated with overtreatment due to screening[7] (as discussed in Chapter 1).

In summary, MRI has potential as a diagnostic adjunct to mammog-

---

[6]By a company known as Metaprobe (Pasadena, California), founded by Thomas Meade.

raphy to eliminate unnecessary biopsies. It may also have a screening role in certain high-risk populations. Ongoing studies may provide the data necessary to define the appropriate applications of the technology. Technological advances may eventually lead to broader or different uses of MRI in the future, but more study and development must occur before that can be considered.

## MAGNETIC RESONANCE SPECTROSCOPY

Proton magnetic resonance spectroscopy (MRS), a method that was originally developed by physical chemists to characterize large molecules in solution, can also be used to measure biochemical components of cells and tissues (Merchant, 1994). Metabolites can increase to abnormal levels in cancer cells and these changes may be detected in tissue samples and also in vivo by MRS. The method is under active investigation as a diagnostic adjunct to mammography and other accepted imaging techniques. It is being studied as an alternate method of analysis for fine-needle aspirates (FNAs; as opposed to cytology) and also as a method for assessment of lesions in vivo to avoid unnecessary biopsies.

Because cytological analysis of FNAs is quite variable depending on the experience and skill of the individuals collecting and assessing the sample, MRS has been studied as an alternate approach to diagnosis by analysis of FNAs. The first study demonstrating the potential of MRS to distinguish benign and malignant lesions by FNA measured choline and creatine levels in 190 samples by visual reading of the spectra obtained by MRS (Mackinnon et al., 1997). More recently, the MRS spectra of more than 150 FNA samples were analyzed by a new computerized statistical classification system. Malignant lesions were distinguished from benign tissue with an accuracy of 93 percent (Mountford et al., 2000).

Studies with tumor specimens obtained by biopsy have validated the ability of the technology to measure the biochemical differences between tumor samples and normal or benign breast tissues (Gribbestad et al., 1999). Recently, several small (10 to 40 women), preliminary studies that used noninvasive MRS have found that the elevated choline content of breast tumors can be detected in vivo as well (Gribbestad et al., 1998; Kvistad et al., 1999; Roebuck et al., 1998). These results suggest that MRS spectra, which are complementary to the images obtained by MRI, could potentially be used to characterize and diagnose breast lesions in a noninvasive manner. However, the high cost and low sensitivity and specific-

---

[7]One of the reasons that the Papanicolaou smear for screening for cervical cancer has been so successful in reducing the rate of mortality from cervical cancer is that the intervention for early lesions is simple, effective, and well tolerated and accepted by women.

ity of the method for the detection of small lesions must be overcome before in vivo breast MRS demonstrates its clinical utility.

## SCINTIMAMMOGRAPHY

Unlike the imaging methods described thus far, in which the transmission of various forms of energy through the tissues is used to generate an image, nuclear medicine approaches rely on the emission of radioactivity from tracers that are injected into the body and that then accumulate in specific tissues. "Scintimammography" in particular uses radioactive tracers to produce an image of tumors and lesions in the breast and elsewhere (Figure 2-7). It may be used as an adjunct to mammography to help distinguish between malignant and benign lesions. The tracers concentrate more in breast cancers than in normal breast tissues by a mechanism that is not fully understood but that may be related to the degree of cellular proliferation and vascular permeability. Several radioactive compounds are being investigated, although only one, technetium-99m sestamibi (MIBI), is approved by FDA for use in breast imaging. Scintimammography images the spatial concentration of the radiopharmaceuticals using a camera that detects gamma rays (a "gamma camera")

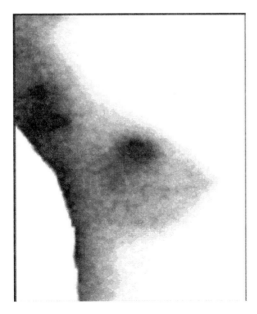

**FIGURE 2-7** Example of scintimammography. Findings: Focal upake in the right breast in the area of a palpable mass. Source: Miraluma™ by duPont Merck Pharmaceutical Company.

and may consist of traditional planar images or three-dimensional images generated by tomographic reconstruction (single-photon-emission computed tomography [SPECT]).

Because it uses radioactive compounds, scintimammography poses radiation health risks akin to those of imaging techniques that use X rays, although the small doses of radioactivity used are generally considered safe except for pregnant women and young children. MIBI imaging is generally more expensive than ultrasound imaging or diagnostic mammography but is less expensive than MRI (Allen et al., 1999).

Unlike mammograms, MIBI scans are not affected by dense breast tissue, breast implants, or scarring (Edell and Eisen, 1999). It has a limited ability to detect cancers smaller than 1 centimeter (cm), however, and MIBI imaging is less accurate for nonpalpable abnormalities than for palpable masses (Ziewacz et al., 1999). Studies indicate that the overall sensitivity of MIBI scans ranges from 75 to 94 percent and that the specificity ranges from 80 to 89 percent (reviewed by Edell and Eisen, 1999 and Stuntz et al., 1999). Based on an analysis of all published data, the Blue Cross/Blue Shield Association (BCBSA) Technology Evaluation Center (TEC) found that scintimammography did not meet its criteria (see Chapter 5) for differentiating between benign and malignant breast lesions in patients with suspicious mammograms or palpable masses (Blue Cross and Blue Shield Association Technology Evaluation Center, 1997). Its analysis of the pooled data found the sensitivity to be 94 percent for the detection of palpable masses but only 67 percent for the detection of nonpalpable lesions. Although one study of 150 women found that MIBI accurately predicted a benign lesion 97 percent of the time (negative predictive value, 97 percent) (Khalkhali et al., 1994), the pooled analysis found such predictions to be accurate for 91 percent of palpable lesions but only 69 percent of nonpalpable lesions. This BCBS TEC analysis predicted that of all the patients who would undergo a MIBI scan, 66 to 73 percent of patients could avoid a negative biopsy but 2 to 8 percent of patients would be exposed to the harms of undetected malignancy. Thus, the panel concluded that the negative predictive value of scintimammography was not sufficient to warrant its adoption as a diagnostic test.

Some clinicians also use MIBI imaging as a follow-up test for women whose mammograms indicate a mass that is "probably benign" and not suspicious enough to warrant a biopsy. Current practice is to recommend that these women have a repeat mammogram in 6 months, but since one-quarter of such women will not comply with the follow-up recommendations, MIBI can give an added level of protection against a delay in breast cancer therapy (Stuntz et al., 1999). In addition, MIBI scans can confirm a benign breast condition in women with palpable lesions whose mammograms or fine-needle aspiration results are inconclusive. MIBI scans can also detect multiple breast cancers that may be missed on a mammogram.

Recent technical advancements may help to overcome some of the current limitations of scintimammography, such as the low resolution of MIBI scans. For example, high-resolution scintimammography (HRSM) increases resolution by using a gamma camera based on a new position-sensitive photomultiplier tube. In one study of 53 patients, it found lesions missed by standard MIBI scans and could detect a lesion as small as 7 mm (Scopinaro et al., 1999). Additional improvements in spatial resolution could further improve the clinical utility of MIBI scans for breast cancer detection. New radiopharmaceuticals may also play a role in the future use of scintimammography. Investigational compounds that show promise for breast imaging include technetium-99m, tetrofosmin and technetium-99m–MDP. These agents may be less expensive and more accurate than MIBI, although more studies are needed to determine this (Stuntz et al., 1999). Other radioactive compounds, such as thallium-201, have also been used to visualize breast tumors, but generally with less favorable imaging traits compared with those of MIBI (Ziewacz et al., 1999).

Scintimammography also has potential for use in functional imaging applications. One example of functional scintigraphic imaging uses SPECT to monitor multidrug resistance (Del Vecchio et al., 1999). Recent research suggests that MIBI can be pumped out of cells that overexpress the multidrug resistance P glycoprotein MDR1, the same mechanism that leads to resistance to chemotherapeutic agents. Rapid MIBI washout rates correlate with treatment failure. Preliminary studies suggest that patients who overexpress MDR1 and who fail breast cancer chemotherapy clear MIBI three times faster. SPECT imaging for the detection of multidrug resistance could potentially allow more individualized treatment planning by identifying those patients likely to fail chemotherapy. P-glycoprotein inhibitors, which may increase the efficacy of chemotherapy regimens in women who overexpress MDR1, are now entering phase II/III clinical trials. These would be most effective in patients who overexpress MDR1, as predicted by MIBI washout rates. Studies with many other molecular markers are also actively under way, but again, one difficulty may be in choosing the appropriate markers for use in assessment and monitoring.

In summary, scintimammography has shown diagnostic potential as an adjunct to mammography, but technical limitations such as resolution have precluded it from becoming more widely used. Although it has FDA approval, the current data do not justify its implementation on a standard basis. Technological improvements and novel radioactive compounds could potentially improve its utility, but at the moment its future is uncertain. The method also has potential for use in functional imaging applications, but further study and development are needed.

## POSITRON EMISSION TOMOGRAPHY

Positron emission tomography (PET) uses radioactive tracers such as labeled glucose to identify regions in the body with increased metabolic activity (Phelps, 2000). Because malignant tissue tends to metabolize glucose in a manner different from that of tissue with benign abnormalities, researchers have used PET to discern malignant from benign lesions in many organs and tissues, including the breast. Preliminary small studies indicate that PET scans have sensitivities between 80 and 100 percent and specificities between 75 and 85 percent, but more studies are needed to assess the clinical utility of PET scans for use in breast cancer diagnosis. In theory, scanning by PET could prove useful for the detection of breast cancers in women with dense breasts, implants, or scars. However, the inability to biopsy lesions that are identified by PET but that are not visible on a mammogram is a major impediment to accurate diagnosis (Stuntz et al., 1999). PET scanners are also quite expensive and not widely available, and the agents used are expensive to make and last only a short time. On the horizon, however, are less expensive, more commercially available PET systems and simpler radiopharmaceutical production methods, both of which could improve the usefulness of PET scans for the detection of breast malignancies (Edell and Eisen, 1999).

Researchers are also exploring the use of radioactive antibodies that target breast malignancies (Goldenberg and Nabi, 1999). These include antibodies to carcinoembryonic antigen and antibodies against other proteins that may be prevalent in breast cancer cells, such as certain growth factor receptors. Although some of these agents show promising sensitivity and specificity for the detection of breast cancer, most of the studies conducted to date have been small and the scans can be difficult to interpret. More clinical studies are needed to determine the roles of these radioactive antibodies in the diagnosis of breast cancer. A primary focus of imaging research in this area is on the development and validation of appropriate markers for breast cancer evaluation.

## OPTICAL IMAGING AND SPECTROSCOPY

Investigators are developing a variety of devices and agents to aid the in vivo diagnosis of breast cancer by optical methods (Alfano et al., 1997). The use of light to image lesions in the breast was first reported by Cutler in 1929 and consisted of simple transillumination, performed by placing a light source against the breast and observing differences in the transmission of light through the tissue. During the 1980s, a digital transillumination system that used two light wavelengths (also known as diaphanography) was developed and tested, but the results were conflicting, and many systems showed low sensitivity and specificity (Moskowitz et al., 1989). Thus, FDA approval was not granted[8] and commercialization of the technology did not go forward.

Past attempts to image tissues with light were severely restricted by the overwhelming scatter that occurs when optical radiation spreads through tissue; however, recent innovations in optical technologies have renewed interest in potential applications for breast cancer detection and characterization (Bosanko et al., 1990; Hebden and Delpy, 1997). Currently, the two main areas of interest in this field are optical spectroscopy to characterize the structure and biochemical contents of lesions and optical imaging (or tomography) to localize as well as characterize the lesions in the tissue. In each case, the procedures are being tested as an adjunct to mammography to distinguish benign and malignant lesions and thus eliminate unnecessary biopsies.

"Optical biopsy" via spectroscopy is one promising technology under investigation as a minimally invasive means of diagnosis of breast cancer (Bown et al., 2000). By exploiting the unique in vivo optical properties of normal and cancerous tissues, optical biopsy techniques may be able to discriminate between a tumor and its surrounding normal tissue in real time. For several years, researchers have been developing an optical biopsy technique known as "elastic scattering spectroscopy" (ESS) for the diagnosis of cancer. The ESS system, which is portable and which is designed for convenient clinical use, involves shining a pulse of light through an optical fiber that is placed in contact with the tissue and then performing spectral analysis on the light that is reflected back through a small volume of tissue. The resultant spectrum is influenced by light scatter due to the cellular and subcellular architectures of the tissues, as well as light absorption by chromophores in the tissue. Computer algorithms are required for the spectral analysis, and artificial neural networks are being tested for this purpose.

Tumors can be detected and cancer can be diagnosed by using spectral measurements because, in addition to significant architectural changes at the cellular and subcellular levels compared with the architecture of normal tissues, tumors may also have altered levels of natural chromophores such as hemoglobin. This approach generates spectral signatures that are relevant to the tissue parameters that pathologists address: the sizes and shapes of nuclei, the ratio of nuclear volume to cellular volume, clustering patterns, vascularity, and so on. ESS analysis is frequently mediated through endoscopes, and a few small clinical studies on the endoscopic application of ESS to bladder cancer and gastrointestinal pathologies have been published (Bohorfoush, 1996; Mourant et al., 1995). The approach is more challenging with solid organs such as the breast,

---

[8]Minutes from the FDA advisory panel meeting, 1991.

but if ESS measurements of breast tissue were reliable, ESS could eliminate many unnecessary surgical biopsies, and the instant diagnosis could improve surgical procedures for breast cancer. Clinical studies are under way to assess the potential of the diagnostic application of ESS with a transdermal needle for the diagnosis of breast cancer. Instant diagnosis by ESS with a needle of the same size used for fine-needle aspiration cytology could reduce patient anxiety (i.e., the anxiety that occurs while waiting for a diagnosis) and, in some cases, permit immediate treatment.

Another potential application of endoscopy in breast cancer diagnosis is known as "ductoscopy." In this case, a fiberoptic endoscope is threaded through the milk ducts of the breast via the nipple orifice. Such an approach can facilitate optical characterization of ductal lesions and could potentially be combined with microsampling methods such as tube currette cytology (Love and Barsky, 1996).

Optical imaging or tomography, which is relatively inexpensive and simple in comparison with many other imaging modalities, is also actively under investigation for a variety of cancers, including breast cancer. The technique uses light in the near-infrared range (wavelengths from 700 to 1,200 nm), which is nonionizing, to produce an image of the breast. Potential advantages of the technology include speed, comfort, and noninvasiveness. An optical scan can be taken in less than 30 seconds by simply placing an image pad over the breast without compression (Chance, 1998). Optical imaging methods offer the potential to differentiate between soft tissues that are indistinguishable by other modalities, and specific absorption by natural chromophores (such as hemoglobin) can also provide biological or functional information. Optical scanning images can also be digitized, thus allowing image manipulation, serial studies, and analysis by computer algorithms. However, hurdles that must be overcome before this technology reaches the clinic relate to accuracy and resolution, which are not yet optimized. In particular, the target-to-background ratios tend to be low. Furthermore, the physiology and thus the optical characteristics of normal and neoplastic breast tissues can be quite variable depending on the age, hormone status, and genetic background of the woman (Thomsen and Tatman, 1998).

Optical imaging systems are being commercially developed by Imaging Diagnostic Systems Inc.[9] (IMDS; Plantation, Florida), DOBI[10] Medical Systems (Mahwah, New Jersey), and Advanced Research and Technology, Inc (ART; Montreal, Canada).[11] The DOBI technology is based on

---

[9]Computed tomography laser mammography (CTLM; www.imds.com/ctlm.htm).

[10]Dynamic optical breast imaging (DOBI; www.dynamicsimaging.com).

[11]Softscan™ laser mammography was developed by ART in cooperation with the National Optics Institute of Canada, which does optical research for organizations such as the National Aeronautics and Space Administration and industrial multinational corporations.

optical detection of angiogenesis in malignant lesions, whereas the IMDS and ART technologies use laser-based technologies to assess various optical properties of breast abnormalities. All three companies are conducting clinical trials for FDA approval for diagnostic use of their devices, but they also plan to pursue a screening approach in the future.

Optical contrast agents (Ntziachristos et al., 2000) that are selectively taken up by tumors in a fashion similar to that for the contrast agents used for MRI may improve the sensitivity and specificity of the technology, but their clinical utility is undefined. By using novel contrast agents that fluoresce after cleavage with specific enzymes, the technology also has the potential to show functional changes associated with cancer initiation and progression, but this application is at an even earlier stage of development (Mahmood et al., 1999). In addition, new types of lasers that emit rapid pulses of energy rather than a continuous wave were recently developed by physicists and may provide additional benefits to the technological advancement of this detection method.

In summary, optical imaging has long been thought to have potential as a means of breast cancer detection, but to date that potential has not yet been realized. Significant technological improvements in recent years may eventually propel this technology into the clinic, but a conclusion cannot yet be reached about its future utility. Optical biopsy methods were proposed more recently, but it is too early in the development stage to assess their clinical potential. Further studies of both applications are needed and are ongoing.

## THERMOGRAPHY

Infrared thermal imaging has been used for several decades to monitor the temperature distribution over human skin. Abnormalities such as malignancies, inflammation, and infection cause localized increases in temperature that appear as hot spots or asymmetrical patterns in an infrared thermogram. Thermography, alternatively termed "thermometry" or "thermology," was pursued for many years as a technique for breast cancer detection. Studies of thermography have focused on a range of potential uses, including for diagnosis, prognosis, and risk indication and as an adjunct to existing technologies; however, the results have been inconsistent and scientific consensus has been difficult to achieve. Thermography was largely abandoned in the 1970s, but technological advances in the intervening years have renewed interest in the technique. The use of infrared imaging is increasing in many industrial and security applications, and the transfer of military technology for medical use has prompted this reappraisal of infrared thermography in medicine. Digital infrared cameras have much-improved spatial and thermal resolutions, and libraries of image processing routines are available to analyze images captured both statically and dynamically.

A breast tumor can raise the temperature of the skin surface by as much as 3 degrees C compared with the temperature of the skin surface of a woman with normal tissue (Foster, 1998). Although this phenomenon is not well understood, likely mechanisms include elevated rates of tumor metabolism and elevated levels of vascularity and perfusion (Foster, 1998; Anbar, 1995). The body dissipates the heat through emitted infrared radiation, which can be detected by infrared cameras; the diagnosis of cancer is based on the difference in temperature relative to that for the contralateral breast, which serves as a built-in control. The procedure is noninvasive and does not require compression of the breast or radiation exposure.

The first published report of breast cancer detection based on temperature measurement appeared in 1956 (Lawson), and through the 1960s and 1970s, thermography was actively studied and used clinically. At one point (before passage of the 1976 Medical Device Amendment requiring FDA approval for devices) between 2,000 and 3,000 thermography clinics were actively operating in the United States (Foster, 1998). In 1977, Stephen Feig published the results of the first large clinical trial (16,000 women) to compare thermography, xeromammography (an early form of mammography), and clinical examination. The sensitivity and specificity of thermography were demonstrated to be 39 and 82 percent, respectively. By comparison, the sensitivity of xeromammography was 78 percent, with a specificity of 98 percent (Feig et al., 1977). Around the same time, the Breast Cancer Detection Demonstration Project was launched with the intent of studying mammography, clinical examination, and thermography. However, thermography was dropped early in the study because of poor results, namely, high rates of false-positive results and a low level of sensitivity (Moskowitz, 1985). Following these studies, thermography of the breast largely disappeared, and the American Medical Association[12] and the Canadian Association of Radiation Oncologists (1998) do not advocate it as a technique for breast cancer detection. However, technological developments in recent years have sparked new interest in the technique.

Modern digital infrared cameras can now image the breast with significantly improved spatial and thermal resolutions (Jones, 1998). Computerized image analysis software is also being developed to analyze and compare images of one breast with those of the other. The goal is to eventually quantitate the parameters of infrared abnormalities, thus cre-

---

[12]American Medical Association, Thermography update, H-175.988, AMA Policy Finder (http://www.ama-assn.org/apps/pf_online/pf_online).

ating an objective measurement of abnormality (Head and Elliott, 1997). A system called dynamic area telethermometry (DAT) has been developed to detect changes in neuronal control of blood flow as evidenced by small changes in heat. Research has shown that malignancy disrupts normal blood flow, and thus, these changes may be evidence of cancer (Anbar et al., 1999).

OmniCorder Technologies has integrated the DAT system with a sensor technology called quantum well infrared photodetector (Anbar et al., 1999) in developing its BioScan system. In December 1999, OmniCorder was granted FDA clearance to use BioScan as an adjunctive technology for the diagnosis of breast cancer.[13] The company has just begun to manufacture systems for distribution and is also conducting trials for other uses such as management of cancer therapy. Computerized Thermal Imaging, Inc., is also developing a system that records thermal images of breast tissues to construct a three-dimensional map of the breast; the system is being tested in clinical trials for FDA approval.[14]

## ELECTRICAL POTENTIAL MEASUREMENTS

Studies indicate that rapid proliferation of epithelial tissue in the breast disrupts the normal polarization of the epithelium. This depolarization involves both the transmembrane electrical gradient and the transepithelial electrical gradient, which are associated with the orientation of the epithelial cells with respect to their apical and basolateral surfaces. The region of depolarization can extend beyond the immediate area of the tumor to the skin surface. Thus, abnormal electrical potential measurements at the skin surface of the breast can be used as an indicator of elevated epithelial proliferation suggestive of carcinogenesis (Cuzick et al., 1998; Faupel et al., 1997; Fukuda et al., 1996). Consequently, this method has been studied for use as a tool for the diagnosis of breast cancer, with the hope of avoiding unnecessary biopsies after mammography.

Biofield Corporation (Roswell, Georgia) was the original developer of the technology that uses electrical potential measurements for the detection of cancer. As a result, the technology is often referred to as the Biofield breast exam (BBE). BBE uses an array of electrical potential sensors placed over both breasts and axillae. Reference sensors are also placed over both

---

[13]OmniCorder Technologies, Inc., The BioScan System, accessed May 2000 (http://www.omnicorer.com/dat.html).

[14]University of Southern California. Study examines non-invasive way to detect cancer of the breast, accessed May 2000 (http://www.usc.edu/hsc.info/pr/1vol3/329/parisky.html).

palms. Following an equilibration period, average voltages are recorded for each of the electrical potential sensors. Differences in electrical potential can be calculated both between sensors on the symptomatic breast and between sensors on the symptomatic breast and the contralateral breast.

One unique feature of BBE is that it gives a single, numerical result that objectively determines whether the lesion is considered malignant or benign. Conversely, tests such as mammography rely on the subjective interpretation of the data by a trained reader. BBE is also relatively inexpensive because it uses very basic equipment and does not require an expert reader. It is noninvasive and not uncomfortable to women, and the procedure can be performed in less than 15 minutes (Faupel et al., 1997).

BBE has been tested primarily as a diagnostic tool for women with palpable breast lesions or nonpalpable lesions identified by mammography or ultrasonography. Two clinical studies of diagnostic BBE have been conducted. All of the women in the studies received a BBE followed by a biopsy. The electrical potential differences between sensors were retrospectively analyzed in light of the biopsy outcomes to determine which weighted sum of measurements best predicted the biopsy outcome. In the first study, which included 101 women, BBE was found to have a sensitivity of 90 percent and a specificity of 60 percent. It was also observed that for cancers measuring less than 2.5 cm, the sensitivity of BBE was 95 percent. The investigators speculated that the test's reduced sensitivity to larger tumors could be associated with the tissue necrosis seen in larger tumors. There were, however, only 19 tumors less than 2.5 cm, so this preliminary calculation of sensitivity for patients with small tumors must be validated (Fukuda et al., 1996). In a second study, which included 661 women at eight different centers, BBE was found to have a sensitivity of 90 percent and a specificity of 55 percent for women with palpable lesions (Cuzick et al., 1998).

Although Biofield has submitted a premarket approval (PMA) application, BBE has not yet been approved by the FDA and so is not used clinically in the United States. However, Biofield has received CE Mark Certification[15] for its diagnostic system, which allows the company to sell

---

[15]Since 1992, the European Parliament has enacted a series of directives intended to provide controls on product design, with the principal objective being to provide a "level playing field" for product safety requirements across the European Community. The Medical Devices Directive was enacted to provide for a harmonized regulatory environment for all medical devices sold within the European Economic Area (EEA). All products that fall within the scope of the directive must meet certain essential safety and administrative requirements and are to be marked CE to show that they comply. Such products may then be freely sold throughout the EEA without being subject to additional national regulations.

the system in Europe. The device was certified as a diagnostic adjunct to mammography or physical examination in younger women with suspicious palpable breast lesions.

## ELECTRICAL IMPEDANCE IMAGING

Transmission of a low-voltage electrical signal through the breast can be used to measure the electrical impedance of the tissues (Figure 2-8). Cytological and histological changes in cancerous tissue, including changes in the cellular and extracellular contents, electrolyte balances, and cellular membrane properties, can significantly decrease the impedance of cancerous tissue (by a factor of approximately 40 relative to that of normal tissue) (Kleiner, 1999). Electrical impedance imaging of the breast is painless, does not compress the breast, and does not use ionizing radiation. The technology also works equally well for women of all ages, including young women with dense breasts and women on estrogen replacement therapy.

TransScan Medical (Ramsey, New Jersey) has developed an electrical

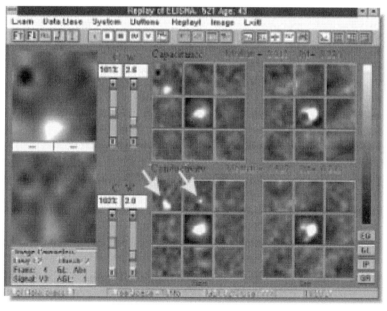

**FIGURE 2.8** Example of an electrical impedance image of the breast. White Spots in the center of the displays are the nipples. The white spots in the outer sectors identified by the arrows were found to be invasive ductal carcinoma on biopsy. Source: TransScan Medical, Ramsey, NJ.

impedance imaging device (the T-Scan 2000) as a diagnostic adjunct to X-ray mammography. The device transmits a 1-volt electrical signal through the breast via an electrode on the patient's arm. A clinician measures the electrical signal at the surface of the breast with a handheld probe containing an array of electrodes. The electrical signal is used to create a real-time, computer-displayed image of the impedance of the underlying breast tissue. Regions of low impedance suggestive of cancer are displayed as bright areas on the computer screen. The combined results of several studies conducted by TransScan Medical indicated that the T-Scan 2000, when used in conjunction with mammography with a targeted population, improved the diagnostic sensitivity by 15.6 percent and the diagnostic specificity by 20.2 percent over those of mammography alone.[16] TransScan Medical has predicted, on the basis of published cancer prevalence estimates and the size of the annual screening population (25 million women in the United States), that the device could increase the number of early cancers detected by 8,000 to 9,000 and decrease the number of negative biopsies by 200,000 to 300,000. In 1999, the FDA granted premarket approval to TransScan Medical for their electrical impedance imaging device, the T-Scan 2000, for use as a diagnostic adjunct to X-ray mammography. TransScan Medical will distribute the T-Scan 2000 within the United States, and Siemens Medical Systems, Inc. (Iselin, New Jersey), has exclusive rights to distribute the T-Scan 2000 device outside of the United States. The company continues to conduct additional studies to further validate the technology.

A spectroscopic electrical impedance tomography (EITS) imaging system has also been evaluated with a very small number of women. Structural features in the EITS images have correlated with limited clinical information available on participants with benign and malignant abnormalities, cysts, and scarring from previous lumpectomies and follow-up radiation therapy (Osterman et al., 2000).

## ELECTRONIC PALPATION

Electronic palpation uses pressure sensors to quantitatively measure palpable features of the breast such as the hardness and the size of lesions[17] (Oncology News, 1999). Manual physical examination of the breast currently contributes significantly to cancer detection, but it is inherently

---

[16]Center for Devices and Radiological Health, FDA, Radiological Devices Panel Meeting, August 17, 1998, accessed April 3, 2000(http://www.fda.gov/ohrms/dockets/ac/98/transcpt/3446t1.rtf).

[17]The clinical assessment of electronic palpation technology: a new approach for the early detection and monitoring of breast lesions, available online(http://www.assurancemed.com/techspec.html).

subjective. Electronic palpation offers the potential to standardize the performance, documentation, and serial monitoring of physical breast examinations. Assurance Medical (Hopkinton, Massachusetts) and Ultratouch (Paoli, Pennsylvania) are developing electronic palpation devices.

Assurance Medical has developed a system that uses an array of pressure sensors mounted in a handheld device that is gently pressed against the breast and moved over its surface (Assurancee Medical, Inc., 1999). The resistance of the breast to the device is measured by the pressure sensors and is used to create a computer-generated image of the hardness of the underlying breast tissue. This image serves as a quantitative, objective measurement of the hardness, discreteness, and size of breast lesions for diagnosis.

The company is seeking FDA premarket approval for use of its device to measure and track the size of known, suspicious lesions. The company is testing the accuracy and reproducibility of its device with 400 women with manually palpable lesions. In that study, trained physicians or nurses first estimate the size of each lesion by manual palpation, and electronic palpation is then used to estimate the size of each lesion. The company hopes to demonstrate that there is less variability between size measurements taken by electronic palpation than by manual palpation. In cases in which the lesion is surgically removed, the electronic and manual palpation measurements are being compared with the size of the lesion as measured by a pathologist to assess the accuracy of the device.

According to the company, preliminary studies suggest that the technology might also be useful for screening. In a study with 137 women in whom 118 lesions were identified by clinical breast examination or mammography, electronic palpation successfully identified 96 of 102 palpable lesions and 12 of 16 nonpalpable lesions, for overall sensitivities of 92 percent for electronic palpation and 86 percent for clinical breast examination. Additional studies are needed to assess the specificity of electronic palpation.

A robotic device (Palpagraph™), developed by UltraTouch, has a single mechanical finger designed to mimic the action of a human finger to map relative breast density. A digital camera and other optical imaging systems create a virtual computer image of each breast consisting of cubic cells between 1 and 4 mm on a side. The robotic mechanism, guided by the virtual image, brings the mechanical finger to the center of each cell on the surface of the breast. For each surface cell, the robotic mechanism applies a series of gentle pulses to the finger, and the response is measured to fill in the underlying virtual cubic cells with density data. The finger lifts away from the breast and moves to the center of the adjacent surface cell until the entire breast, including the axillary areas, has been mapped. An average Palpagraph™ examination will take 10 to 20 minutes and does not involve breast compression. An initial study, which was undertaken in Iran, tested the device in a screening setting with 850 women. The subjects, 90 percent of whom were under age 50, were screened two to three times in 6 months. The sequential palpagrams were compared to find tumors that were growing, becoming more fixed, or becoming more dense. Palpagraphy detected 22 lumps ranging from 2 to 9 mm in diameter that warranted biopsy (those in which the diameter was greater than about 4 mm). Of these lumps, eight were judged to contain malignant cancer. No consistent effort was made to detect the 22 lesions by mammography.[18] The company is now preparing for clinical trials in the United States for FDA approval of the device. The device will be tested first with a population of women referred for diagnostic workup for possible breast cancer, who will be examined by mammography, palpagraphy, and clinical breast examination.

## EXAMPLES OF TECHNOLGIES IN VERY EARLY STAGES OF DEVELOPMENT

### Thermoacoustic Computed Tomography

Thermoacoustic computed tomography (TCT) exposes the breast to short pulses of externally applied electromagnetic energy. Differential absorption induces differential heating of the tissue followed by rapid thermal expansion. This generates sound waves that are detected by an array of ultrasonic transducers positioned around the breast. Tissues that absorb more energy expand more and produce more sound. The timing and intensity of the acoustic waves are used to construct a three-dimensional image of the irradiated tissue (Kruger et al., 1999).

When the incident electromagnetic energy of TCT is visible light, the thermoacoustic effect is also referred to as the "photoacoustic effect." The photoacoustic effect was first described by Alexander Graham Bell in 1861 and has been applied primarily to the spectroscopic analysis of gases, liquids, and solids (Rosencwaig, 1975). Although the thermoacoustic effect has a long scientific history, its application to medical imaging is still in the early stages of development.

TCT does not use ionizing radiation and does not compress the breast. As currently designed, the TCT ultrasonic transducers are arrayed around a hemispheric bowl that is filled with deionized water. The device is mounted beneath a table. To image the breast, the woman lays prone on the table with her breast immersed in the water through a hole in the table. The breast is scanned in approximately 1.5 minutes.

---

[18]Jeff Garwin President, UltraTouch Corporation, personal communication.

One major limitation of traditional X-ray mammography is that it creates a two-dimensional projection of the breast that is highly dependent upon the orientation of the breast, the X-ray source, and the detector. Because TCT images retain three-dimensional structural information, unlike the images obtained by X-ray mammography, the images of a woman's breast obtained by TCT are highly consistent. Because there is less variability in the images, changes should be more apparent and easier to track longitudinally by TCT than by X-ray mammography. Three-dimensional images are, however, potentially more difficult to display and analyze, and therefore, the time and cost required for image retrieval and analysis are potentially greater for TCT than X-ray mammography.

The contrast in a TCT image is determined primarily by the electromagnetic absorption properties of the tissue being imaged (Kruger et al., 1999). Different tissues absorb electromagnetic waves of different frequencies. For radio waves in the range of 200 to 600 megahertz (MHz), there is sevenfold difference between the most and the least absorptive soft tissues. For comparison, there is only a two-fold difference between the most and the least absorptive soft tissues at X-ray frequencies (Kruger et al., 1999). In the range of 300 to 500 MHz, cancerous tissue is two to five times more absorptive than comparable noncancerous tissue, presumably because of the increased water and sodium contents of malignant cells (Chaudhary et al., 1984; Joines et al., 1980, 1994).

The electromagnetic wave pulse, the acoustic properties of the tissue, the geometry of the ultrasonic detector array, and the image reconstruction algorithm determine the spatial resolutions of TCT images (Kruger et al., 1999). To date, the leading developer of TCT, Optosonics, Inc. (Indianapolis, Indiana), has achieved in vivo imaging of the human breast with a spatial resolution of 1 mm up to a depth of 40 mm.[19]

The development of TCT is still in its early stages.[20] To date there have been no large published clinical trials, although Optosonics is planning to conduct an exploratory study with 80 women this year in conjunction with the Indianapolis Breast Center.

## Microwave Imaging

Confocal microwave imaging is a new technique that uses the differential water content of cancerous tissue versus that of noncancerous tissue to detect tumors. The technique transmits short pulses of focused, low-power microwaves into the breast tissue, collects the back-scattered

---

[19]Robert Kruger, Optosonics, Inc., personal communication, March 8, 2000.

[20]The original patent for the "Photoacoustic Breast Scanner" was issued in 1998 (RA Kruger, U.S. patent 5713356).

energy via antennas positioned around the breast, and compounds these signals to produce a three-dimensional image of the breast. Normal tissue is mostly transparent to microwaves; however, the higher water content of malignant tissue and the differences in the dielectric properties of tumor tissue versus those of breast fatty tissue cause significantly more scatter of microwave energy, thus enabling detection of tumors (Meaney et al., 1999). Confocal microwave imaging has several attractive features. It does not require breast compression and does not use ionizing radiation. In theory it will produce a high-contrast three-dimensional image of the breast and should be equally effective for women with dense breasts.

Confocal microwave imaging of the breast is being developed primarily by researchers at the University of Wisconsin-Madison, Dartmouth, and Northwestern University. The work is an extension of other nonmedical applications of focused microwave imaging including groundpenetrating radar for detection of land mines and detection of concealed weapons at airports (Microwave News, 2000).

Many techniques for microwave imaging of the body have been explored by other researchers, including the detection of the passive emission of microwaves by the body, microwave thermography, and active examination of the body by use of narrowband microwaves, which should provide better resolution (Larsen and Jacobi, 1986). The development of these techniques has been constrained by poor resolution, poor penetration to the required tissue depths, excessive power requirements that result in the delivery of potentially unsafe levels of microwaves to the patient, and computationally challenging techniques for image reconstruction (Bridges, 1998; Fear and Stuchly, 1999).

To date, confocal microwave imaging research has emphasized theoretical validation of the technique through computer modeling (Fear and Stuchly, 1999) and measurements of the high-frequency electrical properties of excised breast tissue. As part of the modeling, researchers have considered different antenna arrangements, tumor sizes and placements, breast sizes, and tissue compositions. The results of the modeling suggest that tumors as small as 2 mm should be detectable at a depth of 4 cm. It will probably be several years before the technique is tested with any significant number of women (Hagness et al., 1998).

## Hall Effect Imaging

Hall effect imaging (HEI) is a new general-purpose imaging technique being developed on the basis of the classical Hall effect discovered in 1879 by Edwin Hall (Graham-Rowe, 1999; Wen et al., 1998; Wen, 1999). HEI induces vibrations in charged particles by passing an electric pulse through an object while it is exposed to a strong magnetic field. The vibrating particles produce sound waves that can be detected by ultrasonic transducers and that can be used to create a three-dimensional image of the object.

Different materials vibrate differently according to their electrical properties. As with other emerging imaging technologies including microwave imaging and TCT, HEI is being developed to exploit the electrical properties of tissues in the body, which vary widely with tissue type and pathological state.

Although the Hall effect has been used for many years by nonmedical disciplines, it is unclear whether it will develop into a technique suitable for imaging of humans. HEI is still in its infancy: the first published account of HEI only appeared in 1998. To date HEI has been tested only with excised and simulated tissue.

Perhaps the biggest limitation to the future application of the technology is the cost. As with MRI, HEI will require an expensive, superconducting magnet to produce a sufficiently strong magnetic field. Cost alone would likely limit its usefulness as a breast cancer screening technology, but if the technique is developed, it might be useful for limited, specific populations of women, as has been the case with MRI.

## Magnetomammography

Magnetic source imaging of the breast, magnetomammography (MMG), is a new technique being investigated by using extremely sensitive Superconducting Quantum Interference Device (SQUID) magnetometers.[21] Researchers hope to use SQUID magnetometers to detect magnetic, tumor-specific agents introduced into the body intravenously. This is similar in principle to scintimammography, except that magnetic agents and SQUID magnetometers will replace radionuclides and gamma cameras.

SQUID magnetometers have been used clinically in a limited number of research centers for many years to detect magnetic fields produced by electrical activity in parts of the body such as the brain (magnetoencephalography) and the heart (magnetocardiography) (Clarke, 1994). MMG research is focused on developing an agent that is both magnetic and highly specific to cancerous tissue. At present, no such agent is available, and so MMG remains untested. In theory, MMG should be equally effective for women with dense breasts and would not require breast compression or ionizing radiation.

One limitation of scintimammography, which MMG will similarly have to address, has been its lack of sensitivity to some types of lesions.

---

[21]Robert Kraus, Los Alamos National Laboratory, personal communication.

As with gamma cameras, SQUID magnetometers have poor spatial resolution. The contrast resolution may be sufficiently high to detect small tumors, provided that they have sufficient volume and provided that after injection the ratio of the concentration of the exogenous magnetic agent in the lesion to the background concentration is high. The uptake by cancerous tissue of sestamibi, one of the best agents presently available for scintimammography, is about three times that by surrounding noncancerous tissue, but it has not yet demonstrated efficacy when it is used to detect small, nonpalpable tumors. A further difficulty is that the computational strategies needed to generate MMG images of magnetic sources are much more complex than those needed for scintimammography.

Provided a suitable magnetic agent can be developed, one of the biggest obstacles to be overcome for the implementation of MMG will be cost. SQUID magnetometers are expensive to fabricate and operate. Because they are superconductors, they must be cooled with either liquid helium or liquid nitrogen, neither of which is easily available in all areas of the country. SQUID magnetometers must also often be operated in expensive, magnetically shielded environments because the physiological signals that they are designed to measure are extremely small and easily drowned out by the earth's magnetic field and other background magnetic fields. It remains to be seen whether such special provisions will be required for MMG.

### Three-Dimensional Interactive Visualization

Three-dimensional interactive visualization techniques, including virtual reality, radically alter how individuals interact with computers to understand digital data. Many components of three-dimensional interactive visualization technology have been developed for other nonmedical applications (e.g., target recognition and flight simulators) and could potentially be applied to breast imaging. Several pioneer research groups have already demonstrated improved clinical performance using three-dimensional interactive imaging, planning, and control techniques (e.g., breast MRI). Three-dimensional interactive visualization could potentially be used in breast imaging for visualization, training, procedure planning, procedure support, and prognosis. However, significant improvements in virtual reality technologies are still required, including novel algorithms for breast imaging, before this potential can be realized.

### SUMMARY

At present, mammography is the only technology suitable for screening of the general population for breast cancer. It therefore serves as a "gold standard" with which new technologies will be compared. However, this standard is imperfect, and thus, improvements in the sensitivity and specificity of mammography itself could potentially affect mortality and morbidity from breast cancer and the overall cost of screening. Many technical improvements have been made to FSM since its initial introduction, but it is not known whether these changes have led to better survival rates among screened women. Many have considered digital mammography to be a major technical improvement over traditional FSM, but studies to date have not demonstrated meaningful improvements in screening sensitivity and specificity. Although it could be argued that studies thus far have not directly tested the full potential of FFDM through the use of soft-copy image analysis, difficulties remain with regard to the limited spatial resolution and luminance range of soft-copy display. The technology could potentially facilitate novel techniques such as tomosynthesis and digital subtraction mammography with X-ray-based contrast agents, but the value of these methods has not yet been proven. Digital mammography could also potentially improve the practice of screening and diagnostic mammography in other ways, for example, by facilitating electronic storage, retrieval, and transmission of mammograms. CAD has also shown potential as a means of improving the accuracy of screening mammography, at least among less experienced readers, but again, questions remain as to how this technology will ultimately be used and whether it will have a beneficial effect on current screening practices.

Mammography is particularly limited in young women. Because breast cancer is the principal cause of death for women ages 35 to 50, efforts have been made to identify alternate or complementary screening approaches for young women at high risk. Magnetic resonance imaging and ultrasound have been studied most extensively in this regard and show considerable promise for this select population. To date, however, the data are not yet sufficient to draw sound conclusions with respect to the appropriate screening applications of these technologies. That may change in the near future, as several large studies are ongoing. Ideal detection performance may ultimately depend on multimodality imaging, as no single imaging technology can provide a high signal-to-noise ratio in all circumstances or is able to detect all significant lesions.

Most of the imaging technologies for breast cancer detection described in this chapter are being developed as diagnostic adjuncts to mammography, with the goal of avoiding unnecessary, invasive biopsy procedures. Some, such as ultrasound and MRI, may also be used in conjunction with new minimally invasive therapeutic methods that are under development. Other technologies, such as functional imaging modalities, offer additional promise as both detection modalities and prognostic aids and could potentially shift the paradigm of cancer detection, but advances in this area will require further research to identify the appropriate biological markers to be examined. If and when these developing technologies are adopted for such diagnostic or prognostic applications, they may also be further examined as screening modalities. However, most of the technologies are not far enough along in development to adequately assess or predict their future application or value.

Ultimately, a new technology for early breast cancer detection will be beneficial only if it can lead to a reduction in the morbidity and mortality associated with the disease. Thus, improved methods for early detection of breast cancer may bring new challenges as well as opportunities for intervention. If the information generated by new technologies cannot be acted upon appropriately to improve outcomes, then women are not likely to benefit from the technological advances. Furthermore, as imaging methods become better and better at finding very small, early lesions such as carcinoma in situ, treatment decisions can be difficult to make because so little is known about the malignant potential of these premalignant cells (Tabar et al., 2000). As a result, some women may face the diagnosis of breast cancer and the subsequent therapy for a lesion that may never have become a lethal, metastatic cancer. Research efforts into the biology and etiology of breast cancer must therefore also continue, as discussed in Chapter 3. Moreover, improvements in the understanding of breast cancer progression should lead to treatment advances, and these combined changes could eventually alter both the use and the assessment of imaging tools.

# 3
# Technologies in Development: Genetics and Tumor Markers

The ability to predict who will develop breast cancer is modest at best. Thus, immense efforts have been devoted to identifying hereditary factors that contribute to breast tumorigenesis by studying the DNA of families with a high incidence of breast cancer. In recent years great strides have been made with the discovery of several genes that, when mutated, confer a very high lifetime risk of breast cancer. However, these mutations account for only a small fraction of all breast cancer cases (10 percent or less). In the majority of cases, the hereditary aspects of the disease remain undefined, but a recent study suggests that heritable factors can play a role in some sporadic cases of breast cancer (Lichtenstein et al., 2000), and thus, the search for genetic markers continues. In addition, scientists are also looking for biomarkers in serum, as well as breast tissues and fluids, that may predict the risk for cancer or reveal the presence of cancer.

However, predicting who will develop breast cancer and finding breast abnormalities at an early stage are only the first challenges. The decision-making process that occurs after the identification of a breast lesion can be equally difficult. Breast cancer is a heterogeneous disease at the molecular level, and thus, breast cancers of the same stage can behave very differently (Heimann and Hellman, 2000). As a result, current diagnostic techniques, which rely on morphological traits that have been used for more than 100 years, are considered relatively imprecise for prognosis and for use in making treatment decisions. This recognition has provided the impetus for studying the biological basis and cause of breast cancer, raising the possibility of a future classification system for breast lesions based on molecular mechanisms rather than morphology (Osin et al., 1998).

A better understanding of the biology and etiology of breast cancer may be especially important for assessment of the premalignant and early-stage lesions that are now so commonly identified by screening mammography. These abnormalities are defined by their morphological characteristics, and the probability that they will progress to a life-threatening disease is imprecisely estimated on the basis of indirect epidemiological evidence. Unfortunately, relatively little is known about the biology of premalignant breast lesions, but a variety of technologies are under development or are being used as research tools with the goal of advancing knowledge and applying that new knowledge to improve the means of early detection, diagnosis, and prognosis.

Much of the research on the biology of human breast cancer to date has been done with biopsy tissues obtained in the process of diagnosing a breast abnormality and then preserved in specimen banks. The goal of establishing such banks is to make samples available to scientists studying genetic alterations and changes in gene expression in cancer cells by the methods described in this chapter. One limitation of using biopsy tissues is that they provide only a snapshot in time: at the particular stage of the disease in which they were collected. The chronology of events leading to the initiation of the lesion is difficult to ascertain, and the potential for progression is difficult to assess. Hence, insights into the biology of breast cancer have also been gained through the culture of breast cells in vitro. These model systems may allow a more dynamic examination of the events in cancer progression and modification by protective or promoting factors.

Many public and private initiatives are characterizing the biological basis of cancer. Perhaps the most comprehensive public initiative is the Cancer Genome Anatomy Project (CGAP), which was established by the National Cancer Institute (NCI) in 1997 with the objective of achieving a comprehensive molecular characterization of normal, precancerous, and malignant cells and applying that knowledge to the prevention and management of cancer. The goal of CGAP is to use high-throughput technologies (any technology that uses robotics, automated machines, and computers to process many samples at once) to identify all the genes responsible for the establishment and growth of cancer and to catalog this information in freely accessible databases. Attainment of this goal will require detailed characterization of the distinct genetic alterations that are associated with the transformation to a malignant state, identification of the genes expressed during development of human tumors, and identification and characterization of genetic variations in genes important for cancer.

Recently, NCI also launched the Early Detection Research Network, which will attempt to translate the discoveries of CGAP and others into methods for the detection of cancer at its earliest stages and for the identification of people at risk of cancer before they develop the disease. The network includes nine clinical and epidemiological centers that will focus on providing the network with blood, tissue, and other biological samples; three biomarker validation laboratories that will standardize tests and prepare them for clinical trials; and a data management and coordination center that will develop standards for data reporting and the study of new statistical methods for analysis of biomarkers. Many scientists in this and other organizations are trying to apply new knowledge about the biology of breast cancer, in particular for the development of novel screening, diagnostic, and monitoring tests, as well as new therapeutic approaches.

In many cases, the goals of the technologies described in this chapter are to better characterize biopsy tissues from breast abnormalities that have been identified by imaging methods and thus aid in the diagnosis and decision-making process once a lesion has been found (Table 3.1). Another major goal of this research is to identify the appropriate biological markers to be used for functional imaging methods, as described in Chapter 2. In other cases, such as the analysis of blood samples or breast fluids, the goal is to predict a woman's risk of developing breast cancer or to identify markers of malignancy before the cancer can be detected by traditional imaging methods or physical examinations.

## GERM-LINE MUTATIONS AND CANCER RISK

With the many recent technical advances that make it easier to locate and identify genes and mutations have come increased efforts in the search for disease-causing genes. The current initiatives to sequence the human genome will no doubt further accelerate the study of familial susceptibility to all diseases, including cancer. The ultimate goal of this research is to identify individuals with an increased risk for cancer, who can then take action before cancer develops. Currently, that action primarily entails increased screening and surveillance, but ideally, in the future it should also include preventive strategies.

Traditionally, genes that confer a predisposition for cancer have initially been identified through standard epidemiological studies designed to detect familial clustering of specific cancers. Once family clusters have been identified, a process called "linkage analysis" is used to pinpoint the locations of the mutant genes. Markers throughout the genome are examined for coinheritance with the mutant phenotype because segments of DNA that are located close to a marker on the same chromosome will be inherited with the marker.

**TABLE 3-1** Technologies Under Development for Biological Characterization and Detection of Breast Cancer

| Detection Objective | Techniques | Stage of Development | Current Limitations |
|---|---|---|---|
| Identify germ-line mutations associated with cancer risk | Various genetic tests for BRCA1, BRCA2, p53, and AT DNA arrays | In clinical use<br><br>Preclinical stage | ≤10% of women with breast cancer affected<br>Survival benefit not proven |
| Identify polymorphisms associated with cancer risk | Various sequencing techniques | Used as research tools | Value for predicting cancer risk poorly defined |
| Identify and characterize somatic mutations and epigenetic changes | Fluorescent In Situ Hybridization (FISH), Comparative Genomic Hybridization, Polymerase Chain Reaction (PCR) for loss of heterozygosity (LOH), DNA arrays, DNA methylation asays | Used as research tools | Diagnostic and prognostic values of mutations are poorly defined; tumors are heterogeneous |
| Measure changes in RNA expression in cancer cells[a] | Northern analysis, Reverse transcription-PCR, cDNA array | Used as research tools | Same as directly above; difficult to assess small samples; Need computer algorithms for array data |

| Measure changes in levels of protein expression in cancer cells[a] | Immunohistochemistry (IHC) | Some IHC in clinical use | Same as directly above |
|---|---|---|---|
| | Two-dimensional gel electrophoresis, Mass spectroscopy | All used as research tools | |
| Identify markers of cancer in breast fluids | Nipple aspiration Breast lavage | Used as research tools, early stage of clinical testing | Sensitivity and specificity are low; appropriate markers to be examined are not clear |
| Identify markers of cancer or risk in serum or blood | Various tests for protein markers | Some in clinical use for monitoring disease Others are research tools | Same as directly above |
| | Isolation and analysis of cancer cells in circulation | Early stage of development | |
| Culture of breast cells | Various tissue culture methods | Used as research tools | Primary cultures have been difficult to grow Prognostic value of newer methods unproven |

[a]Potential targets of functional imaging.

## BRCA1 and BRCA2

Two examples of breast cancer genes originally identified in this way are *BRCA1* and *BRCA2*. The search for these breast cancer susceptibility genes began more than 20 years ago (King et al., 1980). By the early 1990s, powerful new tools in molecular biology had been developed, and in 1994, positional cloning was used to identify *BRCA1* on chromosome 17 (Miki et al., 1994). Mutations in this gene are now believed to account for 30 to 45 percent of the familial breast cancer cases and nearly 90 percent of the cases in families with high incidences of both breast and ovarian cancer (Easton et al., 1993; Ford et al., 1994). Because breast cancer in a significant number of families with high incidences of breast cancer appeared to be linked to genes other than *BRCA1*, the search continued for an additional breast cancer gene. In 1995, *BRCA2* was identified on chromosome 13 by focusing on families with a high incidence of breast cancer in both male and female members (Wooster et al., 1995). Mutations in *BRCA2* are thought to account for breast cancer in about 35 percent of families with a high incidence of early-onset breast cancer (Tavtigian et al., 1996).

Although there is no significant homology between the two large genes, the proteins that they encode may have some related activities in cells. Both appear to be multifunctional proteins that have been hypothesized to play a role in DNA repair pathways, cell proliferation, and transcriptional regulation (reviewed by Cortez et al., 1999 and Welcsh et al., 2000). Why germ-line mutations in these genes lead to breast cancer (or ovarian cancer) more frequently than other tumor types remains largely a mystery. However, knowledge of the gene sequences has allowed the development of genetic tests that may aid in determining a woman's risk for breast cancer.

A variety of tests for *BRCA1* and *BRCA2* mutations are now commercially available. The genes can be examined for specific mutations or sequenced in their entirety. Most of the currently available tests are labor intensive, but a recent technological advance known as "DNA microarrays" could potentially allow faster high-throughput analysis of samples. Microarrays, which first emerged in the mid-1990s, consist of thousands of different oligonucleotides spotted onto specific locations on glass microscope slides or silicon chips, which are then hybridized with labeled sample DNA (Figure 3-1). High-density arrays with more than 95,000 oligonucleotides have been used experimentally to identify mutations in exon 11 of *BRCA1* (Hacia et al., 1996). However, the sensitivities and specificities of the various tests have not been fully determined, and thus, their clinical utility remains uncertain.

The decision as to whether a women should be tested for *BRCA* mutations is often made on the basis of the calculated risk that a family may be

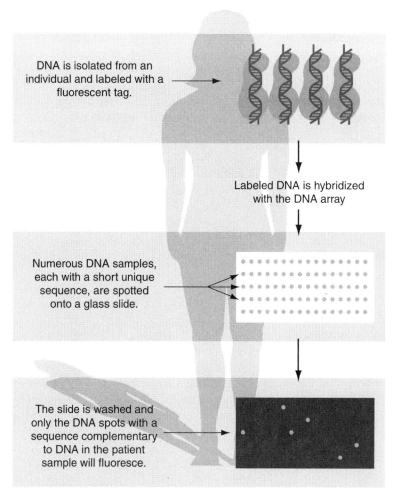

DNA is isolated from an individual and labeled with a fluorescent tag.

Labeled DNA is hybridized with the DNA array

Numerous DNA samples, each with a short unique sequence, are spotted onto a glass slide.

The slide is washed and only the DNA spots with a sequence complementary to DNA in the patient sample will fluoresce.

**FIGURE 3-1**   Example of a DNA array.

carrying a mutation. That risk is approximated by assessing the family history of incidence and age of onset, as well as the family's ethnic derivation (Parmigiani et al., 1998). However, breast cancer is a relatively common disease, so clustering could occur by random chance alone. Furthermore, there is significant heterogeneity among the mutations in these large genes that can predispose individuals to breast cancer, and each of the available tests has limitations in the types of mutations that it can reliably detect. Thus, selection of a particular test and interpretation of the results of that test can be difficult unless an affected relative has already been shown to carry a specific mutation.

Interpretation of negative results is further complicated by the fact that germ-line mutations in other genes may also confer an increased risk for breast cancer (see below). Environmental exposures could also play a role in familial clusters of breast cancer. Thus, a negative result may not be very meaningful to a woman with a strong family history of breast cancer, and it does not necessarily change her individual risk calculated before the test.

A positive test result carries many ramifications for the woman and her family. The ethical, legal, and psychosocial issues surrounding tests for genetic susceptibility are great. Women who carry BRCA mutations must deal with the psychological stress of knowing that they are more likely than women in the general population to develop breast cancer and that they could pass on this susceptibility to their children. Family and other personal relationships can be disrupted, and a woman could potentially face insurance or employment discrimination. A number of state and federal laws restrict some uses of genetic information,[1] but more could be done to ensure the privacy of the information and protection from discrimination. The National Action Plan on Breast Cancer, the National Human Genome Research Institute (HGRI), and others have developed recommendations for further restrictions on the use of genetic information (Department of Labor et al., 1998; Koenig et al., 1998; Rothenberg et al., 1997; Shalala, 1997). These issues are also of great importance to the continuing research on BRCA and other mutations (Fuller et al., 1999).

Genetic testing has not yet been shown to have an impact on breast cancer incidence or mortality, and unfortunately, there are relatively few data to guide a woman's plan of action once she has been identified as carrying a breast cancer susceptibility gene. The possibilities range from participating in standard screening programs, to enrolling in clinical trials for chemoprevention or alternate screening technologies, to bilateral prophylactic mastectomy (Hartman et al., 2000), but none of these interventions has yet been definitively proven to be of benefit among BRCA mutation carriers.

Because of the uncertainties in interpreting negative results, as well as the implications of positive results, genetic testing for breast cancer susceptibility should be accompanied by genetic counseling before and after the test. However, no standard of care for such counseling exists. HGRI includes a branch known as ELSI (ethical, legal, and social issues) that is conducting clinical studies to determine the best approach for the coun-

---

[1]The Health Insurance Portability Accountability Act of 1996 (Public Law No. 104-191, 701, 110 Stat 1936) prevents group health plans from labeling genetic information as a preexisting condition.

seling and education of women undergoing genetic testing. Professional societies, such as the American Society for Clinical Oncology, as well as other organizations like the Breast Cancer Working Group of the Stanford Program in Genomics, Ethics, and Society, have also produced guidelines and recommendations on counseling and genetic testing (American Society of Clinical Oncology, 1996; Koenig et al., 1998).

Such counseling and education are essential for informed consent before the test. Women need to understand the potential risks and benefits of undergoing testing, as well as the accuracy, efficacy, and limitations of the test. Different mutations could show various degrees of penetrance (the likelihood that affected individuals will develop cancer), which could potentially be further modified by other factors in the genetic background or the environment (E.L. Harris, 1999). The estimated cumulative risk of breast cancer by age 70 in the very high risk families originally studied during the search for *BRCA1* was 80 percent (Easton et al., 1993), but some subsequent population-based studies have shown a lower cumulative risk. The risk for the Ashkenazi Jewish population, for example, is estimated to be 56 percent (Struewing et al., 1997).

The tests are offered primarily as a clinical laboratory service by Myriad Genetics Inc., which holds U.S. patents on both *BRCA1* and *BRCA2*. The tests are not subject to Food and Drug Administration (FDA) regulation, and thus, the clinical validity and utility did not have to be documented before entry into the market. Rather, the quality of laboratories that provide genetic testing as a service is regulated under the Clinical Laboratory Improvement Amendments (CLIA) of 1988. CLIA requires the laboratories to demonstrate only that the tests can accurately and reliably measure the analytes that they are designed to assay (Holtzman, 1999). As a result, some advocacy groups such as the National Breast Cancer Coalition and the Alliance of Genetic Support Groups have proposed that the test should be made available only in a research setting. In response to such concerns, the Secretary's Advisory Committee on Genetic Testing (SACGT) was chartered in 1998 to advise the U.S. Department of Health and Human Services (DHHS) on the medical, scientific, ethical, legal, and social issues raised by the development and use of genetic tests. SACGT has recommended FDA review of all genetic tests, with particular attention to tests used for predictive purposes for diseases without an effective intervention. DHHS action on these recommendations is pending.

Myriad Genetics Inc. has recently launched testing services in Canada, Japan, Ireland, and the United Kingdom through exclusive licenses with laboratory service companies in those countries (Cancer Letter, March 2000). In the United States, Myriad recently signed a multiyear agreement with several large medical insurers to include the tests for *BRCA* in its list of covered services for its members (Cancer Letter, February 2000). A number of other major insurers and health care management organizations have taken similar actions. These national and international developments will make the test accessible to many more women, but coverage for counseling and follow-up care does not always accompany coverage for the tests.

Because of the exclusivity of Myriad's licensing agreements and the high cost of testing for *BRCA*, there are concerns that enforcement of Myriad's exclusive licensing agreements will limit access of consumers to the clinical testing provided by other laboratories (Reynolds, 2000). Separate concerns were also raised about the limitations of exclusive licensing with regard to publicly funded research. In response to this concern, some universities have obtained licenses from Myriad to conduct limited testing for research purposes. The company recently agreed to provide testing at a reduced fee to scientists at the National Institutes of Health, as long as the test is performed only for research purposes (Cancer Letter, February 2000). Proponents of the agreement are optimistic that this agreement will lead to increased research activity on the *BRCA* genes that will generate clinically useful information.

### Other Germ-Line Mutations

Approximately 10 percent of all breast cancer cases are thought to be linked to a familial mutation of some sort. The majority can be accounted for by mutations in the *BRCA1* and *BRCA2* genes, but other genes have also been linked to a significantly increased risk for breast cancer. For example, families with Li-Fraumeni cancer syndrome, which is most often due to mutations in the p53 tumor suppressor gene, show increased susceptibility to a variety of cancers, including breast cancer (Malkin et al., 1990). The p53 protein is thought to play a major role in protecting the integrity of a cell's genome by regulating the proliferation and survival of cells harboring damaged DNA. It is estimated that about 1 percent of inherited breast cancers are due to the p53 mutation (Sidransky et al., 1992; Borresen, 1992). Another 1 percent may be due to mutations in the *PTEN* tumor suppressor gene. *PTEN* mutations have been linked to Cowden's syndrome (Liaw et al., 1997), which is characterized by an increased risk for breast and thyroid cancers. Women carrying such mutations have a 30 to 50 percent lifetime risk of developing breast cancer. Because these two syndromes are relatively rare, genetic testing for the associated mutations is limited to a few centers.

Some families with a high incidence of breast cancer have not been shown to harbor a mutation in any of the genes mentioned above, leading scientists to believe that mutations in other, as yet undefined genes may also predispose women to breast cancer. One candidate is the *AT* (ataxia telangiectasia) gene. The *AT* gene, which is mutated in individuals with the rare autosomal recessive disease ataxia telangiectasia, plays a role in protecting cells from ionizing radiation. Because mothers of individuals with AT develop early-onset breast cancer more frequently than would be predicted from the frequency calculated for the general population, it has been hypothesized that heterozygous carriers of the gene may have an elevated risk for breast cancer. Nonetheless, the results of case-control studies conducted to date have not supported this theory (FitzGerald et al., 1997). It may be interesting to note, however, that basic research points to a role for the AT protein in the *BRCA* pathways, as well as the p53 pathway (Cortez et al., 1999; Li et al., 2000; reviewed by Lakin and Jackson [1999]).

## POLYMORPHISMS AND CANCER RISK

Much of the genetic variation among human populations is due to subtle DNA alterations that are shared by many people. Known as polymorphisms, these subtle differences can result in altered protein expression or changes in protein activity that may affect susceptibility to carcinogens and cancer promoters in the environment and that may contribute to the variability in individual responses to treatment. A major goal in studying polymorphisms in women with breast cancer is to more accurately predict which individuals are likely to develop breast cancer or to die from the disease.

Polymorphic sites in many genes have been studied to determine whether they are associated with an increased risk for breast cancer, and a number have been reported to confer elevated risk. A comprehensive analysis of all published studies found four polymorphic sites (in the *CYP19*, *GSTP1*, *TP53*, and *GSTM1* genes) associated with a higher risk for breast cancer (Dunning et al., 1999). However, the investigators noted that there was insufficient statistical power to accurately determine the risk for some sites examined, and there are many more genes and polymorphisms that have yet to be studied. One recent study examined 10 polymorphic sites in the estrogen receptor gene but did not find any association between the polymorphisms and breast cancer (Schubert et al., 1999). Studies are in progress to identify and characterize additional susceptibility alleles, but precise estimation of the risks associated with genetic polymorphisms, as well as investigation of more complex risks arising from gene-gene and gene-environment interactions, will require studies much larger than those undertaken to date. New DNA microarray-based methods may speed the search for relevant polymorphisms in complex diseases like breast cancer by facilitating high-throughput analysis of many genes simultaneously (Hacia et al., 1999).

Polymorphisms that involve single-base-pair differences are called "single nucleotide polymorphisms" (SNPs). Many SNPs, perhaps the majority, do not themselves change protein expression or cause disease, but they may be closely linked on the chromosome to deleterious mutations. Because of this proximity, SNPs may be shared among groups of people with unknown disease-associated mutations and serve as markers for such mutations. Such markers may aid in the identification of the mutations and thus could contribute to the understanding of the molecular changes in diseases such as cancer.

The SNP[2] Consortium Ltd., a nonprofit entity consisting of several major pharmaceutical and technology companies and one large scientific trust, has taken on the challenge of identifying 300,000 SNPs and mapping at least 150,000 SNPs evenly distributed throughout the genome. The project started in the spring of 1999 and is anticipated to continue until the end of 2001. The data generated by this effort are being collected in a database that is freely available to scientists, with liberal licensing provisions for investigators. SNPs will also be deposited in a public database, dbSNP. This database, designed to serve as a central repository for both single-base nucleotide substitutions and short deletion and insertion polymorphisms, was established by the National Center for Biotechnology Information in collaboration with the National Human Genome Research Institute. The SNP Consortium is funding studies to determine the frequencies of at least 60,000 SNP alleles identified through the consortium's research. SNPs that occur in at least 20 percent of a major population (e.g., Caucasians, Asians, or African-Americans) are considered sufficiently common to be useful as genetic markers in the genome.

Recently, another collaboration between Celera Genomics and City of Hope Cancer Center was announced. The two organizations plan to specifically investigate associations between genetic polymorphisms and breast cancer (Cancer Letter, March 2000). In this case, all intellectual property developed through the collaboration will be jointly owned by the two organizations.

## SOMATIC CHANGES IN BREAST CANCER

Initiation of sporadic (nonhereditary) cancers and the progression of

---

[2]The SNP Consortium's members include the Wellcome Trust; 10 pharmaceutical companies including AstraZeneca PLC, Aventis Pharma, Bayer AG, Bristol-Myers Squibb Company, F. Hoffmann-La Roche, Glaxo Wellcome PLC, Novartis Pharmaceuticals, Pfizer Inc, Searle, and SmithKline Beecham PLC; Motorola, Inc.; International Business Machines Corp; and Amersham Pharmacia Biotech. Academic centers including the Whitehead Institute for Biomedical Research, Washington University School of Medicine in St. Louis, the Wellcome Trust's Sanger Centre, Stanford Human Genome Center, and Cold Spring Harbor Laboratory are involved in SNP identification and analysis. Orchid BioSciences performs third-party validation and quality control testing on SNPs identified through the consortium's research.

all cancers occur via accumulation of changes in individual cells within the body. These changes ultimately lead to altered gene expression in those cells and may take many forms, including a variety of genetic alterations in the cell's DNA sequences (i.e., mutations) or epigenetic alterations that leave the DNA sequence intact but that nonetheless modify gene expression. Although many such changes have been observed in breast tumors, the functional relationship between the affected genes and cancer growth is still largely unknown. Indeed, the majority of breast cancers contain so many molecular changes that it is difficult to distinguish between those that are critical for tumor initiation and progression and those that are simply a product of cancer-associated genomic instability. Identification of the critical common events in breast carcinogenesis will therefore be essential for advancing the understanding of breast cancer biology and its etiology and for attaining the ultimate goals of improving means of detection and the ability to establish a prognosis. Most of the techniques described in this section are being used as research tools in studies with biopsy tissues, with the hope that the knowledge gained from this research will eventually be used to more accurately diagnose breast cancer and predict outcomes.

## SOMATIC GENETIC ALTERATIONS

Somatic alterations in cancer cells include genetic changes such as amplification and deletion of DNA sequences, chromosomal rearrangements, and base change mutations. DNA amplification can affect any stretch of DNA, from a single gene (microduplications) to an entire chromosome (aneuploidy). Amplification can result in an increased level of expression of the affected gene(s) and thus is one of the major molecular mechanisms through which the oncogenic potential of proto-oncogenes is activated during tumorigenesis. DNA deletions, on the other hand, result in the loss of genes and the associated gene products. Tumor suppressors are often inactivated in cancer through deletions or insertions. In many cases, base change mutations that alter or inactivate protein function are found on one allele, and the second allele is lost via deletion, a mechanism known as "loss of heterozygosity" (LOH).

A technique known as "fluorescent in situ hybridization" (FISH) can detect common aneuploidies and chromosomal loss or rearrangements as well as microduplications and deletions (Mark et al., 1997). This technology relies on hybridization of chromosomes with labeled DNA probes that are specific for genes or chromosomes. Another related technology is comparative genomic hybridization. In this case, DNA from normal and cancerous cells is labeled with differently colored fluorescent tags that are then simultaneously hybridized to metaphase spreads of normal chromosomes. A gain or loss of chromosomal regions can then be identified by

**TABLE 3-2**   General Chromosomal Locations of Allelic Imbalances
(Gains and Losses) in Premalignant Breast Lesions from Studies
Assessing Loss of Heterozygosity and Comparative Genomic
Hybridization Illustrating Their Tremendous Biological Complexity

| Category | Gains | Losses |
|---|---|---|
| ADH | Unknown | 1q, 2p, 6q, 9p, 11p, 11q, 13q, 14q, 16q, 17p, 17q, Xq |
| ALH | 6q | 11q, 16p, 16q, 17p, 22q |
| DCIS | 1q, 3q, 6p, 6q, 8q, 17q, 20q, Xq | 1p, 1q, 2p, 2q, 3p, 3q, 4p, 6p, 6q, 7p, 7q, 8p, 8q, 9p, 11p, 11q, 12p, 13q, 14q, 15q, 16p, 16q, 17p, 17q, 18q, 21q |
| LCIS | 6q | 11q, 13q, 16p, 16q, 17p, 17q, 22q |

NOTE: ADH, atypical ductal hyperplasia; ALH, atypical lobular hyperplasia; DCIS, ductal
carcinoma in situ; LCIS, lobular carcinoma in situ; p and q, chromosomal arms affected by
the gain or loss.

SOURCE: Allred and Moshin (2000).

the color of the chromosomes. Such current applications could be adapted
for use in the clinical cytogenetic laboratory if they prove to be useful as a
means of identifying markers for diagnosis or prognosis. New sequence
information derived from efforts to sequence the entire human genome,
combined with new high-throughput technologies such as DNA microarrays similar to those designed to detect germ-line mutations and polymorphisms, may also make it easier to detect small somatic mutations in
tumors in the future (Pollack et al., 1999; H. Yan et al., 2000).

LOH studies generally depend on polymerase chain reaction (PCR)-
based methods that analyze polymorphic microsatellite loci[3] as markers
for DNA loss. Many studies have found significant rates of loss of heterozygosity at dozens of genetic loci in individuals with premalignant
disease and early breast cancer (Table 3-2), as well as later-stage cancers,
but to date it is not yet clear whether specific LOH events are associated
with progression to invasive or metastatic cancer (Allred and Moshin,
2000).

## Epigenetic Changes

Scientists have traditionally focused on changes in DNA sequences
like mutations and deletions as the cause for altered cell functions in
human cancer. However, a recent plethora of studies indicates that epigenetic changes that do not alter the sequences but, rather, that result from

---

[3]Microsatellite loci are stretches of repetitive DNA that are located throughout the genome and thus serve as useful markers for genetic analysis.

chemical changes in the DNA, such as methylation, can also be important in altering gene expression during tumorigenesis. The density of cytosine methylation in the promoter regions of genes correlates inversely with gene activity, and many tumor suppressor genes are silenced by aberrant methylation in cancer. Thus, it has been proposed (reviewed by Baylin et al. [1998]) that the identification and characterization of these epigenetic modifications could lead to improvements in means of early detection and the ability to provide a prognosis as they could serve as surrogate markers for altered protein expression. Several PCR-based assays are used to detect epigenetic changes in small tissue samples, suggesting that the technology could be used for early detection applications, but much more work is needed to reach that point. More recently, scientists have developed an array-based method called "differential methylation hybridization," which allows genome-wide screening of gene hyper-methylation in breast cancer cells (P.S. Yan et al., 2000). Although the method has thus far been used to examine only cultured cell lines, results from preliminary studies indicate that analysis of hypermethylation patterns could potentially be used to classify tumors. Another method, known as "restriction landmark genomic scanning," has also recently been used to examine the methylation status of more than 1,000 sites in the genome and has been shown to be able to identify tumor type-specific methylation patterns (Costello et al., 2000).

## RNA Expression

Scientists have long sought to directly characterize gene expression in tumors compared with that in normal tissues and to correlate those differences with disease outcome or treatment response. However, that effort has been limited by a number of technical factors, including lack of gene sequence data and high-throughput technologies, inadequate access to specimen banks with appropriate patient information, and interpretive difficulties due to tumor heterogeneity. New genomic tools, such as complementary DNA (cDNA) microarrays, may offer the opportunity to make new advances.

Gene expression at the messenger RNA (mRNA) level has traditionally been examined by laborious methods such as Northern analysis (RNA-DNA hybridization) or, more recently, by PCR-based methods such as reverse transcription (RT)-PCR, in which only a small number of genes can be examined at one time. DNA microarray technology, in contrast, enables researchers to look at the expression of thousands of genes at once and obtain a tumor "signature." In this case, the microarrays consist of cDNA clones corresponding to different genes. The microarrays are hybridized with differentially labeled cDNA populations made from the mRNAs of the samples to be compared (Figure 3-2). The primary data

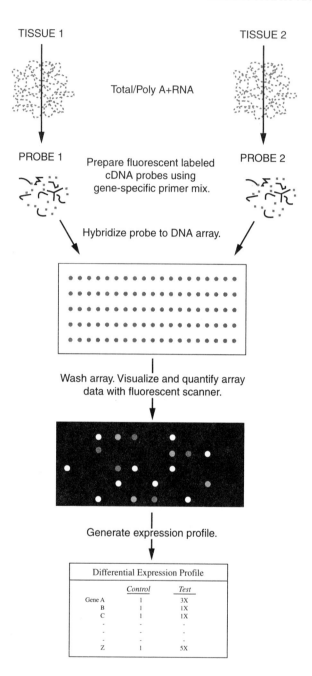

**FIGURE 3-2** Example of a cDNA expression array. SOURCE: Adapted from CLONTECH Laboratories, Inc., 1999.

collected are ratios of label intensity, which are representative of the concentrations of mRNA molecules in each sample. Computer algorithms must then be used to identify differences in gene expression between the samples, as well as "clusters" of gene expression (Eisen et al., 1998). Designing the appropriate algorithms to make sense of all the data generated may in fact be the biggest challenge for this technology.

Breast tumor samples were recently separated into at least two categories on the basis of gene expression clusters (Perou et al., 1999). The investigators also identified expression clusters associated with some of the normal cell types that infiltrate tumors, such as lymphocytes and stromal cells, suggesting that one component of tumor cell heterogeneity could potentially be accounted for by using this technology. However, newer methods of isolating small populations of cells from a tumor sample, such as laser capture microdissection (Emmert-Buck et al., 1996), may improve the accuracy of the technology even more. Such techniques may also facilitate examination of normal breast epithelial tissue and earlier-stage cancers, including ductal carcinoma in situ (DCIS). Thus far, most studies have been done with relatively large tumors (generally greater than 2 centimeters) by using tissue taken from excisional biopsy specimens.

One goal of microarray analysis is to classify tumors on the basis of their complete gene expression patterns. For example, if shared gene expression patterns in breast tumors can be used to establish a prognosis or predict the treatment response with greater accuracy, they will yield classifications directly coupled to treatment and outcome. Much more research is needed before those goals can be attained, but a recent study that used cDNA microarrays did identify two molecularly distinct forms of lymphoma that could not be distinguished by traditional classification techniques. Remarkably, the patient groups with the two subtypes of cancer had significantly different survival times, suggesting that molecular classification could potentially be useful in the future for determining prognosis and the appropriate treatment regimen for this type of cancer, as well as others (Alizadeh et al., 2000). A similar attempt has been made to classify breast tumors at the molecular level. Using microarrays to examine differences in mRNA expression patterns, breast tumors could be classified into subtypes that related to physiological variation, but it is not yet known whether different subtypes are associated with different clinical outcomes or response to therapy (Perou et al., 2000).

The relative levels of mRNA species can be regulated at the stage of gene transcription or RNA degradation. A third stage of regulation, that of pre-mRNA splicing, can also produce variations in the resultant protein sequence and function. This is the stage at which RNA is processed after being produced on the DNA template but before it is exported from the nucleus to be translated into protein. Modulation of the cellular machinery responsible for removing intronic sequences and joining the exons into a readable mRNA transcript can lead to alternative splicing events that produce mRNA "splice variants." Changes in splicing efficiency have been associated with malignant transformation and metastasis, suggesting that splice variants may be useful as tumor markers (reviewed by Cooper and Mattox, 1997). Perhaps the best-studied example of this phenomenon is the cell-surface-adhesion molecule CD44. Abnormal splice variants of this gene have been found in a variety of cancers, including breast cancer, and their presence has been correlated with metastatic potential (Cooper and Mattox, 1997; Kinoshita et al., 1999; Martin et al., 1997; Matsumura and Tarin, 1992). Many splice variants of the estrogen receptor have also been identified in breast cancer and have been hypothesized to play a role in resistance to anti-estrogen therapy (Tonetti and Jordan, 1997). Aberrant splicing can also result from mutations in the sequences at intron/exon junctions. For example, many of the mutations identified to date in the gene encoding the cell adhesion molecule E-cadherin are splice site mutations (Berx et al., 1998).

The variant mRNA species are currently detected primarily by RT-PCR (Matsumura and Tarin, 1992), but if cDNA arrays were designed to include sequences specific for different splice variants, this component of variation in tumor gene expression could also be assessed using the high-throughput technology. In many cases, the resultant protein variants can also be detected in tumor tissue or serum (Kinoshita et al., 1999; Martin et al., 1997), as described below.

### Protein Expression and Function

Knowledge of the RNA expression patterns of cells is not sufficient for determination of cellular behavior. The RNA expression level is not necessarily indicative of protein levels, because protein expression can be modulated at various stages, from the regulation of mRNA translation into protein to the targeting of the protein for degradation pathways. Traditionally, protein levels in tumors have been evaluated by methods such as immunohistochemistry with tissue sections (Figure 3-3). A plethora of proteins in breast tumors has been examined by this approach in the search for prognostic markers. The most commonly used protein markers to date include the estrogen and progesterone receptors and, more recently, the erbB2 receptor, all of which may be considered in the decision-making process for therapy. Although a number of proteins have shown some correlation with breast cancer progression, it has become clear that the identification of a single marker that can accurately predict disease progression is unlikely. In fact, very few tumor markers have been recommended as part of routine clinical care because it is quite difficult to determine the clinical utility of markers. For this reason, inves-

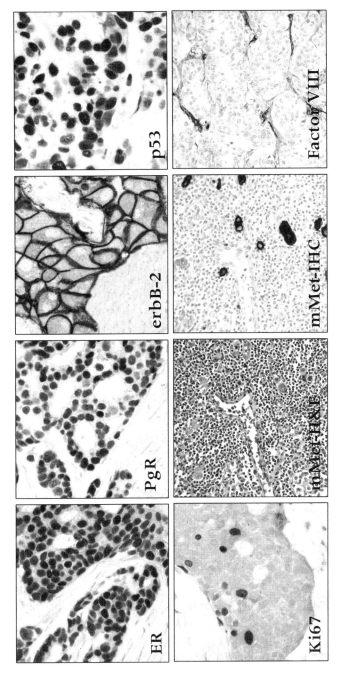

**FIGURE 3-3** Representative examples of prognostic and predictive factors that are commonly assessed in breast cancers by immunohistochemistry, including estrogen receptor (ER), progesterone receptor (PgR), membrane overexpression of the erbB-2 oncoprotein, nuclear accumulation of mutated p53 tumor suppressor protein, Ki-67 proliferation-associated marker, micrometastases (mMET) in lymph nodes (which may be obscure on routine slides stained with hematoxylin-eosin) detected by immunohistochemistry with antiepithelial antibodies that target keratins, and microvascular density with antibodies to the endothelium such as factor –VIII-related antigen. Source: Craig Allred, Baylor College of Medicine, Houston, Texas.

tigators developed a system for assessing the use of tumor markers (Hayes et al., 1996, 1998). The Tumor Marker Utility Grading System established an investigational agenda for the evaluation of tumor markers that is analogous to the system used to evaluate new therapeutic agents, which is quite standardized.

Consideration of the functional state of the proteins could add another level of complexity to protein analysis. Protein function can be regulated on many different levels, including through biochemical modifications such as phosphorylation and glycosylation (addition of phosphate or sugars) and through associations with other proteins. In fact, protein-mediated signal transduction pathways that initiate such critical activities as cell division, cell death, or cell movement can in many cases be activated without the synthesis of new proteins. Thus, a complete understanding of the molecular changes in cancer may require a functional analysis of pathways and circuits in cells and tissues, known as proteomics.

The term "proteome" was first coined in 1994 to refer to all proteins expressed by a genome. Traditionally, such protein analysis has required the labor-intensive method of two-dimensional gel electrophoresis, in which proteins are separated by size in one direction and electrical charge in the second direction. Each protein species migrates to a reproducible spot on the gel, and the proteins at these spots can be isolated and sequenced for identification. However, this method requires large amounts of protein and thus has been limited to cultured cells or homogenized tissues that contain a variety of cell types. Recent technological advances, including laser capture microdissection, new methods for cell sorting and mass spectroscopy[4] and improved bioinformatics may soon allow high-throughput analysis of the specific cell populations within tissues and tumors (Liotta and Petricoin, 2000). For example, one recent study identified a number of differences in the protein profiles of two different cell types in normal breast tissue (Page et al., 1999). Other recent technical advances suggest that the creation of protein arrays (the protein equivalent of DNA arrays) may also soon be feasible (Macbeath and Schreiber, 2000; Service, 2000).

## GROWTH OF BREAST CELLS IN CULTURE

The biology of mammary gland development and tumorigenesis has historically been studied with rodent model systems (Amundadottir et

---

[4]Cyphergen Biostystems, Inc. (Palo Alto, California) has developed a mass spectroscopy technology known as "surface-enhanced laser desorption/ionization" that rapidly analyzes native proteins at the femtomole level without the use of labels.

al., 1996; Russo and Russo, 1996; Welsch, 1987). However, it has been shown that profound differences in the development and transformation of mammary tissue exist between rodent species and humans (Russo and Russo, 1987). It would therefore be advantageous to study normal breast development and function, as well as breast cancer etiology, progression, and treatment, with human mammary cells. A major goal in this area of research is the isolation of specific cell lines derived from a variety of relevant human tissue types, including normal breast epithelium, atypical hyperplasia DCIS, early and late stages of breast cancer, and histologically normal tissue adjacent to the tumor. Such cell lines would allow investigation into the physiological, morphological, and genetic changes that occur during the process of breast tumorigenesis, as well as during subsequent tumor progression. One example of a model human cell line that can be used to study the evolution of breast cancer from premalignant proliferative breast disease is MCF10AT (Dawson et al., 1996; Heppner et al., 1999). The cell line was derived from tissue taken from a patient with hyperplastic growth of the breast epithelium.

Unfortunately, though, primary cultures of human breast epithelial tissue have been notoriously difficult to grow (Bergstraesser and Weitzman, 1993; Smith et al., 1981). A review of the literature suggests that the success rate for the establishment of cell cultures from breast tumors is no more than 10 to 15 percent (Engel and Young, 1978). Thus, much research has been done with a small number of established tumor cell lines that have the limitations of being clonally evolved and generally available only at high passage numbers (Engel and Young, 1978). Furthermore, most of these cell lines were derived from pleural metastases of patients who had been heavily treated with chemotherapuetic drugs. As a result, the cell lines probably represent a very small subfraction of breast tumor cell types. Although valuable information has been gained from these cell lines, much effort has been made to develop more physiologically relevant models.

To date, the success of human mammary epithelial cell (HMEC) culture has been hindered by limited knowledge of the specific factors that are required for the maintenance of epithelial cell function, growth, and differentiation. Although defined media that contain many of the known factors such as steroid hormones and a variety of peptide growth factors have been developed for HMEC culture, none to date have supported the growth of HMECs in primary culture for more than 2 or 3 weeks (Taylor-Papadimitriou and Stampfer, 1992). Furthermore, breast tissue contains several different cell types (stromal fibroblasts, the luminal epithelium lining the ducts and lobules, myoepithelial cells, and adipocytes) whose interaction and communication may be vital for cell growth, survival, and function. New methods for separation of the various cell types from breast tissue have been developed, but thus far, the purified cell populations have been grown in culture only for very short periods of time (Clarke et al., 1994; Monaghan et al., 1995).

Recent advances in tissue engineering, due largely to the commercial availability of extracellular matrix substrata (Hall et al., 1982; Petersen et al., 1992) and an awareness of concepts related to cell communication, have led to the development of a novel cell culture system with the ability to grow primary cell cultures from most breast tissues, both normal and neoplastic (U.S. patent no. 6,074,874).[5] The cultures of normal breast tissue, which have mixed cell morphologies, are long lived as primary cultures and grow and differentiate into organotypic architectures that persist for at least 3 to 4 months. The cultures progress and differentiate from three-dimensional domes or "mammospheres" to de novo luminal branching ducts. Tumor cells under the same culture conditions do not form an epithelial architecture but show a more chaotic behavior.[6] Often, tumor cells manifest autonomous, single-cell behavior and seem to avoid contact with one another. In addition, significant variability among similarly staged tumors has been documented by using time-lapse digital movies of the cell in culture. Studies are under way to determine whether more aggressive tumors demonstrate more aggressive behavior in culture. If such a correlation is found, the technology may perhaps be useful for prediction of metastatic potential, recurrence, and outcomes, but the clinical utility of this technology is currently unknown.

## COLLECTION AND ANALYSIS OF BREAST FLUIDS

Adult breast tissues secrete fluid into the breast ductal system even in the absence of pregnancy and lactation, and this fluid can be aspirated using breast massage and a modified breast pump. A number of studies have been undertaken to determine whether such nipple aspiration fluid (NAF) specimens might be useful for breast cancer screening and diagnosis, but the method is still confined to experimental protocols. Nipple aspiration was first proposed as a potential breast cancer screening technique by Papanicolaou and colleagues in the 1950s when they reported on the diagnosis of a small number of unsuspected cancers as a result of studying NAF specimens from 2,000 women (1958). Cells exhibiting nuclear changes characteristic of hyperplasia, atypia, or malignancy can be observed in NAF, and a more recent prospective study has shown that the incidence and relative risk of breast cancer were positively correlated with increasing severity of the cytological changes (Wrensch et al., 1992). Furthermore, the relative risk of breast cancer associated with hyperplas-

---

[5]Latimer, J.J. Epithelial cell cultures useful for in vitro testing, 1998.
[6]See www.pitt.edu/~rsup/mgb/latimer.html.

tic cells in NAF was similar to the relative risks calculated in other studies for women with hyperplastic changes identified by traditional biopsy methods. Another recent study, in which more than 95 percent of samples were sufficient for cytological evaluation regardless of menopausal status, also found a correlation between abnormal NAF cytology and increased risk of breast cancer (Sauter et al., 1997). However, the current sensitivity (less than 50 percent) of the test is not high enough to reliably determine whether a woman has breast cancer (Sauter et al., 1999). Thus, the proponents of the technology suggest that it could be a useful adjunct to mammography, especially for women for whom mammography has limitations, such as young women at high risk, those with dense breast tissue, or women whose breasts have been irradiated for prior cancers. As in the case of serum markers, this technology would most likely have to be used in conjunction with an imaging method to pinpoint the lesion responsible for the abnormal finding in NAF.

One technical limitation to the clinical use of NAF has been the difficulty in obtaining samples sufficient in volume for analysis from a significant number of women. Although the ability to obtain sufficient samples volumes may increase with practitioner experience, an alternative approach to NAF collection, known as ductal lavage, has also recently been developed (Love et al., 2000). A catheter is used to flush cells from the breast ducts with saline, and the morphologies of the cells are examined by cytology, just as in the NAF procedure. Pro•Duct Health, Inc., is conducting multicenter trials of this approach.

Molecular biology-based assessment of cells obtained by NAF or breast lavage could potentially identify genetic or epigenetic changes, in addition to cellular morphology, that could perhaps be predictive of breast cancer. Such assessment could include examination for chromosomal abnormalities or the use of DNA arrays to identify changes in the DNA of the cells. This approach has more commonly been investigated with other body fluids such as urine and saliva, with mixed results. One difficulty that must be overcome is the extreme sensitivity needed to identify genetic changes in the exceedingly small number of abnormal cells in such samples. One potential approach to overcoming this obstacle may be to focus on mutations in mitochondrial DNA rather than mutations in nuclear DNA (Fliss et al., 2000). Mitochondrial DNA mutations are common in many cancers, including breast cancer, and each cell contains 1,000 to 10,000 copies, making it easier to detect the mutations in small samples. However, this method is at a very early stage of development and has not been studied at all with NAF or breast lavage samples. Another possibility is to culture the collected cells to expand their number, but this can be quite difficult technically.

Collection of breast fluid samples can also facilitate measurement of protein markers such as growth factors and tumor-specific antigens, which are likely to be more concentrated in the breast fluid than in serum. To date, no markers have been demonstrated to reliably predict breast cancer, but several are under investigation.

## SERUM MARKERS AND CELLS IN THE CIRCULATION

Many diseases can be detected and monitored by blood tests, and significant efforts have been made to develop similar tests for the detection and monitoring of cancer. In the case of breast cancer, these efforts have met with limited success. There are two basic approaches to the development of such tests. The first is to measure tumor-specific proteins or other biomolecules in the serum, and the second is to identify and analyze tumor cells themselves in the circulation.

Currently, a few serum markers for breast cancer are mainly used to monitor the course of disease after diagnosis and treatment, although their usefulness in that setting has also been questioned (American Society of Clinical Oncology, 1996; Fitzgibbons et al., 2000; Hayes et al., 1996, 1998). Thus far, the best-established markers are CA 15-3, a polymorphic epithelial mucin, and carcinoembryonic antigen. These markers are unlikely to be used for breast cancer screening or diagnosis because they are accurate only in situations in which the tumor burden is relatively high. Many more potential markers are under development, including growth factors like Her2, oncoproteins such as c-*myc* and mutant p53, cytokeratins, and markers of angiogenesis and bone metabolism (reviewed by Cheung et al. [2000]). This approach is generally dependent on immunological detection techniques such as enzyme-linked immunosorbent assay and radioimmunoassay.

One recent example of a potential new serum biomarker for breast cancer is the riboflavin carrier protein (RCP). Some vitamin carrier proteins are overexpressed in patients with cancer, and RCP was investigated as a serum marker for breast cancer because its expression is induced by estrogen (Rao et al., 1999). The small prospective study found that RCP levels were significantly elevated in women with breast cancer and that the RCP assay could predict the presence of breast cancer with a sensitivity of 92 percent, a specificity of 88 percent, a positive predictive value of 89 percent, and a negative predictive value of 92 percent. However, the results of this very preliminary study have not yet been validated, and the test has not been examined in the setting of breast cancer screening.

Measurement of serum marker levels may also be helpful in determining the risk for breast cancer. For example, two retrospective studies have found significantly higher serum insulin-like growth factor (IGF) type 1 (IGF1) levels in women with breast cancer than in controls, especially premenopausal women (Pollak, 1998). More recently, a study with prospectively acquired blood samples has provided more direct evidence that the serum IGF level is related to the risk of premenopausal breast cancer (Hankinson et al., 1998). However, it remains to be determined whether higher IGF1 levels during the premenopausal years may also influence the risk of breast cancer after menopause.

Methods that rely on the collection and characterization of tumor cells in circulation are still largely in the experimental stages. The cancer cells must first be separated from the normal blood cells in circulation, which outnumber the cancer cells by many orders of magnitude. This can be accomplished by techniques such as flow cytometry or magnetic separation after the cells have been immunologically labeled with molecules that bind to epithelium- or cancer-specific markers on the surfaces of the cells. Once the cells have been isolated, they can be further characterized by the tests described above to measure genetic changes or gene expression.

Because these methods are being developed primarily for use for the monitoring of treatment response and disease progression, it is unclear whether they will ever be sensitive enough for use for "early detection" or how they might be used for screening or early diagnosis and prognosis. In any case, serum markers are unlikely to replace imaging technologies for the diagnosis of breast cancer because current therapy for early disease requires localization of the primary lesion in the breast, which generally depends on breast images.

## OBSTACLES TO BE OVERCOME IN DEVELOPMENT OF BIOLOGICAL DETECTION METHODS

In addition to technology needs, a number of infrastructure needs and other impediments to progress in the development of biomarkers for breast cancer detection have been identified. For example, samples from relatively large tumors obtained by biopsy have traditionally been the specimens most widely available to researchers, but this has limited the study of smaller, earlier lesions. Recently, more effort has been devoted to the development of specimen banks with samples from the entire continuum of malignant and premalignant lesions of the breast, but the small sizes of these lesions make it difficult to share samples for multiple investigations. Attempts have also been made to examine samples obtained by core-needle biopsy or even fine-needle aspirates, but in most cases the technologies are not yet sensitive enough for accurate assessment of these small samples. Because of their small size, materials obtained by needle biopsy are also less likely to be made available to researchers through established tissue banks.

Once the tissues have been collected, other impediments to research can arise. For example, concerns have been raised about informed consent and patient confidentiality (Anderson, 1994; National Bioethics Advisory Commission, 1999). A common approach to obtaining consent is to use a very general consent form that will allow future, unspecified research to be conducted without the need to reacquire consent for every subsequent study. As with all research with human subjects and materials, institutional review boards can then approve or reject specific study designs as they are proposed, but this may lead to variability in the types of studies approved at different institutions. Confidentiality, always a concern in health care and biomedical research with human subjects, could be especially problematic with regard to studies of hereditary genetics (Daly et al., 2000). As a result, NCI has proposed methods for protecting the identities of tissue donors while still maintaining links to data on clinical outcome.[7]

Other organizational challenges also must be overcome to establish and maintain useful specimen banks (Burke and Henson, 1998; Grizzle et al., 1998). Effective use of patient samples depends critically on the ability of the specimen bank to acquire, organize, and disseminate samples and associated information in a timely manner and to standardize sample collection and reporting across different institutions. These activities require substantial monetary support and staff resources, which are often not available at adequate levels . A new high-throughput method know as "tissue microarray" (Kononen et al., 1998)[8] may offer one potential means by which the organization, dissemination, and analysis of tissue specimens could be streamlined and automated, but such an approach would certainly require a broad and general consent form for sample collection.

A recent report by NCI's Breast Cancer Progress Review Group (BC-PRG) concluded that NCI study sections have historically given tissue banking efforts and the associated correlative clinical studies such low priority that they have been unfundable (Breast Cancer Progress Review Group, 1998). The charge to the BC-PRG was to identify and prioritize scientific needs and opportunities critical for progress against the disease and to compare these priorities with the current portfolio of the NCI research program. The group recommended that NCI increase funding support for tissue banks through mechanisms separate from the traditional grants to principal investigators.

Recently, concerns over intellectual property issues associated with

---

[7]http://www.nci.nih.gov/confidentiality.html.

[8]By this method, small cylinders of tissue are punched from 1,000 individual tumor biopsy specimens embedded in paraffin. These cylinders are then arrayed in a large paraffin block, from which 200 consecutive tissue sections can be cut, allowing multiple, rapid analysis of the arrayed samples by immunohistochemistry or in situ hybridization.

biomedical research tools and resources have also been raised. Although some specimen banks freely share samples with investigators, some institutions are beginning to demand a share of any profits derived from technologies that may be developed as a result of research conducted with samples derived from their banks. NCI could potentially alleviate such impediments by requiring specimen banks supported with NCI funding to forego intellectual property right claims to technologies derived from research with their archived samples. There is already precedent for such restrictions. For example, investigators funded through CGAP are required to rapidly add their data to publicly accessible databases and must therefore relinquish any patent rights to their discoveries.

Concerns about funding and intellectual property rights have also been raised in regard to high-throughput technologies. The BC-PRG concluded that the academic research community has inadequate funds to purchase and operate the new high-throughput technologies that are likely to advance the field and recommended increased funding for this purpose, perhaps through shared core facilities. However, patents on gene sequences may keep the price of DNA arrays and related technologies out of reach for many researchers. Some companies may also be limiting the research community's access to new high-throughput technologies through control of the intellectual property rights to future products based on discoveries made with the new technologies.

Another obstacle to be overcome stems from the need for new bioinformatics approaches to make sense of all the data that are being generated by these high-throughput technologies. The field of bioinformatics is relatively new, and thus, the recently developed training programs have not kept pace with the demand for individuals with the necessary experience to tackle these issues. Given the enormous number of genetic and epigenetic changes already identified and the vast heterogeneity within and among breast tumors, this may indeed be the greatest challenge of all.

## SUMMARY

To substantially reduce morbidity and mortality from breast cancer, basic and clinical research must lead to improvements in the understanding of breast tumor biology and etiology as well as improvements in the ability to detect early lesions. To optimize advances made in detection and diagnostic technologies, knowledge about the biology of the lesions detected should ideally play a role in the decision-making process that occurs after detection. In particular, research on the biology of premalignant disease and early breast cancer is crucial for understanding and predicting the progression of breast lesions and for the development of more targeted and effective treatments for those lesions that are likely to become lethal. Such knowledge would also allow women with clinically insignificant lesions to forego unnecessary treatments and the associated side effects.

Identification of meaningful biomarkers of breast cancer could significantly advance the field of functional imaging (as discussed in Chapter 2) and thus lead to improved methods of screening and diagnosis. Better understanding of the genetics and biology of breast cancer can also be expected to open new avenues in the future for assessing the risk of developing cancer as well as aiding in treatment planning once a tumor has been detected. Some of the developing technologies described in this chapter, such as the identification and assessment of biomarkers in serum or breast fluids and tissues, offer promise as screening procedures but will require further study and development before their use as screening modalities can be evaluated. In many instances these technologies could potentially identify fundamental changes in the breast that appear before a lesion can be identified. Thus, they may identify women at high risk of developing breast cancer (or, more importantly, women at high risk of dying from breast cancer). Increased efforts in these areas should also be a priority.

Some of the obstacles to attaining these goals include lack of funding for and accessibility to the resources and tools necessary to move this field forward. For example, much research has focused on late-stage breast cancer due to the predominance of these tissues in the specimen banks and cell line repositories. Thus, the study of early breast cancer has lagged. Furthermore, funding for the establishment and maintenance of specimen banks has traditionally not been a high priority.

NCI has launched several new funding initiatives in the last year aimed at increasing the understanding of breast cancer initiation and progression, in part as a result of its external progress review process. Clearly, much work remains to be done in the field of breast cancer biology. Making sense of the many molecular changes in breast tumors will be extremely challenging, but the end result could potentially have an enormous impact on reducing the burden of breast cancer.

# 4
# Development and Regulation of New Technologies

## DEVELOPMENT: THE PROCESS FOR SELECTING AREAS OF INVESTIGATION FOR CANCER DETECTION

Over the last decade, the activity and investment in research aimed at developing new technologies for early breast cancer detection have increased substantially, in part because of the efforts of advocacy groups and attention given by the U.S. Congress. At the same time, biomedical research has become more complex and capital intensive, requiring enormous investments to develop technologies and to generate and analyze data. Traditionally, basic research and the early stages of medical technology development were the realm of government-funded projects at universities or the National Institutes of Health, whereas private companies were primarily involved in bringing technologies to the market and the clinic. Although that may still be true in some instances, the lines between the various funders and developers of new technologies have blurred, and many new participants have also recently joined the process (see Table 1-1). As in many high-technology industries, the expanding development costs for new technologies and the growing importance of regulatory issues have provided powerful motives for public-private collaboration (National Research Council, 1999).

Many of the decisions about whether to pursue the development of novel and innovative technologies hinge on the perceived balance of opportunity and risk. Opportunity is determined by a combination of technological advances and the presence of an unmet need or interest in the market. Risks include considerations of the time and resources needed to develop technologies when the end results of the research and the profitability of the product are uncertain. In the case of medical technologies in particular, a large part of that uncertainty may be due to the additional processes required for Food and Drug Administration (FDA) approval (covered in this chapter) and adoption by the purchasers, providers, and users of medical care (covered in Chapters 5 and 6). A relative lack of patent protection can further diminish financial incentives and increase the risk for developing new technologies. New medical devices usually have some patent protection, but effective market exclusivity for devices is often shorter than the life of the patent because competitors can "invent around" device patents more easily than around new molecular entities like drugs (Medical Technology Leadership Forum, 1999). On the other hand, the relative lack of effective patent protection for devices provides incentives for other companies to invest in improving technologies already on the market. In fact, the original innovating company is rarely the sole or even the dominant source of further improvements.

## NEW INITIATIVES AND COLLABORATIONS IN MEDICAL IMAGING RESEARCH

The limitations of mammography have been a driving force behind the search for new technologies that can detect breast cancer, eliminate unnecessary biopsies, and provide information that can be used to guide therapeutic decisions. Because of the multidisciplinary nature of technologies for breast cancer detection and diagnosis, a number of collaborative efforts have recently been established or explored (see Table 1-1).

In the spring of 1993, the National Cancer Institute (NCI) held a conference to explore the transfer of novel imaging technologies from the defense, intelligence, space, and energy communities for the purpose of breast cancer detection. The primary focus of that conference was technology transfer specifically for digital mammography and computer-aided detection (CAD). The following year, the U.S. Public Health Service's Office on Women's Health (OWH), along with the Central Intelligence Agency (CIA), NCI, FDA, and other federal agencies, established a working relationship with leaders of the medical imaging community to adapt defense technologies used for missile and target recognition to breast cancer detection. One example of such collaborations was between the University of Chicago and the National Information Display Laboratory, which led to advances in CAD technologies and played a major role in developing the current commercially available CAD software from R2 Technologies, Inc.

Productive interactions such as these led to further interest in applying new technologies to other imaging modalities, such as magnetic resonance imaging (MRI), ultrasound, and nuclear medicine. In the spring of

1996, the Federal Multi-Agency Consortium to Improve Women's Health was established to formalize collaborations between the medical establishment and the nation's defense, intelligence, space, and energy communities. This new consortium included NCI, OWH, FDA, CIA, the National Science Foundation, the National Aeronautics and Space Administration, the U.S. Departments of Defense, Energy, and Commerce, and the Health Care Financing Administration. The initial goal of the consortium was to catalog the state of the art for breast imaging modalities and to identify the scientific and technological needs for application of the technologies to breast cancer detection, diagnosis, and treatment. These needs were then translated into a problem statement[1] of technical specifications that could be understood by engineers, physicists, and other scientists working on imaging technologies. Since its inception, several national public workshops have been held to facilitate technology transfer and to stimulate public-private partnerships for technology development and application to breast cancer (Final Report, 1998).

Similar initiatives that focus more generally on biomedical imaging in oncology have also been launched recently. The first NCI-industry forum and workshop on this topic was held in September 1999[2] following discussions between NCI and the National Electrical Manufacturers' Association (NEMA).[3] The forum had four main objectives: (1) to bring together individuals involved in funding, research, regulation, and reimbursement of imaging technologies; (2) to expand the role of anatomic and functional-molecular imaging in oncology; (3) to develop strategies for application of technical advances in imaging to unmet clinical needs in cancer; and (4) to better understand the processes related to development, adoption, approval, and dissemination of imaging technologies in oncology. A second workshop to continue the dialogue was held in September 2000.[4]

The first large-scale collaborative clinical trials group devoted to the

---

[1]http://www.4woman.gov/owh/bcimage/frames2.htm. Statements were prepared for digital X-ray mammography, MRI, ultrasound imaging, positron emission tomography, and nuclear medicine, computer-aided diagnosis, three-dimensional interactive visualization, and image storage and transmission. The problem statement for each technology describes the current state-of-the art as well as the technological needs and roadblocks to assist researchers unfamiliar with breast imaging in assessing the potential for their own technology, capability, or expertise to help address the stated needs.

[2]For a meeting summary, see http://dino.nci.nih.gov/dctd/forum/summary.htm.

[3]NEMA is a trade organization for more than 600 companies, including 60 that produce diagnostic medical equipment.

[4]For a summary, see http://dino.nci.nih.gov/dctd/forum/summary00.htm.

development of technologies for medical imaging and the conduct of clinical trials to assess them was also launched in 1999. The American College of Radiology Imaging Network (ACRIN)[5] has more than $22 million in funding from NCI for a 5-year period. ACRIN's fundamental objectives are to assess the value of emerging and established medical imaging tools by evaluating their effects on patient outcomes and costs, to increase participation in clinical trials, and to train researchers in conducting clinical trials.

The new multi-institutional consortium is structured to work with other NCI consortia, industry, and insurers. ACRIN has a more "virtual" organization compared with those for other multi-institutional study groups, with participating institutions at many distant sites contributing to an electronic database. The trial infrastructure integrates funding, methodological support, data acquisition and management, informatics, regulatory assistance, quality control, financial management, analysis, and research dissemination. All ACRIN clinical trials must be reviewed and approved by NCI's Cancer Therapy Evaluation Program.

ACRIN's recently approved screening mammography trial will compare full-field digital mammography with conventional mammography. The trial is about to begin, but investigators hope to accrue nearly 50,000 asymptomatic women at approximately 20 sites across the United States for screening mammography with digital machines from four manufacturers (Trex, Fischer, Fuji, and General Electric). The study participants will not be randomized, and all women will undergo both conventional and digital mammography. Two readers will examine the images independently, and decisions for diagnostic workup will be based on the results of both examinations. As designed, the study should have adequate statistical power to determine whether unnecessary recalls for follow-up tests can be reduced by use of digital mammography. The major outcomes measures will include the sensitivity, specificity, positive predictive value, and negative predictive value of digital mammography. Secondary goals are to compare the accuracy of mammography using "soft-copy" image display to that of laser-printed films and to examine the effect of breast density on accuracy. The study is expected to be completed by 2004.

Several initiatives and collaborations aimed at characterizing the molecular biology of cancer and identifying tumor markers have also been launched recently, as described in more detail in Chapter 3. A prime example is the Cancer Genome Anatomy Project of NCI, whose goal is to develop a comprehensive molecular characterization of normal, precancerous, and malignant cells. NCI also recently announced a novel pro-

---

[5]www.acrin.org.

gram that will study the stages of breast development, from normal development of the mammary gland to the metastatic changes of breast cancer.[6] This program encourages multidisciplinary collaborations among such specialists as cell and molecular biologists, bioengineers, geneticists, and pathologists.

## EXAMPLES OF FUNDING MECHANISMS FOR MEDICAL TECHNOLOGY DEVELOPMENT

### National Cancer Institute

Historically, NCI has conducted and funded basic, applied, and clinical and health services research to acquire new knowledge that can be used to prevent, diagnose, and treat cancer (Tables 4-1 and 4-2). Recently, NCI has also developed programs to make its peer review system, which has traditionally been based on hypothesis-driven science, more accessible for technology development. Two years ago, NCI established the Office of Technology and Industrial Relations, with the goal of facilitating expedited technology development and transfer activities. The office oversees the Small Business Innovative Research (SBIR) awards and the Small Business Technology Transfer Research (STTR) grants. The SBIR and STTR programs are designed to support innovative research that has the potential for commercialization. In the case of SBIR awards, the research is conducted solely by small businesses, whereas STTR grants support research conducted cooperatively by a small business concern and a research institution. For the latter, the small business must carry out at least 40 percent of the research project and the partner research institution must perform at least 30 percent of the work.

Support under the SBIR-STTR programs normally includes $100,000 for 6 months for Phase I (proof of concept) and $750,000 for 2 years for Phase II (development). However, the Phased Innovation Award is a new mechanism directed at supporting research on new technologies, from the evolution of the innovative concept to the research development phase. Compared with the traditional two-step grant application process, which can be cumbersome, the Phased Innovation Award allows a single grant application for two previously distinct awards. The new award permits flexible research programs for up to 4 years. To move into the development phase, investigators must achieve measurable milestones.

Areas of focus include cancer imaging and definition of the molecular changes, or signatures, of tumors. A particular focus has been placed on technologies that will permit multiple levels of analysis: in vitro (test

---

[6]http://grants.nih.gov/grants/guide/pa-files/PA-99-162.html.

**TABLE 4-1** National Cancer Institute Extramural Funding for Breast Cancer-Related Research, Fiscal Years 1990 to 1999 (in whole dollars)

| Fiscal Year | Breast Cancer Research[a] | | | Breast Cancer Detection[b] | | |
|---|---|---|---|---|---|---|
| | Grants | Contracts | Total Extramural | Grants | Contracts | Total Extramural |
| 1999 | 325,496,000 | 11,477,000 | 336,973,000 | 58,520,698 | 1,571,010 | 60,091,708 |
| 1998 | 289,621,000 | 10,738,000 | 300,359,000 | 52,642,462 | 636,025 | 53,278,487 |
| 1997 | 269,742,000 | 17,721,000 | 287,463,000 | 51,297,401 | 1,999,580 | 53,296,981 |
| 1996 | 226,720,000 | 5,212,000 | 231,932,000 | 45,967,762 | 4,192,250 | 50,160,012 |
| 1995 | 183,684,000 | 10,293,000 | 193,977,000 | 46,638,799 | 1,583,246 | 48,222,045 |
| 1994 | 171,706,000 | 20,798,000 | 192,504,000 | 40,312,325 | 757,661 | 41,069,986 |
| 1993 | 143,671,000 | 17,836,000 | 161,507,000 | 33,189,587 | 1,704,912 | 34,894,499 |
| 1992 | | | | 19,872,037 | 2,687,428 | 22,559,465 |
| 1991 | | | | 17,063,894 | 1,119,392 | 18,183,286 |
| 1990 | | | | 14,486,403 | 1,928,983 | 16,415,386 |

[a]Includes the three categories indicated, as well as training and basic research and other scientific areas.

[b]Any project involving actual detection of breast tumors (screening, diagnosis, clinical trials), development or refinement of diagnostic techniques or devices, education, or promotion of breast cancer detection.

[c]Anything designed to inhibit the onset of breast cancer, such as drug administration or

tube), in situ (cellular), and in vivo (the whole body). NCI is also developing programs that aim to bring the field of molecular biology together with the imaging community, with the goal of identifying the fundamental molecular changes in tumors. Several program announcements address this area, including developmental grants for diagnostic cancer imaging and the study of novel imaging modalities. NCI has also promoted the study of new imaging agents and probes, especially those that have the potential to better pinpoint the molecular signatures of tumors.

To further spur development of innovative and high-risk technological improvements in cancer detection and treatment, the Office of Technology and Industrial Relations has also developed a nontraditional,

| Breast Cancer Prevention[c] | | | Breast Cancer Treatment | | |
| --- | --- | --- | --- | --- | --- |
| Grants | Contracts | Total Extramural | Grants | Contracts | Total Extramural |
| 27,867,000 | 2,461,799 | 30,328,799 | 85,705,732 | 1,965,658 | 87,671,390 |
| 27,363,273 | 4,701,252 | 32,064,525 | 67,498,736 | 982,960 | 68,481,696 |
| 30,413,527 | 143,282 | 30,556,809 | 77,072,791 | 336,089 | 77,408,880 |
| 20,366,677 | 2,164,405 | 22,531,082 | 77,504,241 | 1,214,610 | 78,718,851 |
| 18,883,694 | 1,556,852 | 20,440,546 | 69,572,849 | 1,887,207 | 71,460,056 |
| 16,039,590 | 3,281,600 | 19,321,190 | 58,987,022 | 4,219,795 | 63,206,817 |
| 20,175,725 | 2,318,649 | 22,494,374 | 53,190,603 | 5,801,301 | 58,991,904 |
| 18,891,894 | 3,822,326 | 22,714,220 | 40,935,757 | 653,008 | 41,588,765 |
| 10,739,031 | 2,582,304 | 13,321,335 | 24,426,247 | 724,750 | 25,150,997 |
| 9,756,434 | 1,398,349 | 11,154,783 | 24,874,428 | 1,853,666 | 26,728,094 |

lifestyle changes.

SOURCES: NCI. Anna Levy, NCI Office of Women's Health; Marilyn Gaston, NCI Inquiry and Reporting Section; Rosemary Cuddy, NCI Division of Extramural Activities.

multidisciplinary program through a new program, the Unconventional Innovations Program.[7] In addition to recruiting new investigators and building multidisciplinary teams, the program is actively engaged in translating technology into other nontraditional domains. The program is modeled after the Defense Advanced Research Projects Agency and emphasizes technology maturation and dissemination.

This program solicits contracts for the development of novel technologies for noninvasive detection, diagnosis, and treatment of cancer.

---

[7]http://www.nih.gov/news/pr/oct98/nci-06a.htm.

**TABLE 4-2** National Cancer Institute Extramural Funding for Breast Cancer Detection Research (Imaging versus Nonimaging), Fiscal Years 1990 to 1999 (in whole dollars)

| Fiscal Year | Imaging | | | Nonimaging | | |
| --- | --- | --- | --- | --- | --- | --- |
| | Grants | Contracts | Total | Grants | Contracts | Total |
| 1999 | 38,099,604 | 916,001 | 39,015,605 | 20,421,094 | 655,009 | 21,076,103 |
| 1998 | 37,587,304 | 93,716 | 37,681,020 | 15,055,158 | 542,309 | 15,597,467 |
| 1997 | 38,884,336 | 1,999,580 | 40,883,916 | 12,413,065 | 0 | 12,413,065 |
| 1996 | 37,993,657 | 2,363,847 | 40,357,504 | 7,974,105 | 1,828,403 | 9,802,508 |
| 1995 | 37,179,948 | 1,566,752 | 38,746,700 | 9,458,851 | 16,494 | 9,475,345 |
| 1994 | 31,135,248 | 590,009 | 31,725,257 | 9,177,077 | 167,652 | 9,344,729 |
| 1993 | 24,500,571 | 1,604,231 | 26,104,802 | 8,689,016 | 100,681 | 8,789,697 |
| 1992 | 16,770,171 | 1,974,525 | 18,744,696 | 3,101,866 | 712,903 | 3,814,769 |
| 1991 | 13,138,486 | 933,272 | 14,071,758 | 3,935,408 | 186,120 | 4,121,528 |

SOURCES: NCI. Anna Levy, NCI Office of Women's Health; Marilyn Gaston, NCI Inquiry and Reporting Section; Rosemary Cuddy, NCI Division of Extramural Activities.

According to the most recent solicitation announcement,[8] the program is "specifically soliciting projects to develop technology systems or systems components that will enable the sensing of defined signatures of different cancerous and precancerous cell types or their associated microenvironment in the body in a way that is highly sensitive and specific, yet non-invasive." The highest priority is for systems that can "either support or provide a seamless interface between sensing/detection and intervention." The stated goal of the program is to "develop technology that will target quantum improvements in existing technologies or entirely novel approaches, rather than incremental improvements to state of the art." The first five awards totaling $11.3 million were issued in 1999 (Table 4-3). Within the next 5 years NCI plans to invest $48 million through this program.

Because of the tremendous need for information systems development in the area of high-throughput biological analysis, NCI is also actively building the Biomedical Information Science and Technology Implementation Consortium (BISTIC)[9] to promote database creation and management that will permit modeling, manipulation, and hypothesis generation. Key components of the strategy include supporting planning grants in national centers of excellence, furthering investigator-initiated research, bolstering the Information Storage, Curation, Analysis, and Retrieval program, coordinating work across the National Institutes of Health (NIH), and building a computing infrastructure. Initially, investments will focus on traditional, low-risk, evolutionary projects, but BISTIC will move toward long-term, higher-risk investments. NCI is also supporting the development of modeling tools to facilitate the identification of new targets for detection and intervention.

In the spring of 2000, NIH combined BISTIC with the Bioengineering Consortium to create the Office of Bioengineering, Bioimaging, and Bioinformatics (OBBB) (Haley, 2000). Recently, legislation required NIH to establish a new institute, the Institute for Biomedical Imaging and Bioengineering.[10] This legislative action has effectively terminated OBBB, which would have operated in conjunction with the current disease-oriented institutions by providing a coordinating infrastructure for bio-imaging and bioengineering initiatives. OBBB did not have grant-making authority or funds itself, in contrast to the new institute, which will have such authority (Softcheck, 2001). However, the field of bioinformatics was not included in the scope and mission of the new institute.

---

[8] http://Amb.nci.nih.gov/UIP.HTM.

[9] http://grants.nih.gov/grants/bistic/bistic2_t.htm.

[10] A bill to create the new NIH Institute for Biomedical Imaging and Bioengineering, H.R. 1795, was signed into law on December 29, 2000, by President Bill Clinton (Haley, 2000).

**TABLE 4-3** NCI 1999 Unconventional Innovations Program Awards

| Summary of 1999 Projects for Noninvasive Detection, Diagnosis, and Treatment of Cancer | Amount Awarded |
|---|---|
| 1. The project will focus on the development of two specific devices, based on current polymer technology, for detection and treatment of cancer; one will be useful for detection of adenocarcinoma of the breast, whereas the other will be used for detection of adenocarcinoma of the colon. | $4.4 million |
| 2. The project will develop a novel optical technique using near infrared for identification of precancer and early cancers. Among other things, it is expected that the end product of the technology will yield a noninvasive (nonintrusive) method of detection for small human breast cancers. | $2 million |
| 3. The project targets the development of a novel system capable of selective transduction (a potential avenue of gene therapy) of target cells in the context of the clinical settings for posttreatment recurrent neoplastic disease and metastatic disease and early subclinical or undetected preneoplastic disease. | $1.8 million |
| 4. The aim of the project is to construct and demonstrate a prototype compact device that may be used in a variety of biomedical applications including in vitro and in vivo spectroscopy and high-resolution imaging, mammography, diagnosis, and radiation therapy. | $1.6 million |
| 5. This project will develop novel carbon nanotube-based biosensor technology and develop a prototype biosensor catheter, suitable for in vitro use, that permits detection of specific oligonucleotide sequences that serve as molecular signatures of cancer cells. | $1.5 million |

SOURCES: http://otir.nci.nih.gov/tech/vip_awards.html, and Richard Hartman, contracting director, NCI, personal communication (July, 2000).

## U.S. Department of Defense

The U.S. Department of Defense (DOD) is the second largest administrator of federally funded breast cancer research in the United States. In addition to managing biomedical research programs that are part of the Army and DOD budget submission, the U.S. Army Medical Research and Materiel Command (USAMRMC) can be directed by the U.S. Congress to undertake special-interest biomedical research programs. One of the congressional research programs managed by USAMRMC is the Breast Cancer Research Program (BCRP), established[11] in 1992 with $25 million ap-

---

[11]BCRP was established by Joint Appropriations Bill 102-328.

propriated for research on breast cancer screening and diagnosis for military personnel and their dependents. In response to requests from breast cancer advocacy groups (Marshall, 1993), the 1993 Defense Appropriations Act provided $210 million for a "peer-reviewed breast cancer research program with the Department of the Army as the executive agent." Appropriations for fiscal years 1992 through 2000 total $1.043 billion. In 1995, $20 million (of the total $150 million appropriation) was earmarked for research in mammography and breast imaging with the goal of applying military technology to mammography to improve its accuracy.

The objective of BCRP is to fund the training of new scientists in the field, infrastructure enhancement, and investigator-initiated research with a balanced portfolio of research on the prevention, detection, diagnosis, and treatment of breast cancer (Table 4-4). Since its inception, the program has funded research at U.S. and international universities, hospitals, nonprofit and for-profit institutions, private industry, and state and federal agencies. BCRP has developed a funding strategy (Institute of Medicine, 1993, 1997) with the goal of complementing awards made by other agencies and has specifically tried to avoid duplication of long-term basic research supported by NIH. Research awards have been made by a two-tiered review process that includes consumer advocates. Peer review panels assess the scientific merit of research proposals, whereas the programmatic reviews determine the contribution of projects to the program goals. BCRP was the first program to use this format for review of grant applications, and since its adoption, NCI has also become more open to the participation of consumer advocates.

BCRP has also initiated new approaches to grant applications through two new awards: the Idea Award and the Concept Award. The intent of the Concept Award is to provide initial funding for a novel concept or theory that could give rise to a testable hypothesis. The one-page Concept Award proposals go through a fast-track submission and review process. Preliminary data are not required, and the award provides $50,000 for 1 year. The Idea Award also does not require preliminary data and is designed to foster innovative ideas and technologies that 'challenge the existing paradigms'. The average grant in this category provides $100,000 per year for up to 3 years.

### Advanced Technology Program, National Institute of Standards and Technology

The National Institute of Standards and Technology (NIST) is an agency of the U.S. Department of Commerce's Technology Administration. NIST works with industry to develop and apply technology, mea-

**TABLE 4-4**　Breakdown of BCRP Funding for Three Categories

| Year | Congressional Appropriation[a] | Prevention | | Early Detection, Prognosis |
| | | No. of Awards | Dollars | No. of Awards |
|---|---|---|---|---|
| 1992-1994 | $235.0 | 10 | $2,654,443 | 97 |
| 1995 | $150.0 | 8 | $2,711,964 | 77 |
| 1996 | $75.0 | 7 | $1,519,845 | 58 |
| 1997 | $108.3 | 9 | $2,678,355 | 69 |
| 1998 | $135.0 | 21 | $7,075,114 | 106 |
| Total | $703.3 | 55 | $16,639,721 | 407 |

NOTE: If both the first and second choices of category for a grant were in the same main category, the funding was counted only once; if the codes were in two different categories, the full amount was counted in both categories.

[a]In millions of dollars.

surements, and standards. It carries out this mission through four major programs, including the Advanced Technology Program (ATP).[12]

The goal of ATP is to stimulate innovation by bridging the gap between the research laboratory and the marketplace. Through partnerships with the private sector, ATP's early stage investments aim to accelerate the development of novel technologies that promise significant and widespread benefits for the nation, in addition to a direct return to the innovators. By sharing the relatively high risks of developing new technologies, ATP can foster projects with greater technical challenges that companies could not or would not take on by themselves.

The ATP has several critical features that set it apart from other government research and development programs:

- Projects focus on the technology needs of U.S. industry, not those of the U.S. government.
- Research priorities are set by industry on the basis of their understanding of the marketplace and research opportunities.
- For-profit companies conceive, propose, cofund, and execute projects and programs in partnerships with academia, independent research organizations, and federal laboratories.
- Strict cost-sharing rules are in place.[13]

---

[12]http://www.atp.nist.gov/atp/overview.htm.

[13]Joint ventures (two or more companies working together) must pay at least half of the total project costs. Large, Fortune 500 companies participating as a single firm must pay at

| Diagnosis, and Dollars | Treatment No. of Awards | Dollars | Total No. of Awards |
|---|---|---|---|
| $52,666,720 | 50 | $26,520,447 | 157 |
| $25,981,647 | 44 | $19,900,740 | 129 |
| $11,034,618 | 61 | $13,759,763 | 126 |
| $22,305,064 | 79 | $29,906,133 | 157 |
| $22,962,976 | 88 | $25,774,586 | 215 |
| $134,951,025 | 322 | $115,861,669 | 784 |

SOURCE: Office of Congressionally Directed Medical Research Programs, Medical Research and Material Command (Stacey Young-McCaughan, Deputy Director).

- ATP does not fund product development. Private industry bears the costs of product development, production, marketing, sales, and distribution.
- Awards are made strictly on the basis of rigorous peer-reviewed competitions. Selection is based on the innovation, the technical risk, the potential economic benefits to the nation, and the strength of the commercialization plan for the project.
- Support does not become a perpetual subsidy or entitlement. For each project goals, specific funding allocations, and completion dates are established at the outset. Projects are monitored and can be terminated for cause before completion.

ATP has funded companies of all sizes, many of which were involved in partnerships with universities and nonprofit organizations. To date, more than half of the ATP awards have gone to individual small businesses or to joint ventures led by a small business. Well over half of the ATP projects to date also include one or more universities as either subcontractors or members of a joint venture. ATP awards are selected through open, peer-reviewed competitions. All industries and all fields of science and technology are eligible. Proposals are evaluated by technology-specific boards that are staffed with experts in fields such as

least 60 percent of the total project costs. Small and medium-sized companies working on single-firm ATP projects must pay a minimum of all indirect costs associated with the project.

biotechnology, photonics, chemistry, manufacturing, information technology, and materials.

ATP has funded several projects that may have a potential effect on breast cancer. Some of these have focused on increasing the efficiency and imaging capabilities of technologies such as X ray, MRI, ultrasound, and other imaging devices while lowering their costs. As one example, ATP awarded $6 million over 4 years to Xerox, in conjunction with Thermotrex Corp., for a proposal to improve the resolution and accuracy of a digital imaging system. ATP has also heavily funded genomic and biotechnology research projects that may have an effect on breast cancer screening, diagnosis, and treatment. For example, ATP awarded Affymetrix and Molecular Dynamics $31 million to develop a 'miniature nucleic acid diagnostic device', which consists of DNA arrays on silicon chips, with the goal of providing a rapid and accurate means of diagnosis of a wide variety of diseases, including breast cancer.

## PRIVATE INVESTMENT

The large, established medical imaging companies devote significant resources to research and development aimed at improving imaging technologies that are already in use and that have broad applications, such as MRI, ultrasound, and X-ray modalities. However, small start-up companies often initially pursue novel technologies, especially those that involve higher risk and potential benefits. About 80 percent of medical device companies are start-ups with less than 50 employees and thus have limited resources at their disposal to generate data and evidence for approval. The devices may cost thousands of dollars each, making distribution of devices for the purpose of conducting clinical trials very expensive. As a result, the timing of some trials may be delayed and the protocols may be restricted. Data collection may also be curtailed by limited patient follow-up or the number of end points assessed (Medical Technology Leadership Forum, 1999).

Investment of venture capital is one way of providing nongovernment start-up monies for the development of new medical technologies. Typically, venture capital firms raise capital, make investments in a small start-up company, and then sell the assets when the product goes into the market. Venture capitalists generally look for a proprietary product with a large market, clearly identified customers, and minimal impediments to adoption and diffusion. In other words, when the perception of risk is low and the returns are expected to be high, investment is more probable.

Traditionally, a venture capitalist's investment timeline was 4 to 10 years. The investment portion of the cycle took about 5 years, with another 3 or 4 years needed to harvest the assets. The expectations for that cycle have changed radically in the last 2 years, largely because of the

Internet, which has spurred enormous investments and exceptional rates of return. On average, it takes an Internet-related business less than 2 years to go public, whereas previously the norm was 3 to 5 years. Because initial public offerings happen much more quickly with Internet-related businesses, investors' money is not locked up as long as it is in traditional investments. In addition, venture capital investors have been earning returns in excess of 100 percent on their Internet-related investments (PricewaterhouseCoopers, 2000). Although these recent trends may not continue in the future, the global economic environment is driving technology research in the private sector. The pace of technological change in general is faster than ever before, compelling companies to make narrower, shorter-term investments in research and development that maximize returns quickly.

These recent investment trends have not been favorable to the health care industry, which typically has a longer investment cycle and more modest returns. Although actual venture capital investments in health care-related companies were at an all-time high in 1999 (Figure 4-1), this increase was largely driven by health care-related Internet endeavors. During the last quarter of 1999, 68 percent of the venture capital cash invested in health care-related companies was devoted to such "e-health" stocks. In 2000, more than 50 percent of venture capital money in health

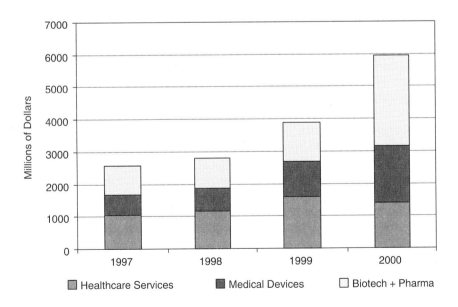

**FIGURE 4-1** Venture capital investments in health care industries, 1997 to 2000. SOURCE: PricewaterhouseCoopers Money Tree™ Survey.

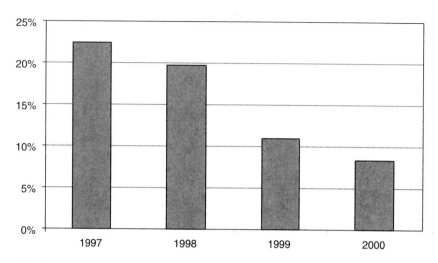

FIGURE 4-2   Health-care related industry investments (includes health-care services, biotechnology, pharmaceuticals, and medical devices) as a percentage of
total venture capital investments, 1997 to 2000. Source: PricewaterhouseCoopers
Money Tree™ Survey.

care was still going to internet-related ventures. Furthermore, the percentage of total venture capital investment going into health care has
plunged from about 25 percent traditionally to about 8 percent by the end
of 2000 (Figure 4-2). Only 2.5 percent of all 2000 venture capital investments was devoted to medical device companies (Figure 4-3).[14]

Venture capital firms may view investment in the diagnostic and
device areas of the health care sector as a high-risk proposition because of
the length of time required to produce data for FDA approval and insurance coverage decisions and because of the uncertainty associated with
those decisions. Unfavorable reimbursement levels and slow adoption
rates for new technologies can add further complications. Technologies
that improve on existing screening and diagnostic modalities may be
viewed as particularly risky with regard to the latter because competition
in the marketplace may lead to inadequate returns on investment.

In 1999, estimated U.S. expenditures on diagnostic imaging and
therapy systems were approximately $5 billion dollars, whereas those for

[14]Data were obtained from PricewaterhouseCoopers Money Tree™ Survey for 1999. The
survey measures venture capital equity investments in the United States on a regional and a
national basis and serves as a barometer of economic health through entrepreneurial developments.

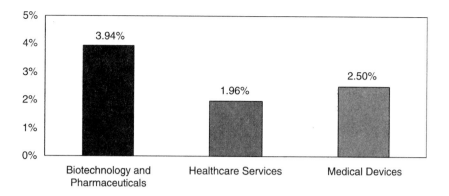

**FIGURE 4-3** Percentage of total venture capital investments in specific health-care industries, 2000. SOURCE: PricewaterhouseCoopers Money Tree™ Survey.

drugs were $120 billion[15] (Table 4-5). Ultrasound and X-ray equipment accounted for about 20 and 30 percent of the total, respectively. However, within each of those categories only a small fraction entails breast imaging equipment (the United States has approximately 10,000 certified breast imaging centers[16]). Because it can cost technology sponsors many millions of dollars to bring a new technology to market, the opportunity for a sizeable return on investment is thus relatively small.

## FDA APPROVAL: PROCESS FOR GETTING NEW TECHNOLOGIES INTO THE CLINIC

FDA is charged with regulating the "safety and effectiveness" of all medical products sold within the United States. Hence, FDA has jurisdiction over all drugs, devices, and biologics, but its approach varies for each category. To understand the specific issues of FDA approval of technologies for breast cancer screening and diagnosis, it is necessary to first look at the general processes used by FDA. Technologies for the early detection of breast cancer will most likely involve either imaging devices or clinical laboratory devices, so the general description of FDA procedures provided here will focus briefly on these categories, which are overseen by the Center for Devices and Radiological Health of FDA.[17]

---

[15]Total retail prescription drug sales in 1999 were $121.7 billion (http://www.nacds.org/ ; accessed December 15, 2000).

[16]See http://www.fda.gov/cdrh/mammography/mqsa_accomplishments.html

[17]www.FDA.gov/cdrh/. Some imaging techniques, such as scintimammography, may require review by FDA's Center for Drug Evaluation and Research because they make use of radionuclide agents.

**TABLE 4-5** Domestic Shipments of Select Product Groups Within the Scope of NEMA's Diagnostic Imaging and Therapy Systems Division (in millions of dollars)

| Sales Billed | 1991 | 1992 | 1993 | 1994 | 1995 | 1996 | 1997 | 1998[a] | 1999[a] |
|---|---|---|---|---|---|---|---|---|---|
| Computed tomography | 453 | 477 | 453 | 372 | 396 | 525 | 543 | 594 | 663 |
| MRI | 717 | 724 | 665 | 691 | 625 | 620 | 592 | 729 | 842 |
| Nuclear imaging | 102 | 194 | 240 | 313 | 337 | 307 | 363 | 360 | 331 |
| Radiation therapy | 488 | 461 | 431 | 388 | 436 | 540 | 576 | 535 | 551 |
| Ultrasound | 708 | 877 | 788 | 784 | 782 | 947 | 1,086 | 1,126 | 1,083 |
| X ray | 1,615 | 1,144 | 1,710 | 1,755 | 1,850 | 1,529 | 1,655 | 1,767 | 1,611 |
| Total | 4,083 | 3,877 | 4,288 | 4,303 | 4,425 | 4,467 | 4,816 | 5,112 | 5,081 |

[a]Based on estimates and projections provided by the NEMA Economics Department.

SOURCES: Current Industrial Reports, U.S. Bureau of the Census, U.S. Department of Commerce.

The Medical Device Amendments of 1976 established a device classification system based on the risk associated with each device and the ability to control that risk.[18] The intent of the amendments was to provide "reasonable assurance" of the safety and effectiveness of medical devices. There are now three classes of devices with each class having increasing levels of FDA review and control (Box 4-1). All medical devices legally marketed before adoption of the amendments were classified into one of these three classes (Class I, II, or III). With the exception of some low-risk devices (most Class I devices, as well as a few Class II devices, are exempt from premarket review), medical devices must now undergo an FDA review before being introduced into the market. There are two major pathways to FDA approval, known as "premarket notification" [510(k)] or "premarket approval" (PMA) application (Box 4-2). Most devices are cleared for commercial distribution in the United States by the premarket notification process [510(k)].

Before undertaking clinical trials for FDA approval, a company must submit a plan explaining how it will conduct the clinical study, including a statement of objectives for the trial, what results are expected, and what risks and precautions may be involved. If FDA[19] considers the request to be sound, it will grant an investigational device exemption (IDE), which allows the device to be used on patients, with informed consent, only for the purpose of gathering data in a clinical trial.[20] In recent years, FDA has also encouraged sponsors to undergo a study protocol review process in which FDA engages in an interactive critique of the experimental design with respect to how a particular study fits into the sponsor's plans for development of the data for marketing approval or clearance (Sapirstein, 2000).

---

[18]Before that, FDA regulated devices under the adulteration and misbranding provisions of the Federal Food, Drug, and Cosmetic Act of 1938 (21 U.S.C.§321 et seq.), but premarket clearance was not required. When FDA learned that a device was unsafe or ineffective, it had to undertake time-consuming and costly legal action to prove that the device was unsafe or that the manufacturer's claims were not true. During the 1960s many new and complex devices entered the market, and FDA found it increasingly difficult to protect patients using this approach (Kahan, 1995). As a result, the Medical Device Amendments Act of 1976 required FDA to set standards for some devices and to undertake premarket clearance for others, although devices with minimal risks are exempt from both requirements.

[19]Institutional review boards (IRBs) may also play a role in determining whether an IDE is granted. A study approved under IDE, with informed consent, still requires IRB oversight.

[20]In the case of in vitro diagnostic studies, it is possible in some instances to perform the study without an IDE, especially if test results are blinded and not used clinically. Informed consent and IRB oversight may still be required, however, particularly if clinical information is linked to patient results.

**BOX 4-1**
**FDA's Three Classes of Medical Devices**

**Class I:** General Controls. Devices in this class consist of those for which general controls, such as those that ensure proper labeling and production, are usually sufficient to ensure safety and effectiveness.

**Class II:** Performance Standards and Special Controls. For devices in this class, general controls are required but are deemed insufficient to provide reasonable assurance of safety and effectiveness. These devices must comply with any applicable performance standards established for the device, and the sponsors must also take any other actions that FDA deems necessary ("special controls") to provide reasonable assurance of a device's safety and effectiveness. Special controls may include special labeling requirements, mandatory performance standards, patient registries, and postmarket surveillance.

**Class III:** Premarket Approval. Class III devices are often life-sustaining or life-supporting devices or are of substantial importance in preventing impairment of human health and thus are often associated with a higher risk. New devices whose risk and reliability are unknown are also automatically placed in Class III until they are found to be substantially equivalent to a device already on the market. Because of the level of risk associated with Class III devices, general and special controls alone are insufficient to ensure the safety and effectiveness of Class III devices. All Class III devices require premarket authorization from FDA, most often in the form of a premarket approval application (see Box 4-2).

SOURCES: Kahan (1995) and HHS Publication FDA 96-4159, U.S. Department of Health and Human Services (1996) (see www.fda.gov).

The evidence gathered for FDA approval must reflect the intended use and labeling of the device. For instance, manufacturers must state whether the device is intended for screening or diagnosis or for a specific population rather than a general population. Approval by FDA may be accompanied by a requirement for additional postmarket analysis to assess performance standards. For example, a company may be asked to measure the sensitivity and specificity of a device in clinical practice for specific populations or under specific conditions.

In 1997, the Food and Drug Administration Modernization Act (FDAMA) responded to industry concerns that the FDA process was burdensome. Under FDAMA, there is generally more flexibility and a more interactive exchange between FDA and the sponsor, allowing more rapid communications with companies.

## EVALUATION OF SCREENING AND DIAGNOSTIC DEVICES

In many ways, film-screen mammography (FSM) does not provide a useful model of the development and approval process for screening and

---

**BOX 4-2**
**Pathways to FDA approval for medical devices**

**Premarket Notification [510(k)]:** A premarket notification is a marketing application submitted to FDA to demonstrate that a medical device is as safe and effective or substantially equivalent to (not superior to) a legally marketed device that was or is currently on the U.S. market (a "predicate device") and that does not require premarket approval. The predicate device may be a Class I or II device or a "preamendment" Class III device for which FDA has not yet called for a premarket approval application. [Class III devices that were commercially distributed before the Medical Device Amendments of 1976 or that are deemed substantially equivalent to such preamendment devices can be cleared via the 510(k) process for premarket notification unless FDA calls for premarket approval applications for such devices.] Most Class I devices and a few Class II devices are exempt from the 510(k) requirement by regulation. (They are not, however, exempt from other general controls.)

**Premarket Approval Application:** The premarket approval application process is required for the approval of higher-risk devices or devices for which no predicate device exists. A Class III device that is not substantially equivalent to a predicate device that was on the market before passage of the 1976 Medical Device Amendments must be approved by the premarket approval applications process. In this case, the sponsor must provide stand-alone evidence of safety and effectiveness, not just a comparison with other devices on the market. An approved premarket approval application is, in effect, a private license granted to the applicant to market a particular medical device.

**Reclassification:** For Class III devices subject to premarket approval, manufacturers may petition FDA to down-classify the device to Class I or II to seek FDA clearance through the 510(k) notification process. However, the data required for reclassification may be as great as those needed to obtain approval via a premarket approval application.

SOURCES: Kahan (1995) and HHS Publication FDA 96-4159, U.S. Department of Health and Human Services (1996) (see www.fda.gov).

---

diagnostic technologies that are under investigation. The first major clinical trial to test the effect of mammography screening on clinical outcome was organized and supported by a health insurance provider (the Health Insurance Plan of Greater New York), not a device manufacturer (Shapiro, 1997). Furthermore, because X-ray mammography was already in clinical use at the time of passage of the Medical Device Amendments of 1976, it was not required to undergo a rigorous FDA approval process to demonstrate safety and effectiveness (rather, it was "grandfathered [for more detail, see below and Chapter 5]). In fact, since its inception, FDA's Center for Devices and Radiological Health has reviewed relatively few cancer screening technologies. Thus, there is a lack of precedent for defining the appropriate experimental strategies for FDA approval of such screening technologies.

In some ways, the approval process for screening and diagnostic devices and tests can be more complicated than that for therapeutics because each device goes through a unique development process and the requirements of FDA can vary considerably for different devices. The stages of development for drugs, in contrast, are more standardized (Table 4-6). A similar paradigm for diagnostic devices has been developed (Table 4-7),[21] but the specific end points of each phase are not well defined.

Therapeutic evaluation is more straightforward because the study end points are well defined. In general, therapeutic interventions generate direct outcomes that can be observed in individuals. In contrast, most patient-level effects of diagnostic devices are mediated by subsequent follow-up or therapeutic decisions. Diagnostic tests generate information, which is only one of the inputs into the decision-making process. Hence, the evaluation of diagnostic tests is fundamentally the assessment of the value of information. "Valuable" information should be obtainable easily and reliably, should be accurate, and should have the potential to influence the process of health care toward better outcomes.

Ideally, screening and diagnostic modalities would be deemed effective if they led to a reduction in disease-specific mortality rates (or perhaps reduced levels of morbidity and an enhanced quality of life). However, FDA approval of detection technologies generally does not focus on clinical outcomes (Houn et al., 2000). The clinical trials necessary to measure such a reduction in mortality must include a large number of subjects, be very long in duration, and thus are very expensive and arduous to undertake. The alternative is to measure the sensitivity and specificity of the modality, assuming that the efficacy and effectiveness of a device are determined by these two values (which may or may not be true).

To some extent, "effectiveness" can depend on the context in which the device will be used. There is often a trade-off between a device's sensitivity and specificity, and choosing which one to optimize may depend on whether it is used for screening or diagnosis, or both. In evaluating a new screening device, it may be more important to have a high sensitivity (the test's ability to detect everyone with cancer), whereas a diagnostic device may require a higher specificity (so that cancer is unlikely in those who do not test positive). If different methods are used for screening and diagnosis, then the high sensitivity of the screening step could be complemented by the high specificity of the diagnostic step. However, if the specificity of the screening device is too low, there will be problems associated with the cost and anxiety generated as a result of too many unnecessary follow-up diagnostic tests.

Safety can also have multiple definitions. For most devices, safety is

---

[21]Constantine Gatsonis, Brown University, manuscript in preparation.

**TABLE 4-6** Trial Phases for Drug Development

| Trial Phase | Design, Objective, and Endpoint |
|---|---|
| Preclinical studies | General safety and effect of the drug is tested in animals and in vitro. |
| Clinical Phase I | Small studies (~10–100 participants) designed to determine the maximum safe dose of drug for use in humans. Drug doses start out very low and escalate as the study progresses. Trial participants are monitored for adverse side effects and drug level. |
| Clinical Phase II | Moderately sized (~50–500 participants) studies designed to establish preliminary estimates of effective drug doses and duration. A primary goal is to determine the appropriate protocol (experimental conditions and end points) for the final phase of testing. The effects of the drug in study subjects are measured in comparison with those in control subjects. |
| Clinical Phase III | Very large studies (several hundred to several thousand participants) designed to definitively determine the effects of drug treatment. Investigators measure drug efficacy and side effects in study subjects compared with those in a control group of subjects. |
| Clinical Phase IV | Very large studies (several thousand participants) designed to assess effectiveness in clinical practice, assess cost-effectiveness, or test new indications for a drug that is already on the market. |

**TABLE 4-7** Paradigm for Developmental Phases of Diagnostic Devices

| Trial Phase | Design, Objective, and Endpoint |
|---|---|
| Stage I (discovery) | Establishment of technical parameters and diagnostic criteria |
| Stage II (introductory) | Early quantification of diagnostic accuracy |
| Stage III (mature) | Comparative assessment of accuracy and outcome in large clinical studies (efficacy). |
| Stage IV (disseminated) | Assessment of the procedure as utilized by the community at large (effectiveness). |

SOURCE: Constantine Gatsonis, Brown University, personal communication, August, 2000

determined by whether use of the device itself can directly cause harm to the patients (for example, by exposing the patient to ionizing radiation). However, in the case of screening and diagnostic devices, harm can also result from missed detection and diagnosis (false-negative results), unnecessary follow-up procedures (false-positive results), or unnecessary treatment (overdiagnosis) as a result of using a device. Does this also fall under the purview of FDA regulations? The answer seems to vary, depending on the device in question, as will be discussed further in the case studies below. For clinical laboratory tests, FDA evaluation specifically does not examine these issues (i.e., an assessment of how the information generated by the test will be used) but, rather, entails only an assessment of the test's accuracy and reliability in detecting the analyte of interest.

In the case of diagnostic and screening modalities for breast cancer, the traditional notion of equivalence between technologies is also difficult to define solely in terms of the average performance of the devices. The clinical evaluation of these technologies is complicated for various reasons. All are imperfect as cancer detection tools and thus are only part of a multipronged diagnostic strategy, which may include invasive procedures such as biopsy. However, given the physical and psychological consequences of biopsy, radiologists, attending physicians, and patients all have varying attitudes regarding the thresholds for follow-up and biopsy. Furthermore, factors such as study population (e.g., age distribution, types and subtlety of lesions, and a screening versus a diagnostic population), reader variability, and technical considerations (e.g., positioning of the breast and display adjustment) can greatly affect the observed performance of a device. Only a study with a very large sample size could control for all these factors, and even then, distinguishing the performance of a device from that of the reader or technologist could be quite difficult.

## CASE STUDIES OF FDA APPROVAL

Numerous breast cancer detection modalities have been reviewed or are under review by FDA. These include palpation aids, mammography, CAD, ultrasound, electrical impedance, scintimammography, MRI, thermography, infrared imaging, biopsy techniques, and ductal lavage (see Chapters 1 to 3). To take a closer look at the FDA approval process for breast cancer detection devices, the remainder of this chapter examines several case studies in greater detail.

### Digital Mammography

Following passage of the Medical Device Amendments of 1976, mammography devices were classified into the Class II category along with most other standard X-ray devices that were already in use. As a result, the clinical efficacy of these devices was essentially "grandfathered" for approval. The required 510(k) reviews for film-screen devices looked only at the technological characteristics of the mammography systems and examined some sample films to ensure that they were "substantially equivalent to" (as good or better than) the pre-1976 devices. Data on the sensitivity and specificity of FSM devices were not required.

However, when full-field digital mammography (FDDM) came onto the scene, FDA took a very different approach to evaluate the safety and effectiveness of the device and to establish its equivalence with standard analog mammography (Table 4-8). In 1995, the Radiological Devices Panel of FDA held its first meeting on digital mammography. At that time, the panel decided that diagnostic comparisons between film-screen and digital mammography (an agreement study) would be sufficient to establish the substantial equivalence of FFDM to FSM, thus avoiding large screening trials, which would be both time-consuming and costly. A guidance document was issued in 1996, in which the agency suggested use of the 510(k) clearance process. Consequently, between 1996 and 1998, the manufacturers undertook multi-institutional studies, each with 500 to 800 women who were scheduled for diagnostic mammography due to a suspicious finding on FSM or a palpable abnormality. The women underwent digital mammography, and the results were compared with those on the original mammogram obtained by FSM. Unfortunately, such a design loaded the test set with both true-positive and false-positive film-screen mammography results, and thus, the results were biased toward FSM in terms of sensitivity and toward FFDM in terms of specificity (Lewin, 1999), making a valid comparison of these measures impossible.

The substantial equivalence of FFDM and FSM could also be established by either comparing the percentage of matches between FFDM and FSM results or looking for agreement between groups of FFDM readers and FSM readers. However, the variability among multiple readings of mammograms is well documented (Beam et al., 1996; Elmore et al., 1994; Thurfjell et al., 1994), and this inherent variability was in fact large enough to obscure any differences between FSM and FFDM readings, thus making the results difficult or impossible to interpret. The other problem with an agreement study is that even if a new technology is superior to the current standard, it would still fail the equivalency requirement because the difference in performance would be considered nonagreement. The Radiological Devices Panel met again in 1998 to discuss alternative study design options, but the members of the panel could not reach a consensus on how to proceed, so in September 1999, the agency issued letters to various FFDM sponsors requesting that they each discuss individual applications with FDA. The letter also suggested alternative pathways to approval, including the PMA application process.

**TABLE 4-8**  FDA Approval Process for FFDM

| Date | Event | Summary |
|------|-------|---------|
| 1976 | Medical Device Amendments | Mammography and other X-ray devices already in use are classified as "Class II." Pre-1976 systems receive "grandfathered" approval. After 1976, systems require 510(k) clearance or PMA application approval. |
| 1995 | First FDA Radiological Devices Panel meeting on digital mammography | Panel decided that to avoid costly and time-consuming large screening trials, diagnostic comparisons (an agreement study) between FSM and FFDM would be enough to establish equivalence. |
| 1996 | Publication of FDA guidance document | FDA suggests the 510(k) approval process. |
| 1996–1998 | Multi-institutional studies undertaken by sponsors | In response to the FDA guidance document for 510(k) clearance, manufacturers conduct comparison studies with 500–800 women with suspicious findings. Test design results in FSM sensitivity bias and FFDM specificity bias. Valid comparison essentially impossible. Variability among multiple readings is also too great to compare diagnostic matches between FSM and FFDM. |
| 1998 | Second FDA Radiological Devices Panel meeting on digital mammography | Discusses need for alternative study design options. No consensus on how to proceed. |
| Sept. 1999 | FDA issues letter to sponsors | Letter sent to various FFDM sponsors requesting separate meetings to discuss individual applications. Letter suggested alternative ways to approval including the PMA application process. |
| Dec. 1999 | Third FDA Radiological Devices Panel meeting on digital mammography | FDA looks at the first individual PMA application: for the General Electric Senographe 2000 D. |
| Jan. 2000 | FDA grants General Electric premarket approval, with conditions | General Electric Senographe 2000 D receives premarket approval for printed film (hard-copy) use. |
| Nov. 2000 | FDA approves General Electric Senographe 2000 D for softcopy use | No other companies' digital mammography systems have been approved to date. |

In January 2000, General Electric's machine, the Senographe 2000 D, was approved for hard-copy use (i.e., with printed film) through the PMA application mechanism. General Electric examined a diagnostic population, as in the original studies, to keep the number of women tested to a minimum. However, in this case the test population was assessed in a screening context, in which the women underwent both FFDM and FSM at the same time and several radiologists read the results on both new mammograms. This approach ensured that the number of cancers detected in the "screen" would be larger than the number detected in a general screening population. The results of the study with approximately 650 women showed that the sensitivity and specificity of FFDM lie within an acceptable range of the values calculated for FSM (i.e., less than a 5 percent difference). The approval order did not specify any post-approval studies, but it did call for expedited approval of the soft-copy modality, which was granted in November 2000. Other manufacturers are gathering data for similar submissions, but to date, none has been successful.

The approval process for digital mammography was complicated, lengthy, and very costly for the developers. Critics have questioned whether a PMA application or extensive clinical data were really necessary, given that the technology of x-ray interrogation of the breast in FFDM is identical to that in FSM, interpretation techniques are similar, and the efficacy of mammography has already been established.[22] When digital detectors for chest X rays were approved, the devices underwent a vastly simpler 510(k) clearance process with little consideration of how the diagnostic images generated would be used or interpreted.[23] Other breast imaging technologies, such as breast MRI and thermography, have also been cleared by this approach. In the case of breast MRI, only the breast coil had to be cleared by the 510(k) process by demonstrating substantial equivalence with MRI devices used to image other parts of the body.[24] No consideration was given to the accuracy of interpreting the images generated by the breast coil. Similarly, the BioScan system, a thermal imaging device manufactured by OmniCorder, was cleared by the 510(k) process for use as a diagnostic adjunct for breast cancer detection.[25] The device was deemed equivalent to other thermal imaging tech-

---

[22]Radiological Devices Panel Meeting Transcript, December 16, 1999.

[23]Chest X rays are not used for screening, and diagnostic chest X rays are generally less difficult to interpret than mammograms.

[24]MRI devices were originally labeled as Class III devices because safety issues with regard to exposures to strong magnetic fields were undefined. More recently, MRI devices were downgraded to Class II.

[25]Several 510(k) applications for thermal imaging devices have been cleared since 1976 for use as adjunct technologies for the diagnosis of breast cancer.

nologies, although none of those technologies had been proved to be valuable for the detection of breast cancer.

According to FDA, however, the inherent "risk" of digital mammography lay in the fact that millions of women rely on mammography for early detection of breast cancer, with implications ranging from breast conservation to saved lives. Thus, in assessing FFDM, FDA stated that it wanted to ensure that the new technology would improve on the successes of FSM or, at the very least, that no loss in sensitivity and no clinically important loss in specificity would occur (usually, FDA requires demonstration of substantial equivalence, not the superiority of new devices). In other words, FDA wanted companies to demonstrate that FFDM would not miss more cancers than the current technology and that the number of unnecessary biopsies in women without cancer would not increase.[26] The ease of handling information acquired digitally was not deemed, in itself, sufficient to support marketing of FFDM unless these two clinical objectives could be met.

The FDA policy and requirements for approval changed multiple times during the approval process. Throughout the discussions the advisory panel struggled with questions of whether digital mammography qualified as a "new" technology and how to define "safety and effectiveness." On the one hand, digital mammography exposes women to a similar level of ionizing radiation as analog film mammography, thus posing no additional direct physical harm to the woman. The difference between FFDM and FSM is the acquisition and display of the images. Whether this significantly changes the "safety and effectiveness" of mammography subsequently determines which approval process [i.e., the 510(k) process versus the PMA application process] is required. In the end, the panel decided to let individual companies decide on their own particular course, with FDA offering guidance. The PMA application process was offered as an alternative because it allows greater flexibility in the study requirements, permitting some questions to be addressed later in the postmarketing period.

In summary, FDA was faced with a challenging evaluation and had good intentions—protecting American women from false-positive findings during breast cancer screening—when it issued its guidance documents for the approval of digital mammography. However, in the end, following those guidance documents led to significant delays in the approval of FFDM, at great expense to the sponsoring companies. The difficulties encountered in attempting to demonstrate the substantial clinical

---

[26]Transcript from an FDA panel meeting (http://www.fda.gov/ohrms/dockets/ac/98/transcpt/3446t2.rtf).

equivalence of FFDM to FSM could have been predicted, given the well-known variability in the interpretation of mammograms. Thus, the initial expectations of FDA for the clinical studies were unrealistic, and indecision on the part of FDA following that realization further contributed to delays in approval.

### Pro*Duct Breast Catheter

The Pro*Duct catheter (Love et al., 2000) is an example of a device that could potentially be used for breast imaging (contrast-enhanced radiography) as well as for biological tests (ductal lavage for collection of breast fluids and cells for analysis). The catheter was recently cleared by FDA via the 510(k) process, with no assessment of how it would be used for breast cancer screening or diagnosis. Clearance was granted on the basis of the indication that it "enables the collection of breast milk duct fluid for cytological evaluation." [27] The product label further stipulates that the "collected fluid can be used in the determination and/or differentiation of normal versus premalignant versus malignant cells." The label specifies that the device should be used only as an "adjunct to standard breast cancer detection methods, including mammography and physical exam." However, the company has not conducted clinical trials to determine the sensitivity and specificity of this technique and has not compared it with other screening and diagnostic methods. Thus, FDA required a precautionary statement in the label to indicate that "sensitivity/specificity data for ductal cytology from well controlled clinical trials is not currently available. The use of the information in clinical practice must therefore be determined on a case by case basis." No guidelines as to how to make such decisions are provided. Furthermore, it is not clear what action should be taken if, in the absence of a mammographic finding, the results obtained by the procedure indicate a malignant or premalignant lesion.

### TransScan Electrical Impedance Imaging

TransScan Medical (Ramsey, New Jersey) initially sought FDA premarket approval in 1997 for its electrical impedance imaging device, the T-Scan 2000 device, as an adjunct to mammography for women with indeterminate lesions. Preliminary discussions with FDA and protocol reviews began as early as mid-1994, and in 1997 the company submitted data from a large, multicenter study with a screening population imaged

---

[27] Angela B. Soito, vice president of regulatory and quality affairs, Pro*Duct Health, Inc., personal communication, September 2000.

both by mammography and with the T-Scan 2000 device. The mammogram and impedance image for each woman were read blindly. The device was not intended to be used for screening, but it was thought that a double-blind study with a screening population would be the most rigorous and unbiased way to evaluate the device. In this setting, the company reported that for women with equivocal mammograms, the adjunctive use of the T-Scan 2000 device improved the sensitivity of mammography by 22 percent and the specificity of mammography by 16 percent. Although the FDA advisory panel considered the device to be promising, it expressed concerns about how it would be used in practice and whether its use would increase the number of biopsies or cause some women with cancer to forego biopsy. As a result, approval of the T-Scan 2000 device was denied, and the FDA panel recommended that the company identify the population that would benefit most from the device and conduct more studies targeted at that population.[28]

TransScan sought FDA premarket approval again in 1998, and in April 1999 the device was approved as an adjunct to mammography for women with equivocal lesions in BIRADS[29] Categories 3 and 4. TransScan submitted data from two additional studies conducted with the targeted population and under conditions more closely resembling those for its intended clinical use. Statistical modeling was used to combine the results of those studies with the results of the original double-blind study. The combined results indicated that the T-Scan 2000 device, when used in conjunction with mammography on a targeted population, improved the diagnostic sensitivity by 15.6 percent and the diagnostic specificity by 20.2 percent over those from the use of mammography alone. The device is not to be used for the assessment of lesions with clear mammographic or nonmammographic indications for biopsy.

TransScan is conducting additional studies to further validate the technology, as required by FDA as part of its premarket approval process. Post-approval studies must look at the clinical use of the T-Scan 2000 device and any consequent changes in sensitivity and specificity, as well as the effects of the menstrual cycle on the performance of the device.[30]

---

[28]Radiological Devices Panel Meeting, Center for Devices and Radiological Health, FDA, November 17, 1997 (http://www.fda.gov/ohrms/dockets/ac/97/transcpt/3353t1.pdf).

[29]The Breast Imaging Reporting and Data System (BIRADS) includes five categories of assessment with increasing suspicion of malignancy, along with standard follow-up recommendations for each category. Category 3 is "probably benign," whereas Category 4 is "suspicious abnormality." For more detail, see Chapter 1.

[30]John Neugebauer, vice president of marketing, TransScan Medical, personal communication, [June, 2000].

## Computer-Aided Detection

CAD was developed with the intent of reducing observational error in the reading of mammograms. CAD systems identify and mark regions of interest in screening mammograms, thus assisting radiologists in locating areas that might warrant closer inspection. In November 1996, the company R2 Technology, Inc., began discussions with FDA regarding clinical issues and protocols that would be appropriate to determine the safety and effectiveness of its M1000 ImageChecker system. As a result of those discussions, three clinical studies with screening populations were designed for premarket approval. Those studies concluded that (1) CAD does not increase the diagnostic workup rate; (2) CAD correctly marks a high percentage of microcalcifications and masses, thus minimizing the rate of false-negative results; and (3) the system generates reproducible results with good sensitivity for the identification of microcalcifications and masses associated with cancer. The Radiological Devices Panel reviewed the application in May 1998, and in June 1998, R2 Technology was granted premarket approval of its M1000 ImageChecker. FDA approved the technology on the condition that a post-approval study be performed to more accurately assess the effect of the device on the rates of true-positive and false-negative results.

In its PMA application, R2 Technology did not list any direct risks to health or safety; however, as an indirect risk, it did mention missed lesions and false-positive results as potential adverse effects. The company does not market the device as a replacement for the radiologist; rather, it is the combined efforts of the radiologist and the device that result in the increased sensitivity. Since there were no direct physical safety issues, the question of effectiveness focused on the radiologist-device combination. In fact, this issue is pertinent for most screening and diagnostic devices, since human interpretation is an essential component of the detection process. The question then becomes whether the approval process should focus solely on the physical device or whether the interpretation and potential consequences of that interpretation should be considered.

## SUMMARY

Over the last 10 years, efforts directed toward the development of new technologies for early breast cancer detection have increased significantly. Many new funding initiatives have been launched, some of which are the direct result of consumer advocacy, and new collaborative efforts have been undertaken. Government funding in particular has recently placed a new emphasis on the translation of science through the development of technology, in contrast to the more traditional focus on basic scientific discovery. Notably, there has been an increase in joint public sector-private sector efforts. This increase in funding opportunities could stimulate progress in the development of new detection technologies.

Private-sector investment in medical imaging technologies is considerably less than private-sector investment in other areas of the health care industry, perhaps because of the perception of risk associated with such ventures. The technology development process in general is complex and costly, and the end results of research are unpredictable, making it a financially risky undertaking. For medical devices, the FDA approval process adds an additional level of risk to the development process (as can coverage decisions, which will be discussed in the next chapter). The requirements for approval have been variable and unpredictable in the past, in some cases increasing the cost of obtaining approval and the length of time needed to enter the market. The subsequent lag in development can conceivably devastate companies that are funded to produce a return on investment in a relatively short time.

Regulation of medical device manufacturers is clearly necessary and beneficial, but also quite challenging. Without regulation, the market could potentially be flooded with unsafe devices. The drawback is that the regulation increases costs and can slow the process of technology release. Problems can arise if decisions regarding regulatory requirements are inconsistent, unclear, delayed, or faulty. For example, assigning technologies to a particular approval pathway [the 510(k) process versus the PMA application process) can have enormous ramifications for the sponsors in terms of the cost of obtaining approval, but these designations have not always been made in a consistent fashion. Similarly, different operational definitions of "substantial equivalence" could have a significant effect on the process of how equivalence is determined. In the case of FFDM, these definitions and designations changed throughout the approval process. Thus, the approval system could be improved by establishing and more clearly defining a requisite level of agreement between technologies and a required level of statistical precision. Given the numerous complexities in assessing new technologies, FDA advisory panels would benefit from the addition of more experts in biostatistics, technology assessment, and clinical epidemiology.

Separate study guidelines for diagnostic and screening purposes are necessary, including delineation of appropriate end points and study sizes. The dominant framework for medical technology development and evaluation has historically been based on therapeutics, whereas early detection relies on screening and diagnostic methods. The evaluation of such methods may be intrinsically different. The "safety" assessment of screening and diagnostic devices examines direct patient harm from use of the device (analogous to therapeutics), but can also include indirect harm from unnecessary interventions that are pursued on the basis of information generated by the device. Similarly, evaluation of the "effectiveness" of screening and diagnostic tests is fundamentally an assessment of the value of the information obtained from the test, in contrast to the direct effects of therapeutics on clinical outcome. Most patient-level effects of these devices are mediated by subsequent therapeutic decisions.

As a result, there are difficulties associated with comparing new technologies to the imperfect "gold standard" of FSM. The intrinsic variability in the production and interpretation of mammograms and other breast images makes it difficult to accurately determine the sensitivity and specificity of imaging modalities. This variability caused major difficulties and delays in the FDA approval process for FFDM, and thus greatly increased the cost and time required to gain approval.

Using measures of accuracy (e.g., sensitivity and specificity) to make approval decisions may be appropriate for most diagnostic devices. In the case of "next-generation" devices (in which technical improvements have been made to a predicate device already on the market), technical advantages such as patient comfort or ease of data acquisition and storage could be considered in determining approval as well. Ideally, all new screening technologies would be compared to gold standard technologies by using the reduction in disease-specific mortality as an end point. However, such an approach is logistically impractical for device companies because of the study size, length, and cost. A more coordinated approach for the testing of new screening technologies, with input and support from FDA, NCI, health insurers, and patient advocates may help to overcome this barrier. If a new device approved for diagnostic use shows potential for screening use and the developers wish to pursue approval of the device for screening, an investigational device exemption should be granted for this use based on measures of accuracy. In addition, conditional coverage (as discussed in Chapter 5) could be provided for the purpose of conducting large-scale screening trials to assess clinical outcomes. This approach would prevent "off-label" adoption of detection technologies that have not been assessed in the screening setting. The recently launched ACRIN trial for the study of digital mammography may provide an example of how screening studies could be conducted under this proposed mechanism.

FDA approval is only the first hurdle that new technologies face once they have been developed. Although both public and physician perception is that FDA approval means that technologies "work" and reimbursement for use of the device should be provided, coverage decisions are rarely that straightforward. For example, FDA approval does not mean that a new device is better than its predecessor or that it is useful for applications for which it has not been evaluated. Approval simply allows a company to sell the device, but ultimately, coverage decisions by third-party payers are likely to determine whether the technology becomes widely used and disseminated. This issue will be examined more closely in Chapter 5.

# 5
# Evaluation and
# Cost Coverage of Technologies

The United States is both the largest market for most new health care technologies and the largest producer of the research and development that generates them. The post-World War II era saw an ever-increasing investment in scientific research in both the public and the private sectors. Increased access to medical insurance coverage through employer-sponsored health benefits and government-sponsored programs such as Medicare and Medicaid made it possible for new medical technologies to be rapidly diffused throughout the medical care system and encouraged continued investment in their development. Initially, physicians essentially controlled the process of technology adoption because a test or procedure ordered by a doctor was deemed medically necessary and was thus eligible for coverage (reviewed by Braslow et al., 1998).

As the costs of health care escalated in the 1970s, the traditional model was questioned and concerns were raised about the lack of professional consensus in medical care as well as the wastefulness of medical interventions and procedures that were of unproven value. Concern was also raised as to whether expensive new technologies were deployed in an efficient manner. Most health economists believe that technology is the single largest driving force behind the long-term rise in health care spending in the United States (Fuchs, 1999; Rettig, 1997). Because the resources for health care are not infinite, there has been increasing pressure to make evidence-based decisions about the use of medical technology, and as a result, the need for technology assessment has risen.

In 1976, an amendment to the Federal Food, Drug, and Cosmetic Act, as discussed in the previous chapter, required approval by the Food and

Drug Administration (FDA) for all medical devices. However, FDA approval does not guarantee that insurers will cover the cost of new technologies in health care. FDA approval permits legal marketing in interstate commerce but does not mandate or imply health plan approval or coverage, which are essential for successful technology diffusion. Such coverage decisions are now often based on critical assessments of the effects of technologies on patient outcomes, and the criteria for these assessments can be far more stringent than those of the FDA (Aubry, 1998). Organizations that assess technologies often ask two related questions: (1) Can the technology positively affect patient outcome, and (2) How does the technology compare with other technologies on the market? Some organizations may also ask whether the technology can achieve results similar to those of products already on the market, but in a more cost-effective manner. A recent report from the Milbank Foundation (2000)[1] found that U.S. purchasers were most likely to use technology assessment data for new technologies that are costly and controversial.

Reimbursement decisions can be highly influential on the adoption of new technologies as well. Coverage decisions determine whether a particular service or product is eligible for reimbursement, whereas the actual rates of reimbursement (the methods and amounts of payment) for covered services and products may vary greatly depending on the specific case, location, insurance carrier, and so on.

As health care purchasers increasingly rely on scientific evidence of improved health outcomes to make coverage and reimbursement decisions, the demand for credible technology assessments will likely increase and the influence of such assessments on the coverage and diffusion of new technologies will grow. The challenge of evidence-based medicine is to develop a health care system that "rewards better outcomes, recognizes value, and encourages efficient use of limited resources" (Eisenberg, 1999, p. 1865).

As in many areas of health care, there will be increasing concern about when to introduce a promising new technology that costs more but that may be more effective. Methods that offer better value (accuracy, sensitivity, or reliability) at a lower cost are likely to be adopted quickly. Technologies that do something entirely new or that clearly offer major improvements are often readily adopted as well. The most difficult coverage decisions will come from technologies that are marginally better but that are also substantially more costly. Unfortunately, many technologies may fall into this category.

---

[1]Health care purchasers in the United Kingdom and the United States (including 13 public officials from 11 states, 4 private-sectors purchasers, 5 representatives of private purchasing coalitions, and 3 consultants) were interviewed by phone over a 3-month period in early 1999.

## OVERVIEW OF TECHNOLOGY ASSESSMENT ORGANIZATIONS AND THEIR ROLES

Early efforts to assess medical technologies so that they would not diffuse too rapidly were initiated by the National Health Planning and Resources Development Act (Public Law 93-641) of 1975. However, this legislation was later repealed because it was viewed as too limiting. From 1975 to 1995, the congressional Office of Technology Assessment (OTA) undertook studies of the methods for technology assessment and carried out several assessments of medical technologies. The National Center for Health Care Technology (NCHCT), established in the U.S. Department of Health and Human Services (DHHS) in 1978, did technology assessments to assist the Health Care Financing Administration (HCFA) with coverage decisions. However, despite its involvement in health technology assessment, the federal government has never really carried out the central technology assessment repository function that was originally envisioned (U.S. Congress, Office of Technology Assessment, 1994). This is in contrast to the situation in many European countries, in which there are either global budgets or some other form of real control by the government (Perry and Thamer, 1999).

Both federal organizations (NCHCT and OTA) have since been dissolved, and technology evaluation activities have increased greatly in the private sector (Perry and Thamer, 1999). Today, health technology assessment is undertaken by a variety of public and private organizations, including insurers and managed care organizations, professional medical societies, health technology companies, academic medical centers, and independent technology assessment institutions (U.S. Congress, Office of Technology Assessment, 1994). The various groups differ in their objectives and process, as is discussed briefly below for some of the major organizations.

### Health Care Financing Administration

HCFA is the federal agency that administers Medicare, Medicaid (in collaboration with the states), and the State Children's Health Insurance Program. In addition to paying for health care, HCFA also performs a number of activities focused on quality, including regulation of laboratory testing (under the Clinical Laboratory Improvement Amendments), surveys and certification of health care facilities, development of coverage policies, and quality-of-care improvements. External advisory panels provide advice or make recommendations on a variety of issues relating to HCFA's responsibilities and activities. As the nation's largest health care provider, the Medicare program directly exerts significant influence on patient access to new medical technologies and also indirectly influences coverage and reimbursement decisions in other sectors of the health care marketplace.

The Social Security Act of 1965 specified broad categories of services covered by Medicare, excluded services, and exceptions to the exclusions. Because the rationale for Medicare's creation was to pay for expensive hospitalization and later for medical care, preventive services were excluded from coverage. The Secretary of DHHS (and predecessor departments) was, however, given authority to add specific items for coverage under Medicare, and the U.S. Congress could always amend the Medicare legislation to include a specific benefit. Mammography, added as a benefit by congressional mandate,[2] is one of only a handful of preventive services that have been added. Experimental drugs, devices, and procedures have traditionally not been covered because they have been defined as not meeting the basic Medicare criterion of being "reasonable and necessary" for diagnosis or treatment.

This changed somewhat in 1995 through an interagency agreement between HCFA and FDA, which established coverage and reimbursement for certain devices and related services in clinical trials carried out under FDA-approved investigational device exemptions (IDEs). Under this agreement, medical devices are categorized by FDA as either Category A (novel, not reimbursable) or Category B ("next-generation" devices, eligible for Medicare reimbursement) (Table 5-1). Category A devices are novel experimental Class III devices (see Chapter 4) that are excluded from Medicare reimbursement. Category B devices are those that FDA has approved for use for one indication but that have been technically altered or are being tested for a new use. They generally fall into Class I or II but may also include some Class III devices that are related to devices that have already been shown to be safe and effective. According to FDA, about 95 percent of device trials involve Category B devices and are thus eligible for reimbursement, although it is not always granted (Institute of Medicine, 2000).

Medicare coverage and reimbursement decisions can be made at the local or national level. Medicare contractors (private insurance companies that contract with Medicare to process claims from beneficiaries, providers, and suppliers) primarily make local decisions with input from advisory committees consisting of local specialists. Carriers and intermediar-

---

[2]Section 4163 of the Omnibus Budget Reconciliation Act of 1990 originally set forth payment limitations and conditions for coverage of screening mammography. A new law signed as part of the Balanced Budget Act of 1997 provides Medicare coverage for annual screening mammograms for all Medicare-eligible women age 40 and over and waives the Part B deductible for screening mammography.

[3]Decisions are always local unless national action is taken.

**TABLE 5-1**   Criteria for Categorization of Investigational Devices under HCFA-FDA Interagency Agreement

*Category A: Experimental*

*Subcategory*

| | |
|---|---|
| 1 | Class III devices[a] of a type for which no marketing application has been approved for any indication or use |
| 2 | Class III devices that would otherwise be in Category B but that have undergone significant modification for a new indication or use |

*Category B: Nonexperimental/Investigational*

*Subcategory*

| | |
|---|---|
| 1 | Devices, regardless of classification, under investigation to establish substantial equivalence to a predicate device (one that is or that could be legally marketed) |
| 2 | Class III devices whose technological characteristics and indications are comparable to those of an approved device |
| 3 | Class III devices with technological ("generational") advances compared with an approved device |
| 4 | Class III devices comparable to an approved device (no significant modifications) but under investigation for a new indication |
| 5 | Class III devices on the market before the current regulatory requirements (1976) but now under investigation |
| 6 | Devices not posing significant risks (Class I or II) for which an IDE is required |

NOTE: Some investigational devices may exhibit unique characteristics or raise safety concerns that make additional consideration necessary. For these devices, HCFA and FDA will agree on the additional criteria to be used. FDA will then use these criteria to assign the device to a category. As experience is gained in the categorization process, this attachment may be modified.

[a]Devices are classified by their inherent risks and benefits on the basis of the level of control necessary to ensure safety and effectiveness. Class I devices present minimal potential for harm to the user and are subject only to "general controls" (e.g., proper registration and labeling and good manufacturing practices). Class II devices are those for which general controls alone are insufficient to ensure safety and effectiveness, so they are also subject to special controls, which may include special labeling requirements, guidance documents, mandatory performance standards, and postmarketing surveillance. Class III is the most stringent regulatory category and includes devices for which safety and effectiveness cannot be ensured solely through general or special controls. Class III devices usually support or sustain human life, are of substantial importance in preventing impairment of human health, or present a potential, unreasonable risk of illness or injury. They require premarket approval, which may include evidence from clinical trials.

SOURCE: Health Care Financing Administration/Food and Drug Administration (1995).

ies still make most coverage and reimbursement decisions,[3] but in recent years, HCFA has attempted to move away from local decisions and more toward national coverage decisions and also toward more evidence-based medical decisions. At the national level, the agency has tried a number of different approaches to coverage policy and may seek input from entities such as the Agency for Healthcare Research and Quality (AHQR; see below); FDA; the U.S. Department of Veterans Affairs-the Civilian Health and Medical Program of the Uniformed Services; the American Medical Association; the National Institutes of Health (NIH); specialty-specific professional organizations; specialty advocacy groups; and health care providers, suppliers, and manufacturers. HCFA is also charged with tracking emerging technologies and patterns of care to determine the applicability of existing coverage policy and to assess the need for policy change, but the process for accomplishing this goal is not yet well established or standardized.

A recent reorganization of HCFA (*Federal Register*, 1999) separated the offices responsible for coverage decisions (i.e., the procedures or devices covered under Medicare) and cost decisions (i.e., the level of reimbursement for those procedures or devices). The Center for Health Plans and Providers determines reimbursement levels, and the Office of Clinical Standards and Quality decides on coverage issues. Requests for coverage review may come from industry, from patients or patient advocacy groups, or from within the agency itself. In making a decision for or against coverage, HCFA may solicit input from a Medicare Coverage Advisory Committee (MCAC) or an external technology assessment organization. The agency may also defer the decision back to the local level.

HCFA has recently proposed two new criteria for making national coverage decisions within the agency and has recommended that contractors use the same criteria to make local decisions (*Federal Register*, 2000). First, the item or service must demonstrate medical benefit, and second, it must demonstrate added value to the Medicare population. To consistently apply these criteria, the following sequential questions would be addressed:

1. Is there evidence that demonstrates that the service is medically beneficial for a defined population?

2. For that population, is a medically beneficial alternative already covered by Medicare?

3. If yes, is the new service substantially more beneficial than the current one that is covered?

4. If the service is equivalent in benefit, will it result in equal or lower costs for Medicare?

The use of external advisory committees is also a new approach that is being undertaken in part to make the process more open and accountable. The mission of MCACs is to serve as an impartial panel that reviews and evaluates the evidence on the effectiveness of services that Medicare is considering for coverage. MCACs review the available data on a new technology, make a judgment on its effectiveness compared with that of the established standard of care, and consider the applicability of the evidence to Medicare patients. MCAC assigns the technologies to one of six categories:

1. breakthrough– (more effective than the current standard of care);
2. as effective as the current standard of care, but with advantages;
3. as effective as the current standard of care, but with no advantages;
4. less effective than the current standard of care, but with advantages;
5. less effective, but with no advantages; or
6. not effective.

The MCAC program is organized into six panels, each of which is composed of 15 voting members, a chair, one consumer representative, and one representative from industry. The six panels cover six broad areas: drugs, biologics, and therapeutics; laboratory and diagnostic services; medical and surgical procedures; diagnostic imaging; medical devices and prosthetics; and durable medical equipment. MCAC also has an executive committee that develops criteria for assessment of effectiveness, develops panel procedures, coordinates panels, develops an annual slate of technology assessments, and approves panel recommendations and then submits them to HCFA. MCAC's executive committee consists of the chair and vice-chair of each panel, as well as one consumer representative and one industry representative.

Two reports by The Lewin Group[4] (1999, 2000) have recently examined the HCFA process for making coverage and reimbursement determinations and the effect of that process on the medical device industry. The group concluded that although the recently redesigned national coverage process is an improvement over the previous process, it can still be unpredictable and time-consuming, especially for novel or breakthrough tech-

---

[4]The Lewin Group was commissioned by the Advanced Medical Technology Association (AdvaMed) to conduct a study on the current situation of the U.S. medical device and diagnostic industry and produce a series of reports on the following topics: the state of the industry, the Medicare payment process and patient access to technology, technology assessment by public and private payers, and the impact of regulation and market dynamics on innovation.

nologies. They further concluded that problems with the Medicare coverage and payment systems can influence provider behavior, impede access to health care technology, and affect the viability of small companies and the direction of innovation in both large and small companies.

## Agency for Healthcare Research and Quality

AHRQ[5] conducts research on health care outcomes, quality, cost, use, and access. AHRQ (formerly the Agency for Health Care Policy and Research) is a U.S. Public Health Service agency in DHHS. One of AHRQ's missions is to provide evidence-based information that can help health care decision makers—patients and clinicians, health system leaders, purchasers, and policy makers—make more informed decisions and improve the quality of health care services. Although the agency does not mandate practice guidelines or standards for the measurement of quality, AHRQ established the Center for Practice and Technology Assessment (CPTA) in 1997 to serve as a single contact for organizations and individuals searching for comprehensive evidence-based reviews of health conditions, treatments, and technologies. CPTA supports several major programmatic activities, including 12 evidence-based practice centers (EPCs)[6] that develop scientific knowledge in health care. CPTA also supports and conducts research grants and evaluation projects that focus on two key areas: (1) methodologies used to conduct systematic, evidence-based reviews and syntheses, such as meta-analysis, cost and cost-effectiveness analyses, and decision analysis, and (2) approaches used to incorporate evidence-based clinical information and recommendations into the health care delivery system. Projects compare alternative strategies to facilitating change in provider behavior and investigate the effects of implementation efforts on health outcomes as well as patient knowledge, behavior, and satisfaction.

The U.S. Preventive Services Task Force (USPSTF) is an independent

---

[5]Authorized by the Healthcare Research and Quality Act of 1999 (see http://www.AHRQ.gov/).

[6]The 12 EPCs are Blue Cross/Blue Shield Association Technology Evaluation Center, Chicago, Illinois; Duke University, Durham, North Carolina; ECRI, Plymouth Meeting, Pennsylvania; Johns Hopkins University, Baltimore, Maryland; McMaster University, Hamilton, Ontario, Canada; MetaWorks, Inc., Boston, Massachusetts; New England Medical Center, Boston, Massachusetts; Oregon Health Sciences University, Portland, Oregon; Southern California Evidence-Based Practice Center-RAND, Santa Monica, California; Research Triangle Institute and University of North Carolina at Chapel Hill, Chapel Hill, North Carolina; University of California, San Francisco, Stanford University, Stanford, California; and University of Texas Health Sciences Center, San Antonio, Texas.

panel of preventive health experts convened by AHRQ who are charged with evaluating the scientific evidence for the effectiveness of clinical preventive services, including screening, and producing age- and risk factor-specific recommendations for these services. Currently, AHRQ provides the technical support for USPSTF through two of its EPCs and oversees implementation of USPSTF recommendations by providing tools for clinicians and health systems to improve the delivery of preventive care.

## NIH Office of Medical Applications of Research

At the request of the U.S. Congress, NIH established the Office of Medical Applications of Research in 1977 (Office of Technology Assessment, 1994). Under the auspices of this office, the Consensus Development Program was established with the goal of reaching general agreement on whether a given medical technology is safe and effective. Panels consisting of physicians, consumers, scientists, and others are asked to weigh the available evidence and form a consensus recommendation on the use of a given technology. The first consensus development conference, held in 1977, was on breast cancer screening. Additional panels have since been convened to revisit the breast cancer screening issue, both in general and for specific age groups.

## State Mandates

State legislatures often require public and private insurers to cover or at least offer coverage for specific medical interventions or procedures. Breast cancer screening is by far the most frequently mandated coverage among screening tests for cancer. Currently, 46 states mandate some form of coverage for screening mammography (Figure 5-1). In comparison, only 22 states mandate coverage for cervical cancer screening, 18 mandate coverage for prostate cancer screening, and 1 mandates coverage for colorectal cancer screening (Rathore et al., 2000). For most states, coverage is required for annual mammograms for women over age 50, but other details vary considerably among the states, especially with regard to the age and frequency of screening. This is due to differences in the selection and use of screening guidelines by each state (see Table 6-1). A recent study found that 23 states used American Cancer Society (ACS) guidelines only, 18 states used ACS as well as other guidelines, and 3 states used only non-ACS guidelines in determining coverage mandates. No state screening coverage mandate reflected the screening guidelines of USPSTF (Rathore et al., 2000).

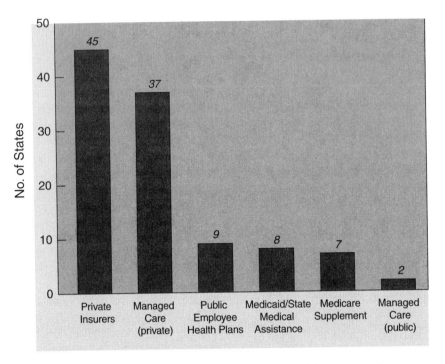

**FIGURE 5-1** States requiring specified insurer to provide coverage for screening mammograms (as of March 31, 2000).

## Private Insurers and Managed Care

The evaluative science of technology assessment has been expanding in the private sector since the 1980s, and commercial health plans increasingly use these assessments, when they are available, to determine evidence-based coverage decisions (Aubry, 1998). In the past, health care insurers, purchasers, and providers relied on ad hoc opinion by experts in making coverage decisions, but virtually all now have formal technology assessment programs or more structured decision-making processes for determination of coverage (Perry and Thamer, 1999). However, different plans use different criteria to determine coverage for new technologies, so the results of the evaluations can vary significantly and thus coverage is far from uniform.

A number of large insurers have established their own staffed technology assessment divisions, including United HealthCare, CIGNA, Humana, and Aetna. One of the oldest and largest commercial health plan programs for assessment of new medical technologies is the Technology Evaluation Center (TEC) Program of Blue Cross/Blue Shield Association (BCBSA). The TEC program, which relies heavily on scientific criteria and which is overseen by a multidisciplinary medical advisory panel, was initiated in 1985 and expanded in 1993 when BCBSA reached an agreement with Kaiser Permanente to collaborate on technology assessment. The program currently annually produces 35 to 40 formal assessments of both diagnostic and therapeutic technologies. The major focus of the evaluations is on health outcomes for patients, but the technologies are expected to meet five criteria (Aubry, 1998), as follows:

1. The technology must have final approval from the appropriate government regulatory bodies.
2. The scientific evidence must permit a conclusion to be made concerning the effect of the technology on health outcomes.
3. The technology must improve the net health outcome.
4. The technology must be as beneficial as any established alternatives.
5. The improvement must be attainable outside the investigational setting.

TEC and BCBSA do not themselves determine coverage. Rather, the scientific reports produced by TEC are available by subscription and are frequently used by Blue Cross and Blue Shield plans, as well as other health plans, as part of their coverage decision-making process. Once a coverage decision is made, the level of reimbursement may vary significantly. This is due to a multitude of factors, including network coverage, certificate language, and negotiated rates within a community.

### Independent Technology Assessment Organizations

The increased interest in evidence-based medicine and technology assessment has also provided incentives to launch private firms that specialize in medical technology assessment. One of the oldest and largest private firms is ECRI, whose Health Technology Assessment Information Service has been designated an EPC by AHQR. Public and private payers, health systems, health care providers, purchasers, government agencies, and other health care constituencies in the United States as well as other countries use ECRI's services and resources, including a technology assessment clearinghouse funded by the World Health Organization. In evaluating emerging technologies, ECRI often uses decision modeling, which is one of the least-used tools for the assessment of new technologies but which is potentially useful when data from clinical trials are sparse.

Other technology assessment organizations include MetaWorks, Inc. (Medford, Massachusetts), which offers meta-analyses of clinical studies, and the Lewin Group (Fairfax, Virginia). In addition, medical professional organizations often develop clinical practice guidelines, and a number have published recommended guidelines for breast cancer screening (see Table 6-1).

## CRITERIA BY WHICH NEW TECHNOLOGIES ARE JUDGED

Health care technology assessment entails the systematic evaluation of the properties and effects of medical technologies, both in absolute terms and in comparison with other competing technologies. The process may involve collection of new primary data as well as collection and pooled analysis of existing data, such as meta-analyses.[7] To date, health outcomes have been measured primarily in terms of changes in mortality or morbidity, but the analysis may also include measures of clinical safety, efficacy or effectiveness, and cost and economic attributes or effects, as well as the social, legal, ethical, or political effects of a medical technology (Goodman, 1998). In the case of coverage decisions, the major focus is on efficacy and effectiveness. Efficacy is a measure of whether a device or procedure has utility among a group of patients in an ideal setting (e.g., a clinical trial). Effectiveness, in contrast, is a measure of the utility of a device or procedure for individual patients in a realistic clinical setting (e.g., community medical practice). Studies of effectiveness are necessary because new technologies may be associated with a complex learning curve for users and a limited range of applicability that make it difficult to duplicate, in the real world of the clinic, results produced with select populations in carefully controlled trial settings.

## RELATIVE MERIT OF DATA FROM STUDIES WITH
## VARIOUS DESIGNS

Technology assessment can entail the examination of data from several studies with various designs that may differ in their strengths and the validity of their results from which investigators can draw conclusions. As a result, organizations that undertake such assessments have developed scales that can be used to rank the evidence from different studies and the strength of recommendations on the basis of the available data (Boxes 5-1 and 5-2).

---

[7]Meta-analysis refers to a group of statistical techniques that combine the results of multiple studies to obtain a quantitative estimate of the overall effect of a particular technology on a defined outcome. This combination may produce a stronger conclusion than that which can be provided by any individual study.

---

**BOX 5-1**
**AHCPR Evidence Grading for Clinical Practice Guidelines**

**Type of Evidence**

I.   Meta-analysis of multiple, well-designed, controlled studies.

II.  At least one well-designed experimental study.

III. Well-designed, quasiexperimental studies, such as nonrandomized controlled, single-group pre-post, cohort, time series, or matched case-control studies.

IV.  Well-designed nonexperimental studies, such as comparative and correlational descriptive and case studies.

V.   Case reports and clinical examples.

**Strength and Consistency of Evidence**

A.   There is evidence of Type I or consistent findings from multiple studies of Type II, III,or IV.

B.   There is evidence of Type II, III, or IV, and findings are generally consistent.

C.   There is evidence of Type II, III, or IV, but findings are inconsistent.

D.   There is little or no evidence, or there is Type V evidence only.

SOURCE: Agency for Health Care Policy and Research, U.S. Department of Health and Human Services (1994).

---

Two basic types of study designs, experimental and observational studies, are used to evaluate technologies (Prorok et al., 1999). The randomized controlled trial is considered by many to be the "gold standard" of experimental designs and is often the method of choice. In a randomized clinical trial, study participants are randomly assigned to either (1) a group that receives the test or treatment in question or (2) a control group that receives a placebo or that does not undergo the procedure being tested. In observational studies, information is collected for groups of individuals who have chosen a particular course of medical intervention or who have a specific condition. They can be prospective, in which data about subsequent events are collected, or retrospective, in which information about past events is collected. Observational studies may include censuses, surveys, case-control[8] studies, or cohort studies.[9] Observational

---

[8]In a case-control study, women who have a particular disease (cases) are compared with women who have similar characteristics but who do not have the disease (controls) by looking back in time to determine the frequency of a particular intervention (such as screening) in the two groups.

[9]In a cohort study, researchers identify a group of subjects of interest and follow them over time to see what happens.

---

**BOX 5-2**
**USPSTF Evidence Grading for Clinical Preventive Services**

**Quality of Evidence**

I.      Evidence obtained from at least one properly designed randomized controlled trial.

II-1.   Evidence obtained from well-designed controlled trials without randomization.

II-2.   Evidence obtained from well-designed cohort or case-controlled analytic studies, preferably from more than one center or research group.

II-3.   Evidence obtained from multiple time series studies with or without the intervention. Dramatic results from uncontrolled experiments (such as the results of the introduction of penicillin treatment in the 1940s) could also be regarded as this type of evidence.

IV.     Opinions of respected authorities, on the basis of clinical experience, descriptive studies, or reports of expert committees.

**Strength of Recommendations**

A.      There is good evidence to support the recommendation that the condition be specifically considered in a periodic health examination.

B.      There is fair evidence to support the recommendation that the condition be specifically considered in a periodic health examination.

C.      There is insufficient evidence to recommend for or against the inclusion of the condition in a periodic health examination, but recommendations may be made on other grounds.

D.      There is fair evidence to support the recommendation that the condition be excluded from consideration in a periodic health examination.

E.      There is good evidence to support the recommendation that the condition be excluded from consideration in a periodic health examination.

SOURCE: U.S. Preventive Services Task Force (1996).

---

designs may be similar in many respects to experimental designs, but their results can be more difficult to interpret and analyze because the comparison groups are not established by randomization and thus the studies are subject to bias. They are often used when a randomized clinical trial is not possible, but the results of observational studies may also complement those of randomized clinical trials. A recent report in the *New England Journal of Medicine* even suggests that when they are well designed, the results of observation studies and experimental studies may be statistically indistinguishable (Concato et al., 2000).

If a screening test is already in common use, it can be very difficult to randomly assign test subjects to screened or unscreened test groups. This was the initial experience with prostate-specific antigen (PSA) screening for prostate cancer in men (Mandelson et al., 1995), although a randomized clinical trial[10] sponsored by NCI is under way to test the ability of PSA screening to reduce mortality from prostate cancer. A similar situation may be developing for lung cancer screening by spiral computed tomography, a relatively new form of computed tomography that has been shown to detect lung cancers at an earlier stage than would otherwise be possible but that has not yet been tested for its ability to reduce lung cancer mortality (Henschke et al., 1999; Newman, 2000). An alternative would be to examine the disease-specific mortality rate among a group of individuals who have chosen to undergo screening with that among a group of individuals who have foregone screening and who have been selected to match, as closely as possible, the screened population in terms of age, risk, and other characteristics (a case-control study). A second alternative would be to compare the disease-specific mortality rates in different geographic regions that have significantly different rates of voluntary screening (a cohort study). In both cases, there is a possibility that the individuals who volunteer for screening are at increased risk for cancer and may therefore be more likely to benefit from a screening program, which is a selection bias (see Chapter 1). In the case of mammography, for which a positive effect of screening has already been shown, it would be both difficult and unethical to randomize women to be screened by either mammography or a new modality. Rather, studies are likely to entail screening by both modalities, but such a design can make it difficult to assign the effects of screening to a single modality.

## SPECIFIC CRITERIA FOR EVALUATION OF SCREENING AND DIAGNOSTIC TECHNOLOGIES

Medical technologies can be divided into two broad categories: therapeutic technologies that cure or prevent a disease and screening and diagnostic technologies that detect an abnormality so that therapy can subsequently be applied. In the latter case, the technology itself does not improve health outcomes, but it may produce a positive effect when combined with an effective therapeutic intervention. Because of this fundamental difference, models of evaluation are not equally applicable to medical technologies in both categories. Therapeutic technologies should be assessed differently than diagnostic and screening technologies, but definition of the assessment criteria and process for the latter category has lagged.

Several investigators have suggested criteria for the evaluation of new diagnostic tests (Lijmer et al., 1999; U.S. Preventive Services Task

---

[10]The Prostate, Lung, Colorectal, and Ovarian Cancer Screening Trial will study 148,000 volunteers.

---

**BOX 5-3**
**Criteria for Determining Whether a Medical Condition Should
Be Included in Periodic Health Examinations**

1.  How great is the burden of suffering caused by the condition in terms of:
    Death                          Discomfort
    Disease                        Dissatisfaction
    Disability                     Destitution

2.  How good is the screening test, if one is to be performed, in terms of:
    Sensitivity              Cost              Labeling effects
    Specificity              Safety
    Simplicity               Acceptability

3.  a.  For primary prevention, how effective is the intervention?
        or
    b.  For secondary prevention, if the condition is found, how effective is the
        ensuing treatment in terms of:
        Efficacy
        Patient compliance
        Early treatment being more effective than later treatment

SOURCE: Fletcher et al., 1997.

---

Force, 1996; Fletcher et al., 1996) (Box 5-3). Key criteria include (1) the use of an appropriate spectrum of subjects (i.e., the subjects in the evaluation should resemble the kinds of people for whom the test might be used in practice); (2) the use of consecutively chosen subjects (to avoid any possibility of selection bias); (3) the use of both the new diagnostic test and the "reference standard" (i.e., the test against which the new test is compared) for all subjects and (4) blinded determination of test results (i.e., the results of the reference tests should not be known when the results of the diagnostic test under study are determined). When an appropriate evaluation of a diagnostic test is carried out in this way, the accuracy of the new test (specifically, its sensitivity and its specificity) can be calculated, as can the positive and negative predictive values (see Box 1-1). These are the key outcomes for diagnostic tests (not efficacy and effectiveness).

The criteria for an appropriate evaluation of a screening test include all the criteria for evaluation of a diagnostic test, but because of differences between screening and diagnosis, several features are unique. First, because most diseases are uncommon, studies that evaluate a new test to be used to screen for a disease such as breast cancer require much larger numbers of people than studies that evaluate a new diagnostic test. Second, the reference standard for a new screening test almost always must include a follow-up observation period to identify any false-negative test results. For example, in breast cancer screening, the reference standard is commonly a combination of mammography, pathological verification of breast cancer (to be certain that the breast cancer diagnoses are correct), and results from 1 year of follow-up to verify the results for subjects with true-negative results and to identify subjects with false-negative results (cancers that were missed on the original examination by both the test under study and the older test, usually mammography). Monitoring over time is an imperfect reference standard, but in screening, it is unrealistic and unethical to subject all participants to histological verification of a negative test result. Because of these two features, evaluation of a new screening test is more difficult than evaluation of a new diagnostic test. However, if a test is to be used for screening, it is critical to evaluate it for that purpose because many good diagnostic tests are poor screening tests.

Traditionally, diagnostic tests should be highly specific, with few false-positive results. For example, it is important that pathological diagnoses of breast cancer not include any false-positive results because such results could lead to unnecessary breast surgery. On the other hand, screening tests should be highly sensitive because they are looking for an uncommon event (for breast cancer, only a few women in 1,000 will have breast cancer at any given time). However, because screening tests are given to such large numbers of people, the numbers and percentages of people suffering false-positive test results is also important, because all these people must have further testing. In addition to added cost and inconvenience, false-positive test results can cause anxiety.

In calculating the sensitivities of screening tests, it is also important to consider the potential for overdiagnosis due to a technology's ability to diagnose early conditions such as ductal carcinoma in situ (DCIS), which may or may not progress to become a lethal cancer (see Chapter 1). If a new technology's sensitivity is calculated by counting all cases of DCIS detected as true-positive results, it will be judged to be superior to an older technology regardless of its effect on a patient's health. The new test will appear to be better because the numerator will include all cancers found, not just those with invasive potential. To deal with this possibility, a method for calculation of a test's sensitivity called the "incidence method" has been developed (Box 5-4).

A key issue in the evaluation of screening is the question of whether a test is efficacious and effective. As pointed out earlier in this chapter and in Chapter 4, neither a diagnostic test nor a screening test alone, in the absence of treatment, can be efficacious or effective. Thus, a particularly vexing challenge is the need to demonstrate that use of a test leads to improved health outcomes in combination with follow-up therapy. Measurement of a test's sensitivity, specificity, and positive and negative pre-

---

**BOX 5-4**
**Detection and Incidence Methods of Measuring Sensitivity**

The traditional method of measuring the sensitivity of a screening test is the *detection method*, in which the sensitivity of a test is calculated as the number of true-positive results divided by the number of true-positive results plus the number of false-negative results. In contrast, the *incidence method* calculates the cancer incidence among persons not undergoing screening and the interval cancer rate (cancers found between screening tests) among persons who are screened. The rationale is that the sensitivity of a test should affect interval cancer rates but not disease incidence. For breast cancer, the sensitivity of a new test would be 1 minus the ratio of the interval breast cancer rate among a group of women receiving the test to the breast cancer incidence among a group of women not screened. The problem with the incidence method of calculating sensitivity is that it does not account for cancers with long lead times. Therefore, ideally, both the detection and incidence methods should be used.

---

dictive values provides end points that are only imperfect surrogate measures for the most critical measures of patient outcome: disease-specific morbidity and mortality. It is not sufficient to demonstrate that a screening test can be accurately and reliably performed. It must also be shown that testing leads to a change in treatment or management of a patient's condition that results in improved health outcomes or a net benefit to the patient (i.e., the benefits must outweigh the harms). Unfortunately, such trials are often slow to produce data and are expensive because of their size and duration. The first randomized controlled trial of screening mammography enrolled 62,000 women, and it took 8 years to publish the first results from the study showing a reduction in breast cancer mortality. Reaching the first consensus on recommendations for screening mammography required additional studies and demonstration projects that lasted many more years (Lerner, 2001).

Because multiple randomized controlled trials have demonstrated the effectiveness of mammography in combination with follow-up therapy, it may not be necessary to require that each new technology developed for breast cancer screening be evaluated in a new randomized clinical trial. Instead, the technology could be evaluated as outlined above, with the reference standard being a combination of mammography, pathological verification of cancer, and follow-up observation. A possible concern with this approach is that the new test may be detecting different types of breast cancer that respond differently to follow-up treatment and that would therefore lead to a different level of effectiveness if evaluated in combination with treatment.

## COST-EFFECTIVENESS

Cost-effectiveness analysis provides a framework for comparison of the economic efficiency of different therapies or programs that produce health. Although sometimes misconstrued as a method for assessing the "cost savings" from health interventions, cost-effectiveness analysis is in fact a measure of the relative value—the amount of health produced per dollar spent—of alternative therapies. In a cost-effectiveness ratio, two interventions are compared. The numerator of the ratio represents the difference in cost in dollars of the two alternatives, and the denominator represents the difference in health effects. The denominator is generally measured in years of life or the number of quality-adjusted life years (QALYs) gained (Table 5-2). The QALY represents a measure that combines survival and health-related quality of life. Because of the extensive gains made in the treatment of symptoms associated with chronic diseases such as diabetes and arthritis, a measure that captures both length of life and morbidity is an increasingly important gauge of the effectiveness of a health intervention. In addition, because all health care is not benign, that is, many diagnostic tests and treatments can initiate a series of untoward health outcomes, QALYs provide additional value in being able to capture the negative effects of health-related quality of life. For example, in the case where an antibiotic therapy were to "cure" an infectious disease but, as a side effect, induced permanent hearing loss, QALYs would record the increased life expectancy positively but could also capture the decrement in health-related quality of life associated with deafness. A major difficulty with this approach is objectively defining quality-

**TABLE 5-2**   Cost, Effects, Utility, and Benefits of Treating Patients with Disease $X$ with Two Alternate Strategies, Treatment A and Treatment B

| Strategy | Treatment Costs | Effectiveness (Life Expectancy) | Utility (Quality of Life) | Utility (Quality-Adjusted Life Expectancy) | Benefits |
|---|---|---|---|---|---|
| Treatment A | $20,000 | 4.5 years | 0.80 | 3.6 QALYs* | $4,000 |
| Treatment B | $10,000 | 3.5 years | 0.90 | 3.15 QALYs | $2,000 |

Incremental cost-effectiveness ratio = ($20,000 - $10,000) ÷ (4.5 years – 3.5 years) = $10,000 per life-year gained.

Incremental cost-utility ratio = ($20,000 - $10,000) ÷ (3.6 QALYs – 3.15 QALYs) = $22,222 per QALY gained.

Incremental cost-benefit ratio = ($20,000 - $10,000) ÷ ($4000 - $2000) = 5

SOURCE: Detsky and Naglie (1990).

of-life measures, particularly when comparing or ranking different aspects of life quality. The results of these analyses can be quite different depending on how quality is defined and measured.

Efficacy (performance of a therapy under ideal conditions) or effectiveness (performance of a therapy under real-life conditions) information for cost-effectiveness analyses is generally gathered from clinical trials or observational studies. The strongest measures of effectiveness come from studies in which the experimental design permits direct linkage of the intervention with changes in survival or quality of life. For screening tests, this linkage can be elusive. For example, although it may be possible to demonstrate that a particular screening test detects a disease earlier in the disease process than another test does, that information alone does not provide adequate information about the effectiveness of the test in either prolonging life or improving its quality. The identification and treatment of tumors at an earlier point in the progression of the disease by screening does not guarantee that the rate of tumor progression will be altered or that the ultimate outcome will be changed. (See the discussion of lead-time and length biases in Chapter 1.) Furthermore, a screening test may detect lesions that would not cause death but would precipitate potentially harmful (or costly) medical follow-up (overdiagnosis) (see Chapter 1).

Cost-effectiveness analyses of screening mammography for the detection of breast cancer have relied upon a relatively extensive literature that has demonstrated that early detection by mammography can extend survival for certain groups of women. Most studies have found that the cost per years of life gained for screening mammography falls within a generally accepted range ($50,000 or less/QALY) (Gold et al., 1996), although the cost-effectiveness varies depending on age, screening interval, and the assumed benefit of screening (percent decrease in breast cancer mortality) (Brown and Fintor, 1993; Rosenquist and Lindfors, 1998).

Recently, questions have been raised about the potential cost-effectiveness of full-field digital mammography (FFDM) compared with that of film-screen mammography (FSM). The cost of the new machines will be significantly greater (General Electric FFDM machines cost ~$450,000 per unit, whereas FSM machines cost ~$70,000 per unit), but to date, the sensitivity and specificity of FFDM have not been shown to be vastly improved over those of FSM. A simulation model for assessing the cost-effectiveness of breast cancer diagnosis in the United States suggests that an increased cost of $20 per digital mammogram could be cost-effective and could produce an overall cost savings, even if the positive predictive value (cases of breast cancer accurately detected) increased by as little as 2 percent, because of the reduced numbers of unnecessary follow-up biopsies (Nields and Galaty, 1998). The investigators noted, however, that the cost-effectiveness of digital mammography as a screening tool is more difficult to model and may require prospective, randomized trials.

A number of studies have also compared various imaging and biopsy techniques to determine the most cost-effective diagnostic modality for women whose mammograms suggest a suspicious lesion. For example, core-needle biopsy and magnetic resonance imaging (MRI) may be cost-effective diagnostic alternatives to open biopsy (Doyle et al., 1995; Hillner et al., 1996; Hrung et al., 1999). However, the model used in the MRI study was extremely sensitive to changes in estimates of the sensitivity and specificity of MRI, which can be quite variable depending on the patient population, the type of imaging technique used, and the diagnostic criteria used (Hrung et al., 1999b). For palpable lesions, fine-needle aspiration and ultrasonography may also be cost-effective alternatives to open biopsy for certain patients (Vetto et al., 1996; Rubin et al., 1997).

Data linking the newer breast cancer detection technologies to reduced breast cancer mortality rates for women are lacking. To conduct a cost-effectiveness analysis of any of the technologies examined in this report, investigators would need to estimate the level of effectiveness of a technology in extending the length of life or would need to estimate the improvements in health-related quality of life that would accompany use of the technology. Cost-effectiveness analyses that are done under speculative circumstances such as these are referred as "what-if" analyses (Siegel et al., 1996). For example, a recent computer modeling study suggests that MRI screening for young women at high risk (on the basis of germ-line mutations or a strong family history) may be cost-effective (Plevritis, 2000a). Computer models that simulate a variety of screening protocols and trial results could perhaps also be helpful in selecting the most promising trial design needed for evaluation of new detection technologies by inferring long-term outcomes from short-term end points (Plevritis, 2000b). This could potentially lead to a reduction in both the duration and the cost of screening trials. Although from a policy perspective such models may provide useful information about the potential efficacy of particular medical interventions, from a coverage perspective they are inadequate, since they are not based on a proven clinical effect from experimental trials.

Cost-effectiveness analysis is most straightforward when an alternative technology gives the same or a better result but at a lower cost. Unfortunately, this is rarely the case. Thus, the issue becomes a question of how much better the outcome is and how much one should spend to get that outcome. In the absence of societal agreement on how much of the gross national product should be spent on health care, it will be difficult to reach a consensus on the use of cost-effectiveness analysis in making coverage decisions. Because the United States does not have a global budget for medical care (in contrast to the situations in Canada and the

United Kingdom), the pressure to decide what should be prioritized for payment with a defined pool of money is lacking, and there is an aversion on the part of policy makers, clinicians, and the public to initiate discussions on such topics.

Physicians, manufacturers, and patients have often opposed considerations of cost-effectiveness in technology assessment (Braslow et al., 1998), but their reasons may differ. Although physicians and patients are to some degree aligned in wanting "the best" no matter what the cost, manufacturers are more influenced by their need to sell their products in the marketplace. FDA and HCFA are not authorized to review the cost-effectiveness of medical devices, and at present, neither HCFA nor private insurers are explicitly using cost-effectiveness analyses in their coverage decisions. However, cost-effectiveness analyses have been performed for some technologies in recent years by private organizations such as the TEC program of BCBSA. This information is supplemental to rather than an integral part of the clinical TEC assessment.

As greater consensus is achieved regarding the best way to incorporate costs into the coverage decision-making process, cost-effectiveness analyses of competing imaging technologies may become increasingly important. This may be particularly true in diagnostic imaging, in which alternative tests may be available for a given condition. Cost-effectiveness is not just an issue of the absolute cost of a technology but is a measure of how that cost and all downstream costs compare to the current standard of care. If a new test is more costly than an established test but detects disease at an earlier stage, when treatment is more effective or treatment costs are substantially lower, the cost-effectiveness ratio of the diagnostic test will be more favorable. What appears initially to be an expensive technology may become a more attractive coverage option for insurers.

## LIMITATIONS OF TECHNOLOGY ASSESSMENT PROCESS

The technology assessment process is complicated by the fact that technology development is often incremental and ongoing. If new technologies came out of the initial research and development phase in complete and final form, technology assessment might be relatively straightforward because new technologies could be evaluated one by one, with the good ones accepted and the poor ones rejected. However, most technologies that ultimately achieve widespread use go through a long period of development, variation, assessment of what they are good for and what they are not good for, and discovery of how to use them effectively (Gelijns and Rosenberg, 1999). During this process, there is a considerable amount of two-way interaction between research and development on the one side and actual experience with clinical use on the other. Physicians who are using the device in practice provide valuable feedback, including aspects that may not have been considered by the manufacturers. This information is different from the information about the efficacy of the device acquired earlier in the process for FDA approval. Thus, the process of technology development and diffusion can be caught in a sort of catch-22 that could potentially prevent technologies from reaching their full potential. Successful diffusion depends on whether a device is covered, but a device may need to be used and improved over time as it diffuses into everyday practice before it is deemed effective enough for general coverage.

Because of this conundrum, the concept of "conditional coverage" has been explored as a potential way to allow new medical technologies to enter the market before a final and definitive yes-or-no decision about coverage is made. Conditional coverage in either the public or private sector refers to limited, temporary coverage under specified conditions to allow collection of data that can be used to determine the value of a technology and to set a definitive coverage policy. Although neither the utility of this form of coverage nor the barriers to its implementation are fully understood, a recent report by the Medical Technology Leadership Forum[11] identified the steps that have already been taken in the public and private sectors to facilitate coverage of experimental technologies and ascertained some remaining barriers to broad application of the concept.

Once a technology is adopted into practice, it can be difficult to restrict its use even if no evidence supports its effectiveness (unless direct harm is documented). It has been estimated that only 20 percent of medical technologies in current use have documented evidence of effectiveness (Braslow et al., 1998). However, vested economic interests, disputes over withdrawal of coverage, and political pressures make it difficult to restrict their use. Even the emergence of newer, better, or cheaper technologies does not necessarily lead to the elimination of older technologies from clinical use (Eisenberg, 1999).

In practice, there are few reassessments of "old technologies" that are already disseminated, despite arguments that this type of activity is greatly needed (Banta and Thacker, 1990). In theory, any technology, whether disseminated or not, could be subject to assessment and reassess-

---

[11]The Medical Technology Leadership Forum is a nonprofit, educational enterprise supported by members representing the broad range of leaders in the medical community. It has engaged in a series of explorations of issues relating to evidence of value for medical technologies, and in July 1999, it convened a summit on conditional coverage of new medical technologies. A panel of experts representing both the public and the private sectors included individuals from NIH, FDA, AHQR, HCFA, academia, the clinical research community, and those who provide and pay for medical services.

ment based on the best available and current scientific data. However, current efforts in technology assessment have focused on new and emerging technologies before they have been disseminated. This is especially true of higher-cost technologies, which also tend to be more controversial and create more pressure for both an assessment and a formal coverage decision. Greater emphasis on technology assessment for both developing and disseminated technologies will require commitment and resources from both the public and the private sectors, but it could make the system more efficient and effective in the long run.

Some of the major challenges to developing and implementing a conditional coverage program include defining an evidence threshold at which new technologies would be considered eligible for conditional coverage, setting guidelines for the timeliness of conditional and subsequent definitive coverage decisions, and assigning financial responsibilities for the process. The criteria used to qualify technologies for definitive coverage decisions may serve as a model for the development of less stringent criteria for conditional coverage. Different decision paradigms would most likely need to be developed for different types of technologies (e.g., drugs versus devices) and would reflect the same issues discussed above with regard to definitive coverage decisions. For example, in the case of cancer screening, the evidence needed for a definitive coverage decision would ideally include reduced disease-specific mortality and morbidity rather than simply the indirect measures of sensitivity, specificity, and so forth, but it can take years to accumulate these data, so the time lines for conditional coverage may be longer.

Local Medicare coverage can be another way of allowing technologies to diffuse slowly, but this approach has its own complexities (Strongin, 1998). In this case, a national coverage decision could be made at a later date on the basis of an assessment of the results obtained in the areas where local coverage was previously approved. However, a negative decision at the national level could then be problematic in the areas in which the technology was formerly covered. Furthermore, because the local decision-making process is not standardized, it can be confusing and frustrating for both patients and providers. It could also raise the question of fairness by those not covered in the initial study area.

## NCI BREAST CANCER SURVEILLANCE
## PROGRAM TO MEASURE EFFECTIVENESS

Technology assessments are perhaps most useful when they reflect everyday medical practice rather than just the experience of the technology developers in controlled environments. The benefit of medical technologies as predicted from controlled clinical trials may not be realized in general clinical practice because there are more variations in both the target population and the way in which the technology is used. Who should do or fund these effectiveness studies, however? What are the incentives? Once a technology has been approved for coverage, a company has very little incentive to carry out large, expensive surveillance studies to assess the effectiveness of disseminated products. In the case of cancer screening technologies, the National Cancer Institute (NCI) has made some effort to fill this gap, in part because of a congressional mandate.

The Applied Research Program of NCI supports research to examine the dissemination of cancer screening technologies, to understand factors that influence that dissemination, and to assess the accuracy of screening at the population level. In addition to extramural research activities, research programs have focused on the evaluation and development of methods and national database resources. The Breast Cancer Surveillance Consortium[12] (BCSC) in particular was established to monitor the effectiveness and impact of breast cancer screening programs and to address issues that can be adequately examined only with a very large sample drawn from diverse geographic and practice settings.

NCI began pilot studies in 1990 to appraise the feasibility of creating a breast cancer surveillance system to determine if screening in community practice resulted in breast cancer mortality rate reductions comparable to those demonstrated in clinical trials. With a mandate from the Mammography Quality Standards Act (MQSA) to create such systems, NCI established BCSC in 1994 to evaluate population-based screening mammography in the United States.[13]

The three major objectives of the Surveillance Consortium are to:

- Enhance the understanding of breast cancer screening practices in the United States through an assessment of the accuracy, cost, and quality of screening programs and the relation of these practices to changes in breast cancer mortality or other shorter-term outcomes, such as stage at diagnosis or survival.

- Foster collaborative research among consortium participants to examine issues such as regional and health care system differences in the provision of screening services and subsequent diagnostic evaluations.

- Provide a foundation for the conduct of clinical and basic science research that can improve understanding of breast cancer etiology and prognosis. The intent is to collect a core set of pathological data on established prognostic indicators and to provide the capability to examine the prognostic potential of other, more investigational indicators.

---

[12]http://www-dccps.ims.nci.nih.gov/ARP/BCSC.
[13]BCSC also works with the International Breast Cancer Screening Network.

The consortium's database contains information on more than 3 million screening mammogram examinations and more than 24,000 breast cancer cases contributed by eight medical centers across the nation. The consortium has made an effort to collect data on women across a wide range of ages and from various racial or ethnic groups.[14] The first major effort of the consortium was to create a standard set of carefully defined variables to facilitate pooling of data with sample sizes sufficient to examine various factors in subgroups for which the number of cancers in any one study is relatively low, such as younger women, women with a family history of breast cancer, or some ethnic or racial groups.

In addition to its intended purpose of evaluating population-based screening mammography in the United States, the database serves as a resource for future research. For example, BCSC studies are examining the hypothesis that the accuracy of screening mammography varies by biological characteristics, the stage of the breast tumor, and the rate of growth of the breast tumor. Furthermore, the BCSC database will provide information on demographic characteristics, risk factors, clinical characteristics, and treatments for women who subsequently develop breast cancer. It will also provide data on a large population-based sample of women at high risk for breast cancer, including those with a family history of breast cancer or benign breast disease. Therefore, this resource may be particularly useful for the identification of patients relevant for research into the population prevalence of genetic and other biological markers for breast cancer risk and prognosis and research into the potential associations of these markers with other known breast cancer risk factors. Data from BCSC will provide estimates of the prevalence of subsequent diagnostic follow-up and information about means of improving the communication of risks and benefits of screening. The mammography registry may also serve as a resource for intervention trials to study ways to improve compliance with recommendations for screening mammography.

## REIMBURSEMENT

Reimbursement rates can vary greatly, depending on the location, health insurance carrier, and other factors, even if coverage decisions are

---

[14]The age distributions of women currently receiving mammography within the database are 8%, 31%, 26%, 19%, and 16% for women ages less than 40, 40 to 49, 50 to 59, 60 to 69, and 70 and older, respectively. The racial makeup of the study population is as follows: white, 67 percent; Hispanic, 7 percent; African-American, 4 percent; Asian and Pacific Islanders, 2 percent; and American Indians, 2 percent. The remaining 18 percent were categorized as "Other/Unknown."

relatively uniform. Reimbursement by Medicare for physician services is determined by three factors: practice expenses, physician work, and professional liability (reviewed by Farria and Feig [2000]). Each component is assigned a numerical value (a relative value unit [RVU]) that represents its relative contribution to the expense incurred in delivering that service. The practice expense component (~41 percent of the total) was initially based on historical Medicare charge data, but a new method based on actual practice expense survey data (derived from 1995 to 1997) is being phased in.

The new system also differentiates the various facilities in which a service can be performed. (Under this new system, the RVU for diagnostic mammography is expected to decrease [Farria and Feig, 2000]). The physician work component (~54 percent of the total) is determined by several factors, including the time required to perform the service, mental effort and judgment, the technical skill required, and stress due to the potential risk to the patient. The malpractice component is based on Medicare procedure charge data from 1991 and data from the American Medical Association, but in the future this component will also be based on actual resource information rather than historical data.

Screening mammography is unique in that it is not reimbursed using RVUs, but rather by a special statutory rule (Farria and Feig, 2000). The payment rate, which is updated annually, is split between a technical fee (68 percent) and a professional fee (32 percent).

In the private sector the payment rate for mammography varies from $42 to $150, but it most commonly falls in the $60 to $70 range (Farria and Feig, 2000). For Medicare reimbursement, the 1999 cap was $66.22 for screening mammography (Figure 5-2). Radiologists have argued that the reimbursement for mammography is too low for the time, effort, and interpretive skill that it requires compared with that required for other imaging procedures (Farria and Feig, 2000; Feig, 2000a,b)[15] (Table 5-3). The additional costs associated with new mammography technologies such as computer-assisted detection and digital detection are not included in the reimbursement rates.

MQSA may add additional financial pressures to mammography facilities. MQSA requires all mammography facilities to meet minimum quality standards for equipment, radiologists, physicists, and technologists. Regulations require extensive records of medical audits and outcome analyses, personnel qualifications, and medical reporting. Thus,

---

[15]In March 2000, the American College of Radiology formally requested that HCFA consider an increase in the physician work component of the RVU for diagnostic mammography for this reason.

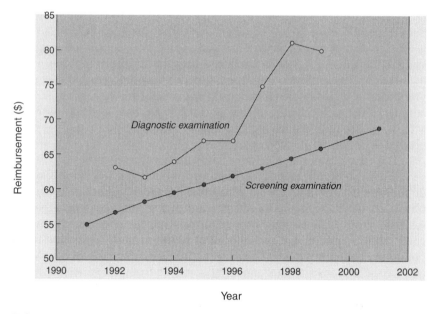

**FIGURE 5-2** Medicare reimbursement rates for mammography. Filled circles = screening examination; open circle = diagnostic examination. SOURCE: Farria and Feig (2000).

MQSA increases costs to facilities, but it does not mandate reimbursement levels to cover those costs. Inspections to ensure compliance with MQSA cost each facility $1,549 annually, and the average annual cost required to reach compliance with MQSA is $18,000 (Inman, 1998). These fees may be particularly burdensome for smaller, lower-volume centers (Inman, 1998; Eastern Research Group, 1996).

If the reimbursement rates for mammography are in fact artificially low, this could also have a negative effect on how new technologies are compared with the current standard of care with respect to cost-effectiveness. HCFA has recently proposed linking both coverage and reimbursement rates to patient outcomes (*Federal Register*, 2000). Since the commercial sphere tends to closely follow the actions of Medicare, if these criteria are adopted by HCFA, they may be used by health plans as well.

From a reimbursement perspective, new technologies that replicate current techniques or that make incremental improvements may have a particularly difficult time compared with those that are completely novel or that offer major improvements over technologies that are the current state of the art. A relevant model for this phenomenon is the ThinPrep Pap Test[16] for cervical cancer screening. After several years of testing, the ThinPrep Pap Test was shown to have a small positive effect on patient

**TABLE 5-3** Medicare Reimbursement for Selected Radiology Procedures, 1999

| Procedure | Professional | | Technical | |
|---|---|---|---|---|
| | RVU | Payment ($) | RVU | Payment ($) |
| Screening mammography[a] | NA[a] | 21.5 | NA[a] | 45.8 |
| Bilateral diagnostic mammography | 0.90 | 31.30 | 1.40 | 48.60 |
| Unilateral diagnostic mammography | 0.74 | 25.70 | 1.14 | 39.60 |
| Breast sonography | 0.71 | 24.70 | 1.13 | 39.20 |
| MRI, unilateral breast | 2.15 | 74.70 | 19.10 | 663.80 |
| Stereotactic core breast biopsy | 2.13 | 74.00 | 6.20 | 270.20 |
| Wire needle localization | 0.73 | 25.40 | 1.40 | 48.60 |
| Aortogram | 0.71 | 24.70 | 13.67 | 474.80 |
| Chest radiograph | 0.29 | 10.10 | 0.67 | 23.30 |
| Foot radiograph | 0.21 | 7.30 | 0.53 | 18.40 |
| MRI of brain | 1.96 | 68.10 | 12.15 | 422.00 |
| CT of abdomen with contrast | 1.68 | 58.30 | 7.42 | 257.70 |
| CT of brain without contrast | 1.13 | 39.20 | 5.13 | 178.20 |
| Three-phase bone scan | 1.35 | 49.60 | 5.18 | 179.90 |
| Barium enema | 0.92 | 32.00 | 1.86 | 64.60 |
| Transvaginal ultrasound | 0.92 | 32.00 | 1.66 | 57.70 |

[a]Screening mammography services for Medicare beneficiaries are not reimbursed by using RVUs but are reimbursed under a special statutory rule (Farria and Feig, 2000).

outcomes compared with standard Pap smears. However, after health plans had agreed to cover it, the level of reimbursement was sometimes half of what the company was requesting. Meanwhile, several other related technologies, such as PapNet,[17] were not able to demonstrate significantly better outcomes, and some are no longer on the market (Brown and Garber, 1999; Hutchinson et al., 2000).

## SUMMARY

Developers of new technologies have major hurdles to clear in seeking coverage and reimbursement. Payers are increasingly looking for evidence of improved patient outcomes in making coverage decisions. That is, if improved outcomes cannot be demonstrated, then coverage may be denied or the level of reimbursement may be low. Given the immense and growing expenditures for medical care, more efforts to incorporate cost-effectiveness analysis as an aid to decision making may also be undertaken in the future. Many new technologies are only marginally better than the current standard of care, but they are also substantially more costly. These are the technologies for which coverage decisions will be the most difficult. In the absence of an ulimited budget for health care, decision makers in the health care industry may be unlikely to endorse spending on technical innovations unless a new device or test offers a real opportunity to lessen the disease burden by reducing morbidity and mortality.

The uncertainty of coverage and reimbursement decisions can have an indirect effect on technology development. Expectations that research firms and investors have about the market for new technologies affect the projects they choose to pursue. Uncertainty about the scientific outcome of research is inevitable, but uncertainty about the market profitability also results from the unpredictability of coverage decisions by public and private health insurers. HCFA coverage policy has been changing and evolving in recent years, adding to the high-risk atmosphere for device developers who face uncertainties about the specific coverage criteria that will be applied to devices. As in the case of FDA approval (discussed in

---

[16]With the ThinPrep Pap Test, the physician collects the cervical cell sample in the traditional manner, but rather than smearing it directly onto a glass slide, the collection device is rinsed in a vial of preservative solution. The cervical cell sample is then dispersed and filtered to reduce the levels of blood, mucus, and inflammation before applying a thin layer of the cervical cells to a glass slide. The slide is evaluated for cellular abnormalities by a cytologist, as usual.

[17]PapNet is a computer-assisted detection system for cervical cancer screening. It was developed to double check Pap smears that were deemed normal by a cytologist.

Chapter 4), the dominant model for HCFA coverage decisions is based on drug development, which is not always applicable to the medical device industry.

Unfortunately, the process of technology development, evaluation, and adoption can also be quite slow and is generally iterative. That is, most technologies that ultimately achieve widespread use go through successive stages of development, variation, and appraisal of actual experience in the marketplace. For screening technologies in particular, proving a reduction in disease-specific mortality and morbidity due to screening is a long and difficult process, requiring large study populations and extended periods of time. It took more than 10 years from the start of the first randomized clinical trial before consensus was reached that mammography actually decreased breast cancer mortality as a result of early detection. For this reason, most new breast cancer detection technologies have been or are being evaluated by diagnostic studies rather than screening studies. However, once a technology has FDA approval for diagnostic use, manufacturers are often likely to advocate use of the technology for screening purposes.

One potential way to avoid this situation would be to use a conditional coverage policy that would provide a mechanism to bring new screening technologies into the clinic, but only in the context of clinical trials for assessment of the clinical outcome. When potential screening devices meet basic standards for safety and accuracy (sensitivity and specificity), FDA, NCI, HCFA, and private insurers should coordinate the oversight and support of clinical trials to assess patient outcomes through approval of an investigational device exemption from FDA and conditional coverage from the insurers. HCFA and private insurers would provide conditional coverage for use of the technologies in approved clinical trials, whereas the technology sponsors and NCI could cover additional costs attributable to the study design. Data review at appropriate intervals by all participants would determine whether the technology is sufficiently effective to obtain approval from FDA and to change the conditional coverage status to approved coverage for the general population (for those deemed sufficiently effective).

Such a mechanism would not only prevent new technologies approved for diagnostic use from being widely adopted as screening tools before their effectiveness for screening is proven, but it would also make it easier for the technology sponsors to conduct the clinical trials needed to gather the necessary data on outcomes. Data on diagnostic sensitivity and specificity are simply not adequate for assessment of the potential screening value of either newer technologies or technical improvements to established technologies. However, screening trials that could evaluate the effects of recently introduced breast cancer detection technologies on patient outcomes have not been designed thus far.

When FSM was introduced, FDA approval was not required, and it represented a "void-filling" technology. As a result, new technologies face a much different level of assessment that will likely include comparison with mammography. The adoption process will be complicated in other ways as well. These issues will be revisited in Chapter 6.

# 6
# Dissemination: Increasing the Use and Availability of New Technologies

A positive coverage decision from Medicare or private insurers does not guarantee adoption of new technologies. Even after the hurdles of approval, coverage, and reimbursement have been cleared, the adoption and dissemination of new technologies will ultimately depend on whether consumers and providers find them acceptable. Many factors can influence the extent to which new devices or procedures are used. For example, health care providers must be educated about the new technology and are unlikely to use it unless they believe that it will be beneficial for their patients. Providers also need to be reimbursed at a level that will allow them to recover the costs of using the technology. In this regard, "big-ticket" technologies may have a more difficult time with adoption than low-price items.

It is essential to educate women about new screening and diagnostic technologies as well. Women are not likely to undergo medical procedures unless they believe that the potential benefits outweigh the potential risks. Medical technologies must also be readily available in their own communities if women are to take advantage of them. Even in the case of a highly accurate breast cancer screening tool, it would be truly effective only if it was widely available and acceptable to women and used routinely by them.

The developers of new technologies will undoubtedly face questions about each of these issues during the adoption process. Much is already known about the adoption and dissemination of film-screen mammography, and this knowledge may prove instructive for the developers of other developing technologies. Experience from current mammography programs suggests that outreach to women, education of women and providers, and access to facilities and services may be as important as technical factors in saving lives.

## HISTORY OF DISSEMINATION OF MAMMOGRAPHY

Mammography provides a good example of how social, cultural, and political factors, in addition to experimental data, can influence the dissemination of medical technologies into clinical practice because even the best scientific information is subject to interpretation (reviewed by Lerner, 2001).

Although the use of X-ray imaging for the detection of breast cancer was first suggested in the early years of the 20th century, mammography did not begin to emerge as an accepted technology until the 1960s (see Figure 1-1). Between 1930 and 1960 a number of technical innovations were introduced to produce higher-quality images that were more reproducible and easier to interpret. Subsequently, the developers of the technology promoted its use, and some physicians began ordering mammograms to help with the diagnosis of complicated cases in which the physical examination was inconclusive.

The early reports of mammography's ability to detect small cancers coincided with increased public education efforts on the part of organizations like the American Cancer Society (ACS), which had launched a "war on breast cancer." Before the introduction of mammography, ACS encouraged women to perform breast self-examinations and to seek medical attention for any breast lumps that they found. The advent of mammography was seen as a potentially powerful new weapon in this war. Even in the absence of clinical trials to test the value of breast self-examination or mammography, earlier detection was intuitively thought to be a good thing.

As the results of the first randomized controlled trial for the assessment of mammography as a screening tool were published over a number of years, the real potential of mammography to reduce breast cancer mortality seemed to have been realized (about 30 percent fewer deaths among screened women than among unscreened controls for women over age 50). The screening technology then began to diffuse more widely, in large part because of a demonstration project (a noncontrolled study) organized by the National Cancer Institute (NCI) and ACS. When preliminary results suggested that screening resulted in breast cancer detection at an earlier stage, the press and anticancer organizations like ACS enthusiastically spread the news. Anecdotal stories of women, both famous and unknown, whose cancers had been detected by mammography added to the belief that screening was a great success. Women finally felt that they had some control over a terrifying disease.

By the late 1970s, mammography had diffused more widely into common clinical practice, but it had also become a source of considerable controversy. Advocates of the technology were enthusiastic about its ability to detect smaller, potentially more curable cancers, but critics questioned whether mammography, particularly for women age 50 and younger, actually caused more harm than benefit. Initial fears about the potential dangers of radiation exposure have largely been put to rest (although some questions remain for specific groups of women [see Chapter 1]), but concerns continued to build about the lead-time and length biases of screening and the possibility of overdiagnosis due to screening mammography (see Chapter 1). Most importantly, the analysis of the data from the original screening trial showed that the decreased death rate was statistically significant only among women age 50 and older. Many statisticians and some clinicians had recommended additional randomized trials for women between the ages of 40 and 50 rather than the demonstration project, but the organizers of the project had rejected this suggestion. Now it was the controversy over screening of women in this age group that received considerable attention from the press.

In an effort to help resolve the debate about the use of mammography in younger women, the National Institutes of Health (NIH) convened an expert panel for a consensus conference in 1977. The panel agreed that annual screening mammography of women over age 50 was appropriate but recommended that women ages 40 to 49 receive a screening mammogram only if they had previously had breast cancer or had a strong family history of breast cancer.

In the 1980s NCI, the American College of Radiology, and 11 other medical organizations followed the lead of ACS in recommending routine screening mammograms for younger women based on the findings of the demonstration project. Dissent reemerged in 1993, however, when NCI withdrew its support for this policy because of the growing amount of data available from a series of randomized controlled trials of mammography that included women in their 40s. Another NIH consensus panel was convened in 1997 in an attempt to resolve the issue. The panel again concluded that there was not enough evidence to support routine screening mammography for women in their 40s, but the controversy only escalated and many organizations continued to recommend screening for women in their 40s (see below and Table 6-1). Even the U.S. Senate joined in the fray, voting 98 to 0 to encourage NCI's National Cancer Advisory Board to reject the consensus panel's conclusions.

In retrospect, several commentators have pointed out that the experts on opposing sides of the screening debate have not really disagreed about what the data showed (a 16 to 18 percent reduction in breast cancer mor-

**TABLE 6-1**   Breast Cancer Screening Guidelines from Various Organizations (

Organization

| Age | ACS | ACR | AMA | NCI |
|---|---|---|---|---|
| 20-39 | Monthly BSE; CBE every 3 years. Women at higher risk should consult with their physician about beginning mammography screening before age 40. | Same as ACS | Same as ACS | No recommendation Women at higher risk should consult with their physician about beginning mammography screening before age 40. |
| 40-49 | Monthly BSE; begin annual mammography and CBE at age 40. Women at higher risk should consult with their physician to determine their mammography schedule in their 40s. | Same as ACS | Same as ACS | Mammography every 1–2 years for women in their 40s at average risk of breast cancer. Women at higher risk should consult with their physician to determine their mammography schedule in their 40s. CBE every 1–2 years. |
| 50+ | Annual mammography and CBE, monthly BSE. | Same as ACS | Same as ACS | Mammography every 1–2 years for women ages 50 and older |

NOTE: Abbreviations: ACS, American Cancer Society; ACR, American College of Radiology; AMA, American Medical Association; NCI, National Cancer Institute; AAFP, Ameri-

| AAFP | USPSTF | ACOG | ACP |
|------|--------|------|-----|
| Monthly BSE, CBE every 1–3 years for women ages 30–39 | Insufficient evidence to recommend for or against routine mammography or CBE or the teaching of BSE. | Same as ACS | No recommendation |
| Monthly BSE, annual CBE | Insufficient evidence to recommend for or against routine mammography or CBE or the teaching of BSE. | Monthly BSE, annual CBE, mammography every 1–2 years | Recommends against screening for women under age 50 |
| Monthly BSE, annual CBE, and mammography | Mammography with or without CBE every 1–2 years. Insufficient evidence to recommend for or against routine mammography or CBE for women ages 70 and older. | Monthly BSE, annual CBE, and mammography | Mammography every 2 years for women ages 50–74. Recommends against screening for women over age 75. |

can Academy of Family Physicians; USPSTF, United States Preventive Services Task Force; ACOG, American College of Obstetricians and Gynecologists; ACP, American College of Physicians; BSE, breast self-examination; CBE, clinical breast examination.
SOURCE: U.S. Preventive Services Task Force (1996).

tality, about half as great as that among older women) but, rather, how the data should be interpreted and acted upon. Opponents argued that 2,500 healthy women under age 50 would have to receive regular screening to extend one life, leading to many unnecessary interventions in women without any actual breast disease. They also were concerned by the lag time (10 years or more) between screening initiation and decreased mortality in women under age 50. The controversy continues today, even though mammography has been more thoroughly evaluated than any other screening test.

## EVIDENCE ON USE AND ACCEPTANCE OF MAMMOGRAPHY BY WOMEN

The use of screening mammography has increased greatly over the past decade (Blackman et al., 1999; Makuc et al., 1999; U.S. Department of Health and Human Services, 2000) (Figure 6-1). The percentage of women age 50 and over who reported having a recent mammogram rose to 69 percent in 1998, up from 61 percent in 1994 and 27.4 percent in 1987 (U.S. Department of Health and Human Services, 2000). However, despite this overall increase, many women do not follow the screening guidelines advocated by a variety of medical institutions by getting mammograms at the recommended intervals. One recent study found that 27 percent of women had the age-appropriate number of screening examinations, whereas 59 percent of women had been screened within the previous 2 years (Phillips et al., 1998). For 1998, the estimated number of U.S. civilian noninstitutionalized women over age 40 who reported that they had not received a mammogram within the past 2 years was 19.4 million, representing 33 percent of that population (Table 6-2). In comparison, the number of women in this age group who reported that they had not received a Pap test as a screen for cervical cancer in the past 3 years (the recommended screening interval) was 14.5 million, or 24.7 percent of that population. The percentage of women who had "recently" received a Pap test may be higher because of the longer screening interval, but other factors could also contribute to the difference. For example, Pap testing can be performed during a physical examination and thus does not require an additional visit, as mammography does. Notably, women between the ages of 40 and 49 are more likely to undergo screening for cervical cancer than for breast cancer, whereas the opposite is true for women over age 65.

Despite the generally positive attitude of most women toward screening mammography (Baines et al., 1990; Gram et al., 1990), some barriers clearly exist. Many reasons have been cited for the lack of breast cancer screening at recommended intervals, including limited access to health

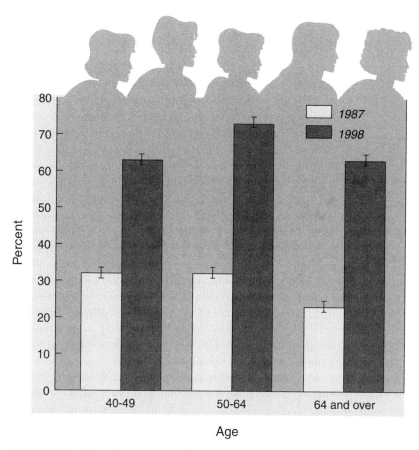

**FIGURE 6-1** Use of mammography by women 40 years of age and over, 1987 and 1998. Percent of women having a mammogram within the last two years. SOURCE: U.S. Department of Health and Human Services, 2000 (www.cdc/gov/nchs/products/pubs/pubd/hus/hus/htm). Data are based on the National Vital Statistics System, National Center for Health Statistics..

care and health insurance, lack of education and physician referral, pain or discomfort from the procedure, fear of what could be found, beliefs that mammograms are necessary only when symptoms arise, and inconvenience because of the location of the test facility (Baines et al., 1990; Rimer et al., 1989; Vernon et al., 1990). Some women with disabilities have also found mammography facilities to be inaccessible to them (Haran, 2000), and a report by the Centers for Disease Control and Prevention (CDC) found that women over age 65 with functional limitations were

**TABLE 6-2**   Number of U.S. Women (ages 40 and older) in 1998 Who Had Not Undergone Recent Screening Tests for Breast and Cervical Cancer, by age

| Age Group | Number of women without a Pap test in the last 3 years, in millions[a] (percent) | Number of women without a mammogram in the last 2 years, in millions [a, b](percent) | Estimates of the total civilian noninstitutionalized female population, in millions |
|---|---|---|---|
| 40 and older | 14.5 (24.7) | 19.4 (33.0) | 58.8 |
| 40–49 | 3.1 (15.1) | 7.5 +/− 0.25 (36.6) | 20.5 |
| 50–64 | 4.0 (20.3) | 5.2 +/− 0.20 (26.4) | 19.7 |
| 65 and older | 7.5 (40.3) | 6.7 +/− 0.22 (36.0) | 18.6 |

[a]The screening interval for the given type of cancer that is recommended by USPSTF (with the exception of mammography for women aged 40 and over, which is not currently recommended by USPSTF)

[b]Values are means +/− standard errors.

SOURCE: Diane Makuc, Ph.D., Director, Division of Health and Utilization Analysis National Center for Health Statistics, 1998 data.

less likely than other women their age to have ever had a mammogram (Centers for Disease Control and Prevention, 1998).

Some of the major issues pertaining to the use of mammography are discussed below and were described in more detail in a recent Institute of Medicine (IOM) report, *Ensuring Quality Cancer Care* (Institute of Medicine, 1999). The authors of that report concluded that the underuse of screening mammography to detect breast cancer early, in conjunction with lack of adherence to diagnostic standards and treatment regimens, leads to reduced survival rates and, in some cases, compromised quality of life.

A great variety of interventions targeted toward women have been developed with the intent of increasing breast cancer screening rates, including multimedia educational interventions and peer counseling. Studies have shown that diverse campaign strategies directed toward women are needed to alter the screening behaviors of different groups of women, especially among medically underserved populations (Abbott et al., 1999; Wismar, 1999). The rate of mammography use varies by factors such as age, socioeconomic status, education, and ethnicity (U.S. Department of Health and Human Services, 2000) (Figure 6-2). For example, women between the ages of 50 and 65 are more likely to undergo screening mammography than women over age 65, even though the risk for and incidence of breast cancer are considerably higher among women in the latter age group (Table 6-2; see also Table 1-4).

A higher level of education and higher socioeconomic status are also

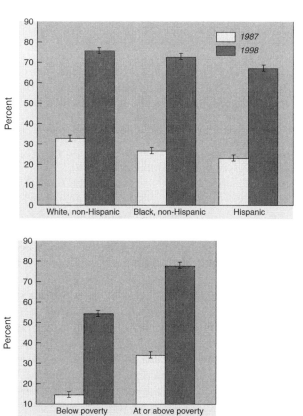

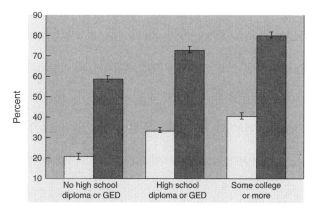

**FIGURE 6-2**  Use of mammography by women aged 50 to 64 according to various attributes (1987, 1998).  Percent of women having a mammogram within the last two years.  SOURCE:  U.S. Department of Health and Human Services, 2000. (www.cdc/gov/nchs/products/pubs/pubd/hus/hus/htm).  Data are based on the National Vital Statistics System, National Center for Health Statistics.

associated with a more frequent use of mammography (Katz and Hofer, 1994). Investigators have noted sizeable increases in the numbers of poor women as well as women whose family incomes are at or above the federal poverty level who have received screening mammograms. Poor women, however, are still less likely than women with higher incomes to receive screening. Among women whose family incomes were below the poverty threshold in 1998, 53 percent reported that they had recently received a screening mammogram, whereas 72 percent of women whose family incomes were at or above the poverty line reported that they had recently received a screening mammogram.

Very few studies have directly examined the breast cancer screening behaviors of immigrant women, but the available data suggest that the rates of screening among first-generation immigrants are significantly lower than the rates among women in other groups of the population (Wismar, 1999). Language and cultural barriers can make it difficult for immigrant women to obtain information about screening tests, and immigrants often have limited access to health care and insurance, a major reason why women are not screened. Having a regular source of health care (with or without insurance) is also significantly correlated with the use of screening mammography, independent of age, ethnicity, socio-demographic status, or other variables (Mandelblatt et al., 1999).

The U.S. Department of Health and Human Services recently set a breast cancer screening goal in the report *Healthy People 2010*.[1] The report suggests that by the year 2010, it is reasonable to expect that 70 percent of all women over the age of 40 will have had a recent mammogram (within the last 2 years).

## IMPEDIMENTS OF EFFECTIVE DIFFUSION OF MAMMOGRAPHY

### Lack of Provider Compliance with Screening Recommendations

CDC found in a recent study that a significant fraction of women between the ages of 50 and 75 do not receive recommendations for screening mammography from their physicians (May et al., 1999). A review of the medical records for more than 1,000 women (ages 50 to 75) attending three clinics in an urban university medical center found that only 66 percent of the women received a recommendation for screening mam-

---

[1]Healthy People is a national health promotion and disease prevention initiative that brings together national, state, and local government agencies; nonprofit, voluntary, and professional organizations; businesses; communities; and individuals to improve the health of all Americans, eliminate disparities in health, and increase the number of years of healthy life and improve the quality of life (see http://www.health.gov/healthypeople/).

mography from their doctors. Another study found that older women reported less physician encouragement for screening than younger women (Grady et al., 1992).

Physician referral is one of the strongest predictors of mammography use, and the most frequently cited reason for not having a mammogram is that a woman's physician did not recommend one (Fox and Stein, 1991; Grady et al., 1992; Lane et al., 1996). Consequently, a number of strategies have been designed and tested for their ability to increase the number of physician-ordered screening mammograms. A recent meta-analysis examined the effectiveness of these various interventions intended to increase the rate of mammography use among women by encouraging physician recommendations for screening (Mandelblatt and Yabroff, 1999). The interventions were divided into three categories: behavioral, cognitive, and sociological. Behavioral interventions included a reminder or office system prompts. Cognitive interventions identified provider attitudes toward screening and breast cancer and provided focused educational material directed at increasing the rate of compliance with ordering of mammography. Sociological intervention strategies included nurse-based interventions or reorganization of the clinic. The results demonstrated that all types of provider-targeted interventions (behavioral, cognitive, and sociological) could increase the rate of mammography use (6 to 21 percent over that for controls) in a fashion similar to what has been observed for patient-targeted interventions (Yabroff and Mandelblatt, 1999). However, most studies analyzed changes in mammography use at only a single point in time, so it is difficult to discern the long-term effects of the interventions. If the programs do not lead to increases in the rates of regular screenings, the observed change in the rates of screening mammography may not translate into reductions in breast cancer mortality.

Contrary to intuition, combined strategies that targeted both patients and providers or that used multiple approaches (e.g., behavioral and cognitive approaches) did not appear to be more effective than single approaches or provider-targeted interventions alone (Mandelblatt and Yabroff, 1999). The reasons for this surprising finding are not known, but may include undefined effects on patient-provider communication and behavior. Alternatively, the results may indicate limitations of the studies and the analysis.

## Inconsistent and Conflicting Guidelines

Practice guidelines for screening mammography have been developed by many different scientific and professional organizations (U.S. Preventive Services Task Force, 1996). Although some groups like the U.S. Preventive Services Task Force (USPSTF) use explicit evidence-based methods, in most cases the recommendations for screening have been based on a combination of expert opinion and a review of published studies. As a result, the guidelines vary with respect to the age at which screening should begin, how often a woman should be screened, and when screening should be discontinued (Table 6-1). This has led to some confusion on the part of both patients and providers and has generated considerable controversy. The guidelines have changed over time as new studies have been published, but there is not a universal consensus on the value of screening for women under age 50 or women over age 70 (see Chapter 1). Furthermore, the age range of 50 to 69 years, for which screening recommendations are most uniform, is to a large extent based on artificial boundaries chosen for study purposes. For any individual woman, these boundaries may not represent a real biological point at which the ratio of benefits to risks sharply increases or decreases. Among a population of women, this ratio is likely to change along an age continuum rather than at discrete boundaries. As a result, when interpreting the guidelines, women and their physicians may find it quite challenging to make appropriate, informed decisions about when and how often the woman should be screened for breast cancer.

## Health System Issues

A lack of health insurance is clearly linked to lower rates of screening mammography (Hoffman, 1998). The type of insurance coverage that a woman has may also play a role in a woman's decision to undergo screening for breast cancer. For example, individuals covered by managed care plans have higher rates of cancer screening than those covered by fee-for-service plans (Potosky et al., 1998), although the gap may be narrowing. Among Medicare beneficiaries, those with private supplemental insurance are more likely to be screened for cancer than those with Medicare alone (Potosky et al., 1998), even though Medicare provides coverage for screening.

For women with adequate health insurance, screening mammography may still be unavailable if facilities are not readily accessible where they live (Katz and Hofer, 1994; Mandelblatt et al., 1995). Women living in both rural and inner-city settings are less likely to undergo cancer screening than those living in other urban locations, which often have more mammogram facilities.

Similar issues come into play with regard to monitoring women with abnormal screening results. As discussed in Chapter 1, a screening mammogram alone cannot definitively identify breast cancer. Abnormal findings on a mammogram must be followed up with additional diagnostic tests. In addition, early detection through screening for breast cancer is not beneficial unless appropriate medical interventions can reduce the numbers of deaths from breast cancer. However, many women do not receive appropriate follow-up care in the form of diagnostic tests and treatments for the same reasons noted earlier for a lack of screening (reviewed by the Institute of Medicine, 1999).

In 1990, the Breast and Cervical Cancer Mortality Prevention Act mandated the establishment of the National Breast and Cervical Cancer Early Detection Program because a significant number of women did not have access to screening mammography. Since its inception in 1991, the program has grown to cover all U.S. states and territories and annual funding has increased from $30 million to $167 million. The program targets hard-to-reach women who lack health insurance, with a focus on screening at recommended intervals. Approximately 60 percent of the budget is allocated for screening services, with the remaining 40 percent devoted to education and outreach, including special promotional events, culturally specific brochures, home visits, church-based presentations, and provider education. In all areas of its work, the program seeks to collaborate with a variety of public and private organizations.

The breast cancer screening and diagnostic services available through the program include clinical breast examinations, screening and diagnostic mammograms, breast ultrasound, fine-needle aspiration, and breast biopsy. The program's policy on new technology requires that when new and improved methods of detection become widely available and are shown to be most effective they should replace the methods currently in use. Screening is offered at a myriad of institutions and centers, including local health departments, federally funded community health centers, hospital-based clinics, and mobile mammography vans, but at present, the program serves only 12 to 15 percent of eligible women.

Funding for treatment of cancers detected through the program were initially not included, but federal legislation that results in the provision of funding for such coverage was recently passed.[2] The Breast and Cervical Cancer Treatment Act gives states the option of providing Medicaid reimbursement for treatment of cancers detected through the CDC screening program, with federal and state governments sharing the costs. The bill must now be considered by each state legislature for adoption.

## Financial Issues

A number of radiologists have raised concerns about reimbursement rates for mammography. Mammography is often seen as a money-loosing activity in radiology departments (Brice, 2000; Feig, 2000a,b; Kolb, 2000), and many believe that the current reimbursement rates do not

---

[2]The bill was approved by the U.S. Congress and signed by President Bill Clinton in October 2000.

cover the actual total expense of providing the service (see the section on Reimbursement in Chapter 5). Others have argued that more efficient management, at least in high-volume centers, could improve the financial status of mammography facilities (Brice, 2000). If reimbursement does not meet the costs of providing mammography services, it could potentially lead to problems with access because facilities may close if they are not financially solvent. A recent study of seven university-based breast care centers found that all seven had lost money on the professional component of mammography. Other breast-related procedures also lost money, but the high volume of mammography made it more problematic for the centers (Brice, 2000). Likewise, a survey of mobile mammography facilities found that less than half were financially profitable or breaking even (Debruhl et al., 1996).

To date, there have been few documented cases of breast screening facilities closing because of financial difficulties, but some anecdotal cases of breast screening facility closings have recently been reported (Brice, 2000). Even if facilities are not closing, preliminary results from a recent survey of the Society of Breast Imaging (SBI)[3] membership suggest that the capacities of screening facilities are not keeping pace with the increasing demand for mammography services. Half of the respondents indicated that waiting times for mammography appointments had increased at their facilities. Nine percent of respondents reported that their facilities will actually decrease their volume of breast imaging in the coming year for a variety of reasons, with reimbursement rates, rising costs, and lack of equipment or personnel topping the list.

Because of the perceived financial difficulties of mammography facilities, several options to make breast imaging more efficient and economically viable have been suggested (Feig, 2000b; Kolb, 2000), including the following:

• streamlining the appointment processes for screening and follow-up procedures;
• batch reading of mammograms;
• making more efficient use of the radiologist's time by shifting all tasks that are not directly related to interpretation or consultation to other personnel;
• accepting only self-paying patients to avoid reimbursement caps;
• performing more interventional procedures such as biopsy and aspiration, which have higher reimbursement rates; and

---

[3]SBI is a national organization consisting of more than 2,000 radiologists who interpret the results of breast imaging studies. The survey of SBI members was carried out by ACS and the American College of Radiology. The results are based on 635 responses.

• renegotiating hospital contracts to balance losses from mammography with downstream profits from surgery, radiation therapy, and oncology treatment of cancers detected by mammography.

## Training Issues

Mammography is one of the most technically challenging radiological procedures (U.S. General Accounting Office, 1998a,b). Ensuring the quality of the image is not easy, and reading the image is difficult because no criteria can absolutely distinguish benign and malignant lesions. As a result, the more experienced radiologists detect a greater percentage of breast cancers (Elmore et al., 1998b). Regulations promulgated under the Mammography Quality Standards Act require each facility to have a training program that meets a set of initial personnel training requirements and to maintain the continuing education and continuing experience of its staff.

With the increased use of mammography during the 1980s, the need for improved training of more radiologists became apparent, and mammography became a separate category on the oral examination of the American Board on Radiology (ABR) in 1989. In the early 1990s the number of breast imaging questions on the written examinations of ABR increased to equal that for each of the other nine subspecialty categories. In 1999, SBI assumed a leadership role in breast imaging education by developing both a residency and a fellowship training curriculum (Feig, 1999b). This undertaking was in response to a request made by the Curriculum Committee of the Association of Program Directors in Radiology that each subspecialty society develop goals and objectives, and a graded curriculum that can be mastered reasonably well by the residents within the allotted training time. The SBI Residency Training Curriculum contains extensive and detailed lists of key concepts in 14 subject areas and recommends that residents be familiar with several texts. The SBI Curriculum Committee concluded that the program should require 3 full-time-equivalent months in breast imaging, interpretation of a minimum of 1,000 mammograms, and performance of breast ultrasound and needle localization.

Despite the increased emphasis on training in mammography, the number of individuals undertaking specialty training may not be sufficient to meet the growing demand for breast screening services (Eklund, 2000). Nationally, the number of mammography fellowships has decreased by about 25 percent over the last 5 years (American College of Radiology survey) (Box 6-1), and a recent survey of radiology residents found that only 4 percent accepted fellowships in women's imaging in 1999 (Goodman et al., 2000). Although the current demand for trained mammographers has not been thoroughly examined or quantified, anec-

**BOX 6-1**
**Current Mammography Fellowship Programs in the U.S.**
**(as of July, 2000)**

**Breast Imaging Fellowships**
Baylor University Medical Center
Indiana University School of Medicine
Johns Hopkins University
Mallinckrodt Institute of Radiology
Massachusetts General Hospital
Rush-Presbyterian-St. Lukes Medical
    Center
Thomas Jefferson University Hospital
University of Michigan
University of North Carolina at
    Chapel Hill
University of Pennsylvania Medical
    Center
University of Texas M. D. Anderson
    Cancer Center
William Beaumont Hospital

**Mammography Fellowships**

Beth Israel Medical Center (New York)
Columbia Presbyterian Medical Center
Duke University Medical Center
Henry Ford Hospital
Medical College of Virginia of the
    Virginia Commonwealth University
Montefiore Medical Center
New York Hospital Cornell Medical
    Center
Princess Margaret Hospital
Q E Z Health Sciences Center
Saint Barnabas Medical Center
Stanford University Medical Center
University of Alabama Hospital

University of California, Los Angeles,
    School of Medicine
University of California, San Francisco
The University of Chicago Hospitals
The University of Illinois College of
    Medicine at Peoria
The University of Minnesota School of
    Medicine
University of Montreal
University of Texas Southwestern Medical
    Center at Dallas
University of Toronto
University of Virginia Health System

**Women's Imaging**
Beth Israel Deaconess Medical Center
    (Massachusetts)
Brigham and Women's Hospital
Case Western Reserve University
Magee-Women's Hospital–University of
    Pittsburgh Medical School
Medical College of Wisconsin
The University of Maryland Medical Center
University of Texas Southwestern Medical
    Center at Dallas
University of Utah School of Medicine
Wake Forest University School of Medicine
Western Pennsylvania Hospital

**Breast and Body Imaging**
Memorial Sloan-Kettering Cancer Center

**Breast Imaging and Women's Imaging**
Emory University School of Medicine

SOURCE: The Society of Breast Imaging (www.sbi-online.org/fellowships.htm).

dotal reports from the field indicate that it is becoming increasingly difficult to fill vacant positions (Brice, 2000). There are similar reports that too
few mammography technologists are being trained to meet the demand.
According to the American Society of Radiologic Technologists, 1,800
technologists took the national mammography examination[4] in 1999, less
than half the number who took the test in 1997 (Martinez, 2000).

## Legal Issues

A study by the Physician's Insurers Association of America (1995)
found that allegation of error in the diagnosis of breast cancer is now the
most prevalent reason for medical malpractice lawsuits among all claims
against physicians and is associated with the second highest indemnity
payment rate[5] As mammography use has increased, both the number of
malpractice suits filed and the sizes of the awards or settlements have
increased. Radiologists are the specialists most frequently sued in malpractice suits involving breast cancer, and within the radiology community, concerns have been raised over trends in malpractice litigation and
their potential effect on the practice of radiology (Berlin, 1999). Pathologists who interpret biopsy samples for the diagnosis of breast cancer have
also raised similar concerns (Skoumal et al., 1996).

In addition to the increase in the number of claims that results natu-
rally from an increase in the number of mammograms performed, at least
two additional factors may contribute to the rise in the number of malpractice claims for failure to diagnose breast cancer. First, the legal doctrine is in the process of change: the advent of the "loss of chance" doctrine (Box 6-2) has lowered the hurdle to a legally acceptable claim.
Second, jury verdicts in medical malpractice claims—and insurance settlements based on predictions of jury decisions—may reflect a change in
public expectations.

The negligence basis (Box 6-3) of the medical malpractice system in
general is often criticized. There is only a weak correlation between the
cases in which a malpractice claim is filed and those in which expert

---

[4]This examination was first offered in 1992. In addition to students taking the examination upon completion of their degrees, many of the people taking the examination in the
first years in which it was offered were already working in the field. Thus, the noted decrease may be only partially due to the declining number of students enrolling in technologist training programs (Jerry Reid, Executive Director of the American Registry for Radiologic Technologists, personal communication, December 2000).

[5]The current Medicare reimbursement relative value units do not reflect the higher malpractice costs and risks of mammography compared with those for other radiology procedures (Farria and Feig, 2000). See Chapter 5 for more detail.

---

**BOX 6-2**
**Loss of Chance Legal Doctrine**

Suppose a diagnostic test indicates that a patient has cancer and has an approximately 40 percent chance of survival with the appropriate treatment. To make a factually clean case, the clinician clearly violates the standard of care and fails to notice the cancer (or just fails to inform the patient of the cancer). Six months later, the same patient has the diagnostic test repeated and the cancer is detected. At this point, the patient has only a 10 percent chance of recovery. A malpractice suit could theoretically be based on one of the following legal definitions:

**Traditional "more-probable-than-not" standard:** The cause element of a medical malpractice tort claim requires that the negligent act of the physician "more probably than not" caused the patient's death. This standard requires expert testimony asserting a 51 percent chance or greater that the clinician was responsible for the patient's death. Therefore, in the example described above, the clinician cannot be held liable. More probably than not, the clinician is not responsible for the effects of the cancer: the clinician's negligent failure to diagnose only deprived the patient of a 30 percent chance of survival.

**Loss of chance:** The "loss-of-chance" doctrine allows patients to recover damages for medical treatment that "more probably than not" fails to meet the standard of care but that deprives the patient of a chance of survival that is less than 50 percent. In other words, the negligence on the part of the clinician must still be proven according to the traditional causation standard, but the damages are redefined as the loss of the chance of survival, not the death itself. Under "loss of chance" the claim can be either retrospective or prospective with respect to the timing of the harm.

**Retrospective:** The retrospective category is more straightforward. In the example described above, the patient subsequently dies of cancer, and the patient's estate files a claim against the clinician for a 30 percent loss of a chance of survival.

---

assessment identifies negligence (Brennan, 1996). Because the concept of "standard of care" is quite vague, even "the finest panel of medical reviewers" may not be able to classify "the majority of cases... as either due to medical negligence or not due to such negligence" (Rubin, 1997). Furthermore, juries often idealistically believe that medical technologies should be used whenever a patient might possibly benefit, even if the probability is quite low (Havighurst, 1998).

Most medical malpractice claims for breast cancer are due to missed diagnoses. Given that breast cancer is a potentially fatal disease that can strike a relatively young population, the potential severity of any failure to diagnose breast cancer (or the perception thereof) may also increase the likelihood of a favorable verdict or settlement. According to Brennan (1996), the severity of a patient's disability, not the occurrence of an adverse event or an adverse event due to negligence, is predictive of pay-

---

**BOX 6-3**
**Definition of a Tort Claim**

Medical malpractice claims use traditional negligence analysis from torts law. According to legal doctrine, to mount a successful claim the patient or plaintiff must demonstrate each of the following four elements:

**Duty:** Individuals have an obligation to act with reasonable care toward others only in limited situations. In the malpractice arena, the physician-patient relationship unquestionably places this duty on the physician.

**Breach:** (failure to provide the appropriate professionally established "standard of care"): The physician must fail to deliver the appropriate "standard of care" as defined by the professional practices of the relevant medical community.

**Cause:** The injury incurred by the plaintiff must have been caused by the physician's failure to deliver the appropriate "standard of care" (e.g., a physician who fails to notice an obvious sign of cancer is not liable for the death of a patient if the patient dies of an unrelated cardiac arrest shortly thereafter).

**Damages:** The patient must suffer some cognizable harm. The valuation of this harm is the monetary sum awarded by the jury.

---

ment to the plaintiff. Thus, the perceived severity of a "delayed" breast cancer diagnosis may be more predictive of a jury's verdict than the occurrence of a true medical "error" in the initial interpretation of a mammogram.

It is unclear whether the increase in malpractice claims for missed breast cancer diagnosis has had a negative effect on the availability of mammography services, as has been suggested by some. If the risk and financial burden of malpractice claims are deemed too great, some facilities may choose to discontinue their services. Likewise, if young radiologists in training view the field of mammography as too risky with respect to malpractice, they may choose other specialties, with a subsequent decline in the number of trained mammographers. However, to date there is no documented evidence that either of these phenomena is occurring.

## POTENTIAL FOR RISK-BASED SCREENING

Since the time of the first randomized clinical trial conducted to evaluate screening mammography, questions have been raised about whether risk stratification could be used to identify populations for which screening would be most beneficial. The goal of risk profiling is to identify groups with a significantly higher or a significantly lower risk for breast cancer than that for the general population and to develop different screening strategies based on that risk. Such an approach could, in theory, increase both the efficacy and the cost-effectiveness of screening programs.

The current breast cancer screening recommendations are already based on age (because the risk of cancer increases with age) and gender (only women are screened).[6] Attempts to base screening strategies on more specific characteristics such as family history or age at menarche or first pregnancy have largely been unsuccessful because the known risk factors for breast cancer are associated with comparably low relative risks (2 or less; see Box 1-2 for a definition of relative risk). Investigators have retrospectively evaluated data from clinical trials and case series studies to determine the proportion of cases that would have been identified if women had been selectively screened on the basis of certain risk factors for breast cancer. Unfortunately, these studies found that screening based on risk stratification could not be used to identify the majority of breast cancer cases (reviewed by Smith, 1999).

More recently, new attempts have been made to develop risk-based guidelines to aid the decision-making process for women who fall into age categories for which the general screening guidelines are inconsistent or controversial (Gail and Rimer, 1998). Models for the calculation of risk may help women and their physicians make decisions about the age at which screening should begin (for women under age 50), how often a woman should be screened, and when screening should be discontinued (for women over age 70).

With technological advances in screening and diagnostic methods has come renewed interest in developing specialized screening programs for women at different risk levels. For example, several large studies are under way to evaluate the use of magnetic resonance imaging to screen high-risk women (see Chapter 2). Much of the effort has focused on women with dense breast tissue, a characteristic associated with an increased risk for breast cancer (Byng et al., 1998), as well as the reduced accuracy of screening mammography (Mandelson et al., 1995). Breast density is highest at menarche and declines with menopause and increasing age, but there is considerable variation in breast density among women at any given age. For example, among postmenopausal women, those on estrogen replacement therapy are likely to have denser breast tissue than those who forego such therapy (Laya et al., 1996). One impediment to the stratification of women on the basis of breast density is a lack of standardization for density classification, in part because of the inability to incorporate volume measurements in standard mammograms. If this difficulty

---

[6]Although men can and do develop breast cancer, the incidence among men in extremely low compared with that among women. Thus, screening of men for breast cancer is not recommended.

can be overcome, then screening protocols could potentially be optimized by studying different approaches, such as the use of magnetic resonance imaging and ultrasound as adjuncts to mammography or other alternative screening techniques with large screening populations.

## NEW ISSUES THAT ARISE WITH ADOPTION OF EMERGING TECHNOLOGIES

New technologies may provide additional choices for women and their physicians, allowing an individualized approach to screening and diagnosis that depends on a woman's specific needs and characteristics. At the same time, new technologies may add layers of complexity to the decision-making processes associated with screening and diagnosis. The current practice guidelines for breast cancer detection and diagnosis are already quite complex (see Figure 1-4), and the incorporation of new technologies will likely make it even more challenging to establish practice guidelines and to define a "standard of care."

Economic considerations also accompany the adoption of new technologies. For example, if the rate of reimbursement for mammography is artificially low, as has been suggested by some directors of breast screening facilities, cost comparisons with new technologies will unfairly favor mammography. Furthermore, many new technologies may first be introduced as an adjunct to mammography (to improve its sensitivity or specificity, or both) and will therefore be used in a more limited fashion and have a smaller market compared with that for mammography. As more breast cancer detection technologies become available, competition among new technologies and with established technologies will likely increase, in effect further reducing the size of the market and thus limiting the profit expectations of developers. Equal access may also become an issue when new imaging technologies prove to be effective but are also significantly more expensive. If the adoption of expensive new technologies is limited to resource-rich health care settings, many underserved segments of the population may be denied access and disparities in the health of different groups may actually increase after their adoption. The effect that the recent advertising of new imaging technologies to the general public (on television and in print media) will have on patient demand and dissemination is as yet unknown, but it is likely to be significant.

## SUMMARY

Use of screening mammography has increased greatly in the last decade, but it has not been universally adopted and accepted by women. Many eligible women have never had a mammogram, and of those who have been screened, a significant number do not undergo screening at the recommended interval. Because mammography is less than an ideal test, women have expressed a variety of concerns about undergoing screening by this procedure, such as discomfort from the procedure and fear of what could be found, including false-positive results.

Much of the controversy over mammography has focused on the recommendation for screening mammographies for women between the ages of 40 and 49, but more lives may be lost because women over age 50 do not get regular mammograms and follow-up care (Aronowitz, 1995). Physician recommendation is the single most important factor that determines whether women are screened, but outreach to and education of women are also important for improving the screening rate. Access to screening facilities, including geographic proximity and payment for the procedure, is an issue for many women as well. Currently, the CDC screening program, established with the intent of improving access for underserved women, reaches only 12 to 15 percent of eligible women.

As the number of women eligible for screening mammography increases (because of the changing age distribution of the U.S. population) and more women adopt the practice of routine screening, there will be increased demand for trained mammographers and certified screening facilities. Whether the medical care system is prepared to meet these needs is not clear, but some concerns have been raised in this regard. Although data are unavailable to confirm or refute such concerns , some suggest that the potential threats to future screening services may include the financial difficulties of some screening facilities, high rates of medical malpractice claims for missed breast cancer diagnosis, and anecdotal reports of a downward trend in the numbers of individuals enrolled in training programs in breast imaging.

Lessons learned from the adoption and dissemination of mammography may be informative as new technologies become available. However, because mammography was a "void-filling" technology, the adoption process for new technologies is likely to be quite different. New technologies may offer novel opportunities for breast cancer detection, but their adoption will ultimately depend on whether they can provide added value to current technologies and survive competition in the marketplace. If they can, screening and diagnostic procedures may become more tailored to individual women's needs, but at the same time, deciding on the appropriate course of action for a particular woman may become more complex.

# 7

# Findings and Recommendations

The purpose of the study described in this report was to review breast cancer detection technologies in development and to examine the many steps in medical technology development as they specifically apply to methods for the early detection of breast cancer. The findings and recommendations presented in this chapter are based on the evidence reviewed in previous chapters. Detailed discussion and references can be found in those chapters and are merely summarized here.

Much of what is known about early breast cancer detection comes from studies of screening mammography. Early detection is widely believed to reduce breast cancer mortality by allowing intervention at an earlier stage of cancer progression. Clinical data show that women diagnosed with early-stage breast cancers are less likely to die from the disease than those diagnosed with more advanced stages of the disease. Mammography has been shown both to detect cancer at an earlier stage and to reduce disease-specific mortality.

However, screening mammography cannot eliminate all deaths from breast cancer and can actually have deleterious effects on some women, in the form of false-positive or false-negative results and overdiagnosis or overtreatment. Thus, there is clearly room for improvement in the screening and diagnosis of breast cancer. The tremendous toll of breast cancer on U.S. women, combined with the inherent limitations of mammography and other detection modalities, has been the driving force behind the enormous efforts that have been and that continue to be devoted to the development and refinement of technologies for the early detection of breast cancer. Most of the progress thus far has led to incremental improvements in traditional imaging technologies, but clinical trials have not been undertaken to determine whether these technical improvements have further reduced breast cancer mortality. To date, it appears that no quantum steps forward have been taken in the field of breast cancer detection, and so a great deal of work remains to be done, particularly in the field of cancer biomarkers.

The pathway from technical innovation to accepted clinical practice is long, arduous, and costly. There are many participants in the process, in addition to the developers of new technologies. A variety of public and private organizations and policy makers play a role in evaluating medical technologies at various points along the way, making decisions that ultimately determine whether they will be adopted and disseminated. In evaluating the potential of new technologies, policy makers consider many factors, including clinical need, technical performance, clinical performance, economic issues, and patient and societal perspectives. Because technical innovations often first get introduced into the system in rather crude form, it can be difficult and problematic to judge them solely on the basis of their early versions.

## FINDINGS

### The use and effect of mammography (Chapter 1)

1. Mammography is used to detect, localize, and characterize breast abnormalities, especially cancer. It is routinely used for breast cancer screening and diagnostic follow-up.

2. Mammography is federally regulated, including standards for equipment, personnel, reporting, and rates of reimbursement for the procedure.

- It is the only medical imaging procedure used for breast cancer screening and the only procedure regulated in this way.
- The Mammography Quality Standards Act is central to the regulation of device quality and clinical practice of mammography.

3. The evidence definitively indicates that screening mammography, when properly performed at recommended intervals and combined with appropriate interventions, can reduce, but not eliminate, breast cancer mortality. This conclusion is based on evidence of efficacy in clinical trials and evidence of effectiveness in the general population.

- In randomized clinical trials, screening mammography reduced the rate of mortality from breast cancer mortality by ~25 to 30 percent for women ages 50 to 70 and ~16 to 18 percent for women ages 40 to 49.

• The time lag between initiation of screening and documentation of a significant reduction in breast cancer mortality in these trials is longer for women under age 50 (10 to 12 years) than for women over age 50 (~5 years).

• Most randomized clinical trials excluded women over age 70, even though the risk of breast cancer increases with age and thus is more prevalent among women in this age group. Recent observational studies suggest that mammography is also beneficial for women over age 70, but further documentation of benefit is important.

• Mortality from breast cancer in the United States has been decreasing over the last decade, and some of this reduction is consistent with the effect of screening.

• Mortality from breast cancer has been decreasing in some other industrialized countries as well, and studies from the United Kingdom and Finland indicate that, in practice, screening programs can decrease breast cancer mortality.

4. There is clearly room for improvement in the screening and diagnosis of breast cancer because of both technical and biological limitations of the current methods.

• It is technically difficult to consistently produce mammograms of high quality, and interpretation is subjective and can be variable among radiologists.

• Mammography does not detect all cancers, including some that are palpable.

• As many as three-quarters of all breast lesions biopsied turn out to be benign.

• Mammograms are particularly difficult to interpret for women with dense breast tissue. The dense tissue interferes with identification of abnormalities associated with tumors, despite the increased risk of breast cancer in these women. This leads to higher rates of false-negative and false-positive findings among these women.

• Optimal screening intervals are not well defined. Some tumors may develop too quickly to be identified at the current screening intervals.

## Evolving imaging technologies (Chapter 2)

1. Since the 1960s there have been many technical improvements in film-screen mammography that have allowed for more consistent detec-

tion of breast cancers at an earlier stage than that possible by physical examination.

• Investigators have not systematically studied whether the improvements already realized have further augmented the survival benefits seen in the earlier randomized screening trials.
• Technical improvements have greatly reduced the dose of radiation necessary to obtain quality mammograms, and most experts agree that the potential benefits of mammography outweigh the risks from radiation. Nonetheless, the risk from radiation may not be uniform across all women. (For example, women with certain germ-line mutations may be at higher risk, but current data are not definitive.)

2. A number of promising new imaging technologies have been developed, and some are already in use as adjuncts to mammography for the diagnosis of breast cancer. Some may have particular potential for augmenting the benefits of mammography in certain subsets of women (e.g., women with dense breasts).

• Technologies approved by the Food and Drug Administration (FDA) include ultrasound, magnetic resonance imaging (MRI), scintimammography, computer-aided detection and diagnosis, thermography, electrical impedance imaging, and full-field digital mammography (FFDM). Many additional technologies are at earlier stages of development.
• FFDM represents a technical advance over traditional film-screen mammography, but studies to date have not demonstrated a meaningful improvement in sensitivity and specificity. However, these studies have not been designed to test the full potential of FFDM with the use of "softcopy" interpretation (on a computer screen rather than on film). The technology could also potentially improve the practice of screening and diagnostic mammography in other ways, for example, by facilitating electronic storage, retrieval, and transmission of mammograms.
• Computer-aided detection has the potential to improve the accuracy of the interpretation of screening mammography, at least among less experienced readers, but questions remain as to how this technology will ultimately be used and whether it will have a net beneficial effect on current screening practices.
• MRI shows promise for the screening of women at high risk (those with *BRCA* mutations or a strong family history of breast cancer who want to begin screening at an earlier age and who are thus more likely to have dense breast tissue). Preliminary results of MRI studies are encouraging, and computer modeling suggests that MRI screening of high-risk

women may be cost-effective, but more study is needed to define its use and value for this population. It also has shown potential as a diagnostic adjunct to mammography, especially for women in whom the sensitivity of mammography is not optimal, such as those with dense breasts or breast implants.

• Ultrasound has traditionally been used to differentiate between cystic and solid lesions. More recently, it has been used to distinguish between benign and malignant solid lesions as well. With newer ultrasound techniques, the vascularity of tumors can be assessed and microcalcifications can be detected. Recent technical advances have renewed interest in the development of the technology for screening purposes as well, particularly for women with dense breast tissue.

• MRI and ultrasound imaging may facilitate new minimally invasive methods for the ablation of early lesions, and such methods are under investigation. The development of more acceptable interventions for early lesions could reduce some of the problems associated with "overtreatment," but clinical trials are needed to assess the potential of these new technologies.

3. Several new image-guided biopsy techniques offer a less invasive alternative to open surgical biopsy for many women.

4. There are difficulties associated with the comparison of new technologies with the imperfect "gold standard" of film-screen mammography.

• There is inherent variability in the production and interpretation of mammograms and other breast images.

• This variability makes it difficult to accurately determine the sensitivity and specificity of imaging modalities.

• This variability caused major difficulties and delays in the FDA approval process for FFDM and thus greatly increased the cost and time required to gain approval.

5. Improved imaging technologies that allow clinicians to detect more lesions at an earlier, preinvasive stage may or may not lead to reduced breast cancer mortality, and may lead to more overtreatment of women unless they are coupled with biologically based technologies that can determine which lesions are likely to become metastatic and lethal.

• A better understanding of the biology and etiology of breast cancer will be critical for increasing the net benefit of screening protocols.

### Technologies based on the molecular biology of breast lesions
### (Chapter 3)

1. The malignant potential of early-stage lesions (invasive and noninvasive) is not well understood.

- It is likely that some early lesions have very little potential to cause the death of the patient, and labeling these women as cancer patients and treating them for breast cancer may lead to increased morbidity without decreasing breast cancer mortality. The magnitude of this dilemma is not known, but the prevalence of ductal carcinoma in situ (a preinvasive lesion that may or may not progress to invasive or metastatic cancer) has quadrupled since the adoption of screening mammography.
- Currently, methods for the classification of lesions detected by mammography are based on morphology, and the ability to determine the malignant and metastatic potential of breast abnormalities from this classification is crude at best.

2. Technologies that might help define the biological nature of lesions found by imaging technologies and that might also help advance the field of functional imaging are being developed. These include culture of breast cancer cells in vitro, measurement of protein expression in cancer cells, identification of markers of cancer cells (or their secreted proteins) in blood, and the identification of tumor genotypes.

- In many instances these technologies could potentially identify fundamental changes in the breast that appear before a lesion can be identified. Thus, they may identify women at high risk of developing breast cancer (or, more importantly, women at high risk of dying from breast cancer).
- The distinction between "early breast cancer" and "high-risk breast tissue" is important but still imprecise.

3. Technologies not based on traditional imaging modalities could potentially contribute to improved patient outcomes in several ways:

- They could distinguish between lesions that require treatment because of a high potential for malignancy and those that do not (e.g., some forms of carcinoma in situ, or even some very slow growing or low grade invasive carcinomas).
- They could identify women who should undergo more frequent screening or who might benefit from newer imaging modalities.

• They could identify women who should explore a "risk reduction" strategy that will affect all breast cells. (However, current strategies for risk reduction are less than ideal. Improved understanding of the biology could also lead to better prevention strategies.)

4. Certain germ-line mutations such as *BRCA1*, *BRCA2*, p53, and *PTEN* mutations are the only markers identified thus far that have some of these characteristics (specifically, the last two bullets under item 3 above).

5. Further progress in this field will be dependent on the establishment, maintenance, and accessibility of tissue specimen banks, as well as access to new high-throughput technologies and bioinformatics.

• Access to these resources continues to be problematic for many reasons.
• More could be done to ensure the privacy of genetic information and protection from genetic discrimination.

## Development of new technologies: requirements and barriers (Chapter 4)

1. The potential barriers to the development of new technologies include the high economic risk of the development and approval process, the length of time that it takes to get a new technology onto the market, and the size of the market.

• The technology development process is complex and costly, and the end results of research are unpredictable, making it a financially risky undertaking.
• For medical devices, the requirements for FDA approval and insurance coverage have been variable and unpredictable, adding additional levels of risk to the development process.

2. In the private sector, investment in breast cancer imaging technologies is less attractive than investment in other areas of the health care industry. The reasons for this appear to be multifactorial and include the following:

• Relatively less return on investment because of limits on rates of reimbursement coupled with regulatory requirements that increase costs for mammographic examinations.

- Delays in FDA approval and confusion about the requirements for approval of new imaging technologies.
- Increasing requirements for evidence of efficacy to obtain a positive technology assessment and thus insurance coverage.
- The relatively small size of the potential market for new breast cancer detection devices is small (the United States has about 10,000 certified breast screening centers).
- Effectively less patent exclusivity for devices and diagnostics than for drugs (because of the nature of the technology).

3. Government funding of research in the health care sector has traditionally focused primarily on basic scientific discovery.

- Recently, a new emphasis on the translation of science through the development of technology has received considerable attention, including the creation of joint public- and private-sector initiatives.
- Technical advances in computer-aided detection and diagnosis and digital mammography are examples of the successes of such initiatives.

4. Based on the findings of the National Cancer Institute's (NCI's) Breast Cancer Review Group, NCI has launched several new funding initiatives in the last year aimed at increasing the understanding of breast cancer initiation and progression.

5. Investment from public resources for the development of new imaging technologies for early detection has been substantially increased as a result of U.S. Department of Defense Breast Cancer Research Funds.

- The program has included innovative and nontraditional approaches to grant application and peer review.
- The initiation and continuation of this program have largely been due to the efforts of advocacy groups.

### Evaluation of the effects of new imaging technologies on patient outcomes (Chapter 5)

1. Early randomized trials of screening mammography were the first to demonstrate that early detection of any cancer would reduce mortality from that cancer. Unfortunately, no similar evaluations on the effectiveness of newer technologies on health outcomes have been performed during the past 15 years.

- The evidence for the benefit of screening mammography was based on the use of technologies that are very crude compared with those in use today.
- The net effect of technological changes could be either positive (more accurate detection, leading to lower breast cancer mortality) or negative (capable of identifying more lesions but not changing mortality and thus leading to greater morbidity and higher costs for screening).

2. Screening trials that could evaluate the effects of recently introduced technologies on patient outcomes have not been designed.

- Data on sensitivity and specificity are necessary but not sufficient to assess the potential value of the newer technologies for screening purposes.
- Thus far, all new technologies have been or are being evaluated by diagnostic studies rather than screening studies, even if they ultimately are intended to be used for screening.
- Adoption of new detection technologies for screening purposes before assessment of their effects on clinical outcomes has been common and very problematic for other diseases.

3. The dominant framework for medical technology development and evaluation has historically been based on therapeutics, whereas early detection relies on screening and diagnostic methods. The evaluation of such methods may be intrinsically different.

- The stages of development for drugs are more standardized, and therapeutic interventions generate direct outcomes that can be observed in patients.
- Most patient-level effects of diagnostic devices are mediated by subsequent therapeutic decisions. Diagnostic tests generate information, which is only one of the inputs into the decision-making process. Hence, the evaluation of diagnostic tests is fundamentally the assessment of the value of information.
- The development process for devices is iterative. That is, most technologies that ultimately achieve widespread use go through successive stages of development, variation, and appraisal of actual experience in the marketplace.

4. NCI's Breast Cancer Surveillance Consortium was established in 1994 to study the effectiveness of breast cancer screening practices in the United States through an assessment of the accuracy, cost, and quality of screening programs and the relation of these practices to changes in breast cancer mortality or other shorter-term outcomes, such as stage at diagno-

sis or survival. A secondary goal of the program is to provide an infrastructure for the conduct of clinical and basic research.

5. The first large-scale collaborative clinical trials group devoted to medical imaging (American College of Radiology Imaging Network) was launched in 1999 with $22 million in initial support from NCI. One of its first studies will evaluate the sensitivity and specificity of digital mammography for the detection of breast cancer in asymptomatic women. This could become a stable infrastructure for the evaluation of patient outcomes as new imaging technologies are tested for screening use.

6. Recently, there has been an increased interest in using cost-effectiveness analysis to assess new technologies. A number of cost-effectiveness analyses of breast cancer detection technologies have been carried out, including computer modeling of screening technologies, whose effect on patient outcome (disease-specific mortality) has not been demonstrated. The assumptions regarding the effect of a technology on mortality have not been uniformly accepted. The result of cost-effectiveness analysis is also dependent on what stage of development the analysis of a new technology is carried out. To date, a consensus has not been reached as to how to use the information generated by the analyses. Neither the Health Care Financing Administration (HCFA) nor other third-party payers use cost-effectiveness analysis to make coverage decisions.

## Diffusion of technologies (Chapter 6)

1. Use of screening mammography has increased greatly in the last decade, but it has not been universally adopted and accepted by women.

• The percentage of women age 50 and over who reported having a recent mammogram rose to 69 percent in 1998, up from 27 percent in 1987. However, an estimated 12 million women in this age group have not had a mammogram within the last 2 years.
• Access to screening facilities is an issue for some women. Currently, the Centers for Disease Control and Prevention (CDC) screening program reaches only 12 to 15 percent of eligible women without health insurance. Treatment of cancers identified through the screening program was not initially covered, but federal legislation allowing Medicaid coverage of treatment was recently passed. Adoption of this new program by individual states is pending.
• Of those women who have been screened, a significant number do not undergo screening at the recommended interval.
• Physician recommendation is the most important factor in determining whether women are screened.

• Women over age 65 are less likely to undergo screening mammography, although the risk and incidence of breast cancer are higher among women in this age group. Physicians are less likely to recommend screening to older women, perhaps because of the lack of consensus guidelines and data on the effectiveness of screening for women in this age group.

• Mammography is less than an ideal test. Women express concerns about discomfort from the procedure, inconvenience of scheduling an annual test, and fear of what could be found, including false-positive results. (However, fear of cancer and the inconvenience of annual tests may be characteristic of any screening test.)

2. As the number of women eligible for screening mammography increases (because of the changing age distribution of the U.S. population) and more women adopt the practice of routine screening, there will be increased demand for trained mammographers and certified screening facilities.

• The current screening facilities may already be operating at or near full capacity, as waiting times for appointments appear to be increasing over the last 2 years.

• There are anecdotal reports that inadequate numbers of mammographers and mammography technologists are being trained to fill the current and future needs. Quantitative data to substantiate these concerns are not currently available.

• Radiologists and health care administrators have expressed concern that the reimbursement rate for mammography is too low to cover the actual costs of the procedure (including the cost of meeting federally mandated requirements promulgated under the Mammography Quality Standards Act) and that this situation could lead to a reduction in screening services. Quantitative data are currently unavailable to confirm or refute these assertions.

3. When film-screen mammography was introduced (before FDA regulation of medical devices), it was a "void-filling" technology.

• New technologies face a different level of evaluation that will likely include comparison with mammography.

• If the rate of reimbursement for mammography is in fact artificially low, then cost comparisons with new technologies will unfairly favor mammography.

• Many new technologies may be first introduced as an adjunct to mammography (to improve its sensitivity or specificity, or both, and its positive predictive value).

- New technologies may provide additional choices for women and their physicians, allowing an individualized approach to screening and diagnosis depending on a woman's specific needs and characteristics. At the same time, new technologies may add layers of complexity to the decision-making processes associated with screening and diagnosis, making it more challenging to establish practice guidelines and to define a "standard of care."

4. Currently, mammography is one of the few screening tests that are reimbursed.

- Preventive services are not routinely covered by HCFA because the U.S. Congress deliberately crafted the Medicare statute to preclude preventive services, reflecting the practice of commercial insurers at the time.
- Congress and state legislatures have mandated coverage for mammography (as well as some other preventive services, including screening tests for cervical, prostate, and colon cancers).

### The "ideal" screening tool

1. All of the tests available for the screening and diagnosis of breast cancer have different strengths and limitations. The ideal test would combine the following characteristics:

- The test should present a low risk of harm from screening
- The test should have high degrees of specificity and sensitivity (low rates of false-positive and false-negative results).
- The test results should have uniform high quality and repeatability.
- Interpretation of test results should be straightforward (objective).
- The test should be simple to perform.
- The test should be noninvasive.
- The test should be able to find breast cancer at a stage that is curable with available treatments.
- The test should have the ability to distinguish life-threatening lesions from those that are not likely to progress.
- The test should be cost-effective (usually considered <$50,000 per quality-adjusted life year saved).
- The test should be widely available.
- The test should be acceptable to women.

2. The "ideal" breast cancer screening tool has not yet been developed.

3. Because each technology has different strengths and limitations, a multimodality approach that includes multiple tests in one examination may, in theory, be the best way to optimize the characteristics listed above.

## RECOMMENDATIONS

The committee's recommendations fall into two general categories: those that aim to improve the development and adoption process for new technologies (Recommendations 1 to 5) and those that aim to make the most of the technologies currently available for breast cancer detection (Recommendations 6 to 10).

**1. Government support for the development of new breast cancer detection technologies should continue to emphasize research on the basic biology and etiology of breast cancer and on the creation of classification schemes for breast lesions based on molecular biology.** A major goal of this research should be to determine which lesions identified by screening are likely to become lethal and thus require treatment. This approach would increase the potential benefits of screening while reducing the potential risks of screening programs.

• Funding should focus on the development of biological markers and translational research to determine the appropriate uses and applications of the markers, including functional imaging.
• Research on cancer markers should focus on screening as well as on downstream decisions associated with diagnosis and treatment.
• Funding priorities should include specimen banks (including specimens of early lesions), purchase and operation of high-throughput technologies for the study and assessment of genetic and protein markers, and new bioinformatics approaches to the analysis of biological data.

**2. Breast cancer specimen banks should be expanded and researcher access to patient samples should be enhanced.**

• Health care professionals and breast cancer advocacy groups should educate women about the importance of building tumor banks and encourage women to provide consent for research on patient samples.
• Stronger protective legislation should be enacted at the national level to prevent genetic discrimination and ensure the confidentiality of genetic test results.
• The National Cancer Institute (NCI) should devise and enforce strategies to facilitate researcher access to the patient samples in specimen banks. For example, the costs associated with the sharing of samples with collaborators should be included in the funding for the establishment and

maintenance of the specimen banks, and specimen banks supported by government funds should not place excessive restrictions on the use of the specimens with regard to intellectual property issues.

**3. Consistent criteria should be developed and applied by the Food and Drug Administration (FDA) for the approval of screening and diagnostic devices and tests.**

• Guidance documents for determination of "safety and effectiveness," especially with regard to clinical data, should be articulated more clearly and applied more uniformly.
• Given the complexity of assessing new technologies, the FDA advisory panels could be improved by including more experts in biostatistics, technology assessment, and epidemiology.

**4. For new screening technologies, approval by the Food and Drug Administration (FDA) and coverage decisions by the Health Care Financing Administration (HCFA) and private insurers should depend on evidence of improved clinical outcome. This pursuit should be streamlined by coordinating oversight and support from all relevant participants (FDA, NCI, HCFA, private insurers, and breast cancer advocacy organizations) at a very early stage in the process.** Such an approach should prevent technologies that have been approved for diagnostic use from being used prematurely for screening in the absence of evidence of benefit. Technology sponsors generally lack the resources and incentive to undertake large, long-lasting, and expensive screening studies, but a coordinated approach would make it easier to conduct clinical trials to gather the necessary outcome data. The proposed process should provide for the following:

• FDA should approve new cancer detection technologies for diagnostic use in the traditional fashion, based on evidence of the accuracy (sensitivity and specificity) of new devices or tests in the diagnostic setting. In the case of "next-generation" devices (in which technical improvements have been made to a predicate device already on the market), technical advantages such as patient comfort or ease of data acquisition and storage could be considered in the determination of approval.
• If a new device that has been approved for diagnostic use shows potential for use as a screening tool (based on evidence of accuracy) and the developers wish to pursue a screening use, an investigational device exemption should be granted for this use and conditional coverage should be provided for the purpose of conducting large-scale screening trials to assess clinical outcomes.

- Trials should be designed and conducted with input from FDA, NCI, HCFA, the Agency for Healthcare Research and Quality, and breast cancer advocacy organizations. Informed consent acknowledging the specific risks of participating in a screening trial would be necessary.

- HCFA and other payers should agree to conditionally cover the cost of performing the test in the approved clinical trials, whereas NCI and the technology's sponsors should take responsibility for other trial expenses. Participation by private insurers would be particularly important for the assessment of new technologies intended for use in younger women who are not yet eligible for Medicare coverage. Although this expense may initially seem burdensome to private insurers, the cost of providing tests within a clinical trial would be much less than the costs associated with broad adoption by the public (and the associated pressure to provide coverage) in the absence of experimental evidence for improved clinical outcome.

- Trial data should be reviewed at appropriate intervals, and the results should determine whether FDA approval should be granted (for those deemed sufficiently effective) and coverage should be extended to use outside of the trials. (A prior approval for diagnosis would remain in place regardless of the decision for screening applications.)

- The ideal end point for clinical outcome is decreased disease-specific mortality. However, given the length of time required to assess that end point and the fact that early detection by screening mammography has already been proven to reduce breast cancer mortality, a surrogate end point for breast cancer detection is appropriate in some cases. As a general rule, a screening technology that consistently detects early invasive breast cancer could be presumed efficacious for the purposes of FDA approval. Detection of premalignant or preinvasive breast lesions, however, cannot be assumed to reduce breast cancer mortality or increase benefits to women, and it is not an appropriate surrogate end point for FDA approval, given the current lack of understanding of the biology of these lesions.

**5. The National Cancer Institute should create a permanent infrastructure for testing the efficacy and clinical effectiveness of new technologies for early cancer detection as they emerge.** The NCI Breast Cancer Surveillance Consortium and the American College of Radiology Imaging Network may provide novel platforms for this purpose through the creation of databases and archives of clinical samples from thousands of study participants.

**6. The Health Care Financing Administration should analyze the current Medicare and Medicaid reimbursement rates for mammography, including a comparison with other radiological techniques, to de-**

termine whether they adequately cover the total costs of providing the **procedure.** The cost analysis of mammography should include the costs associated with meeting the requirements of the Mammography Quality Standards Act. A panel of external and independent experts should be involved in the analysis.

**7. The Health Resources and Services Administration (HRSA) should undertake or fund a study that analyzes trends in specialty training for breast cancer screening among radiologists and radiologic technologists and that examines the factors that affect practitioners' decisions to enter or remain in the field.** If the trend suggests an impending shortage of trained experts, HRSA should seek input from professional societies such as the American College of Radiology and the Society of Breast Imaging in making recommendations to reverse the trend.

**8. Until health insurance becomes more universally available, the U.S. Congress should expand the Centers for Disease Control and Prevention screening program to reach a much larger fraction of eligible women, and state legislatures should participate in the federal Breast and Cervical Treatment Act by providing funds for cancer treatment for eligible women.** The Centers for Disease Control and Prevention should be expected to reach 70 percent of eligible women (as opposed to the current 15 percent). This objective is based on the stated goals of the U.S. Department of Health and Human Services' *Healthy People 2010* report, which by the year 2010 expects 70 percent of women over age 40 to have had a recent (within the last 2 years) screening mammogram.

**9. The National Cancer Institute should sponsor large randomized trials every 10 to 15 years to reassess the effects of accepted screening modalities on clinical outcome.** These trials would compare two currently used technologies that are known to have different sensitivities. Breast cancer-specific mortality would be the principal outcome under evaluation. Such studies are needed because detection technologies and treatments are both continually evolving. Hence, the benefit of a screening method may change over time.

**10. The National Cancer Institute, through the American College of Radiology Imaging Network or the Breast Cancer Surveillance Consortium, should sponsor further studies to define more accurately the benefits and risks of screening mammography in women over age 70.** As the age distribution of the U.S. population continues to shift toward older ages, the question of whether these women benefit from screening mammography will become increasingly important.

# Glossary

**Absolute risk**: a measure of risk over time in a group of individuals; may be used to measure lifetime risk or risk over a narrower time period.

**Adjuvant therapy**: the use of another form of therapy in addition to the primary surgical therapy. It usually refers to hormonal therapy, chemotherapy, or radiation.

**Allele**: any one of a series of two or more different genes that occupy the same position (locus) on a chromosome.

**Amplification**: a process by which genetic material is increased.

**Aneuploidy**: a genetically unbalanced condition in which a cell or an organism has a number of chromosomes that is not an exact multiple of the normal chromosome number for that species.

**Angiogenesis**: the formation of new blood vessels.

**Antigen**: a substance that induces the immune system to produce antibodies that interact specifically with it.

**Ataxia telangiectasia**: an autosomal recessive disorder of the nervous system; affected individuals are sensitive to radiation and have a higher risk of cancer.

**Atypical hyperplasia**: proliferation of cells showing atypical nuclear form, especially as scattered cells.

**Autosomal**: a non-sex-linked form of inheritance (the gene is not found on the X or Y chromosome).

**Bias**: a process at any stage of inference tending to produce results that depart systematically from the true values.

**Bioinformatics**: use of computers and specialized software to organize and analyze biological information and data.

**Biomarker**: see *tumor marker*.

**Biopsy**: excision of a small piece of tissue for diagnostic examination; can be done surgically or with needles.

**Blind study**: a study in which the identity and relevant characteristics of the study subjects are concealed from the investigators.

**BRCA1**: a gene located on the short arm of chromosome 17; when this gene is mutated, a woman is at greater risk of developing breast or ovarian cancer, or both, than women who do not have the mutation.

**BRCA2**: a gene located on chromosome 13; a germ-line mutation in this gene is associated with increased risk of breast cancer.

**Breast lavage**: a procedure in which a small catheter is inserted into the nipple and the breast ducts are flushed with fluid to collect breast cells.

**Breast self-examination**: monthly physical examination of the breasts with the intent of finding lumps that could be an early indication of cancer.

**Carcinogen**: any substance or agent that produces or incites cancer.

**Carcinogenesis**: the production or origin of cancer.

**Carcinoma in situ**: a lesion characterized by cytological changes similar to those associated with invasive carcinoma, but with the pathological process limited to the lining epithelium and without visible evidence of invasion into adjacent structures.

**Catheter**: a tube passed through the body for evacuating or injecting fluids into body cavities.

**cDNA**: complementary DNA synthesized by RNA-directed DNA polymerase using RNA as a template; may be used as a probe for the presence of a gene code.

**Cell culture**: the growth of cells in vitro for experimental purposes.

**Chromophore**: any chemical that when present in a cell displays color.

**Chromosome**: chromosomes carry the genes, the basic units of heredity. Humans have 23 pairs of chromosomes, one member of each pair is from the mother and the other is from the father. Each chromosome can contain hundreds or thousands of individual genes.

**Clinical breast examination**: a physical examination of the breasts, performed by a doctor or nurse, with the intent of finding lumps that could be an early indication of cancer.

**Clinical outcome**: the end result of a medical intervention, e.g., survival or improved health.

**Clinical trial**: a formal study carried out according to a prospectively defined protocol that is intended to discover or verify the safety and effectiveness of procedures or interventions in humans. The term may refer to a controlled or uncontrolled trial.

**Clone:** a group of identical DNA molecules derived from one original length of DNA sequence.

**Comparative genomic hybridization**: method used to identify gain or loss of chromosomal material in cells.

**Computed tomography:** an imaging test in which many X-ray images are taken from different angles of a part of the body. These images are combined by a computer to produce cross-sectional pictures of internal organs.

**Computer-aided detection**: use of sophisticated computer programs designed to recognize patterns in images.

**Contralateral**: originating in or affecting the opposite side of the body.

**Contrast agent**: a substance that enhances the image produced by medical diagnostic equipment such as ultrasound, X ray, magnetic resonance imaging, or nuclear medicine or and imaging-sensitive substance that is ingested or injected intravenously to enhance or increase contrast between anatomical structures.

**Core-needle biopsy**: procedure in which a hollow needle is used to remove small cylinders of tissue from a suspected tumor.

**Cost-effectiveness analysis**: methods for comparing the economic efficiencies of different therapies or programs that produce health.

**Cytogenetics**: the study of cytology in relation to genetics.

**Cytology**: the study of formation, structure, and function of cells.

**Detection**: finding disease. Early detection means that the disease is found at an early stage, before it has grown large or spread to other sites.

**Detection method**: the traditional method of measuring the sensitivity of a screening test, in which the sensitivity is calculated as the number of true-positive results divided by the number of true-positive results plus the number of false-negative results.

**Diagnosis**: confirmation of a specific disease usually by imaging procedures and from the use of laboratory findings.

**Diagnostic mammography**: X-ray-based breast imaging undertaken for the purpose of diagnosing an abnormality discovered by physical exam or screening mammography.

**Digital mammography**: see *full-field digital mammography*.

**DNA:** abbreviation for deoxyribonucleic acid. DNA holds genetic information for cell growth, division, and function.

**Duct:** a hollow passage for gland secretions. In the breast, a passage through which milk passes from the lobule (which makes the milk) to the nipple.

**Ductal carcinoma in situ**: a lesion in which there is proliferation of abnormal cells within the ducts of the breast, but no visible evidence of invasion into the duct walls or surrounding tissues; sometimes referred to as "precancer" or "preinvasive cancer."

**Effectiveness**: the extent to which a specific test or intervention, when used under *ordinary* circumstances, does what it is intended to do.

**Efficacy**: the extent to which a specific test or intervention produces a beneficial result under *ideal* conditions (e.g., in a clinical trial).

**Elastography**: the measurement of the elastic properties of tissue.

**Electrical impedance imaging**: a procedure by which images are generated by transmitting a low-voltage electrical signal through the tissue.

**Electrical potential measurements:** a method that measures and records altered electrical gradients in tissues.

**Electronic palpation:** use of pressure sensors to quantitatively measure palpable features of the breast such as the hardness and size of lesions.

**Endoscopy:** inspection of body organs or cavities with a flexible lighted tube called an endoscope.

**Epidemiology:** science concerned with defining and explaining the interrelationships of factors that determine disease frequency and distribution.

**Epigenetics**: the study of mechanisms that produce phenotypic effects by altering gene activity without altering the nucletide sequence.

**Epithelial tissue**: those cells that form the outer surface of the body and that line the body cavities and the principal tubes and passageways leading to the exterior. They form the secreting portions of glands and their ducts and important parts of certain sense organs. The cells rest on a basement membrane and lie close to each other, with little intercellular material between them.

**Etiology**: the study of the causes of a disease.

**Exon**: the portions of the DNA sequence in a gene that specify the sequence of amino acids in a polypeptide chain, as well as the beginning and end of the coding sequence.

**Experimental study**: a clinical study in which subjects are randomly assigned to different intervention groups.

**False-negative result**: a test result that indicates that the abnormality or disease being investigated is not present when in fact it is.

**False-positive result**: a test result that indicates that the abnormality or disease being investigated is present when in fact it is not.

**Familial clusters**: a disease occurring in a family more frequently than would be expected by chance.

**Fine-needle aspiration:** a procedure by which a thin needle is used to draw up (aspirate) samples for examination under a microscope.

**Flow cytometry:** any technique for sorting, selecting, or counting individual cells in a suspension as they pass through a tube; applied especially to techniques involving the detection of a cell-bound fluorescent label and often used in cancer research as well as in screening for chromosomal abnormalities.

**Fluorescent in situ hybridization:** an experimental procedure for localizing a specific gene or DNA sequence within a chromosome based on binding of a complementary, fluorescently labeled segment of RNA or DNA to it.

**Full-field digital mammography:** similar to conventional mammography (film-screen mammography) except that a dedicated electronic detector system is used to computerize and display the X-ray information.

**Gamma camera:** an imaging instrument that records the spatial distribution of radioactive compounds in the human body.

**Gel electrophoresis:** a method for separating proteins or nucleic acid fragments that is carried out in a silica or acrylamide gel under the influence of an electric field.

**Gene:** a functional unit of heredity that occupies a specific place or locus on a chromosome.

**Genetic marker:** a genetic change in cells that is indicative of cancer or malignant potential, or a piece of DNA that lies on a chromosome so close to a gene that the marker and the gene are inherited together. A marker is thus an identifiable heritable spot on a chromosome. A marker can be an expressed region of DNA (a gene) or a segment of DNA with no known coding function.

**Genome:** an organism's entire complement of DNA, which determines its genetic makeup.

**Germ-line mutation:** an inherited mutation found in all cells in the body.

**Heterogeneous:** exhibiting variable characteristics.

**Heterozygosity:** the state of having different alleles at a specific locus in the genome.

**High-throughput technology:** any approach using robotics, automated machines, and computers to process many samples at once.

**Histology:** the study of the microscopic structure of tissue.

**Hyperplasia:** an increase in the number of cells in a tissue or organ, excluding tumor formation.

**Imaging agents:** any substance administered to a patient for the purpose of producing or enhancing an image of the body; includes contrast agents used with medical imaging techniques such as radiography, computed tomography, ultrasonography, and magnetic resonance imaging, as well as radiopharmaceuticals used with imaging procedures such as single-photon emission computed tomography and positron emission tomography.

**Immunocytochemistry or immunohistochemistry:** a laboratory test that uses antibodies to detect specific biochemical antigens in cells or tissue samples viewed under a microscope; can be used to help classify cancers.

**Immunology:** the study of immunity to diseases.

**Incidence method:** method of measuring the sensitivity of a screening test; calculates the cancer incidence among persons not undergoing screening and the interval cancer rate of persons who are screened.

**In situ:** in position, localized.

**Intron:** an apparently nonfunctional segment of DNA, ranging in size from less than 100 to more than 1,000 nucleotides, which is transcribed into nuclear RNA but which is then removed from the transcript and rapidly degrades.

**Invasive cancer:** cancers capable of growing beyond their site of origin and invading neighboring tissue.

**Invasive ductal carcinoma:** a cancer that starts in the ducts of the breast and then breaks through the duct wall, where it invades the surrounding tissue; it is the most common type of breast cancer and accounts for about 80 percent of breast malignancies.

**Invasive lobular carcinoma:** a cancer that starts in the milk-producing glands (lobules) of the breast and then breaks through the lobule walls to involve the surrounding tissue; accounts for about 15 percent of invasive breast cancers.

**Lead-time bias:** the assumption that identifying and treating tumors at an earlier point in the progression of the disease will necessarily alter the rate of progression and the eventual outcome.

**Length bias:** the assumption that screening tests are more likely to identify slowly growing tumors than those with a fast growth rate.

**Li-Fraumeni syndrome:** a dominant cancer syndrome in which gene carriers have a higher risk of several cancer types, including breast cancer.

**Linkage analysis:** study of the association between distinct genes that occupy closely situated loci on the same chromosome. This results in an association in the inheritance of these genes.

**Lobular carcinoma in situ:** abnormal cells within a breast lobule that have not invaded surrounding tissue; can serve as a marker of future cancer risk.

**Localized cancer:** a cancer that is confined to the place where it started; that is, it has not spread to distant parts of the body.

**Loss of heterozygosity:** loss of one allele at a specific genetic locus via deletion, usually accompanied by a point mutation in the remaining allele.

**Magnetic resonance imaging:** method by which images are created by recording signals generated from the excitation (the gain and loss of energy) of elements such as the hydrogen of water in tissue in a magnetic field.

**Magnetic resonance spectroscopy:** the study of the alteration and interaction of magnetic sublevels, in which the relevant wavelengths include long microwaves through radio-wave frequencies.

**Malignant:** a tumor that has the potential to become lethal through destructive growth or by having the ability to invade surrounding tissue and metastasize.

**Malignant transformation:** changes that a cell undergoes as it develops the ability to form a malignant tumor.

**Mammogram:** X-ray image of the breast.

**Mammography:** technique for imaging breast tissues with X rays.

**Mass spectroscopy:** a method for separating molecular and atomic particles according to mass by applying a combination of electrical and magnetic fields to deflect ions passing in a beam through the instrument.

**Medicaid:** jointly funded federal-state health insurance program for certain low-income and needy people. It covers approximately 36 million individuals including children; aged, blind, and/or disabled people; and people who are eligible to receive federally assisted income maintenance payments.

**Medicare:** a program that provides health insurance to people age 65 and over, those who have permanent kidney failure, and people with certain disabilities.

**Menarche:** the initial menstrual period.

**Menopause:** permanent cessation of menstrual activity.

**Messenger RNA:** the molecule, also called mRNA, that carries the information from the DNA genetic code to areas in the cytoplasm of the cell that make proteins.

**Meta-analysis:** the use of statistical techniques in a systematic review to integrate the results of the included studies.

**Metastasis:** the ability of cancer cells to move from one part of the body to another, resulting in the growth of a secondary malignancy in a new location.

**Methylation:** the attachment of a methyl group ($CH_3$) to cytosine residues of eukaryotic DNA to form 5-methylcytosine.

**Microarray**: thousands of different oligonucleotides spotted onto specific locations on glass microscope slides or silicon chips, which are then hybridized with labeled sample DNA or RNA.

**Microcalcifications**: tiny calcium deposits within the breast, singly or in clusters; often found by mammography. They may be a sign of cancer.

**Modality**: a method of application or use of any therapy or medical device.

**Molecular markers**: changes in cells, at the molecular level, that are indicative of cancer or malignant potential.

**Monoenergetic x-rays**: a beam of X rays whose photon energy is found to lie within a very narrow band.

**Morbidity**: injury or illness.

**Morphology**: science of structure and form without regard to function.

**Mortality**: the death rate; ratio of number of deaths to a given population.

**Mutation**: a change either in the base sequence of DNA or in the order, number, or placement of genes on or across chromosomes that may result in a change in the structure or function of a protein.

**Neoplasm**: new growth; a tumor.

**Nipple aspiration**: use of suction to collect breast fluid through the nipple of nonlactating women.

**Northern analysis:** an electroblotting technique for detecting a specific RNA molecule, in which RNA is transferred to a filter and is hybridized to radioactively labeled RNA or DNA.

**Observational study**: a clinical study in which information is collected on groups of individuals who have a specific condition or who have chosen a particular course of medical intervention.

**Occult tumors**: undetected and without symptoms.

**Oligonucleotide**: a small DNA or RNA molecule composed of a few nucleotide bases.

**Oncology**: the branch of medicine dealing with tumors.

**Optical imaging**: use of light, usually in the near-infrared range, to produce an image of tissue.

**Overdiagnosis**: labeling an abnormality as cancer when it in fact is not likely to become a lethal cancer.

**p53**: a tumor suppressor gene commonly mutated in cancer.

**Palpable tumor**: a tumor that can be felt during a physical examination.

**Phenotype**: the physical characteristics or makeup of an individual.

**Photonics**: the technology of generating and harnessing light and other forms of radiant energy whose quantum unit is the photon. The science includes light emission, transmission, deflection, amplification, and detection by optical components and instruments, lasers and other light sources, fiber optics, electro-optical instrumentation, related hardware and electronics, and sophisticated systems.

**Polymerase chain reaction:** a process for amplifying a DNA molecule up to $10^6$- to $10^9$-fold.

**Polymorphism:** the regular and simultaneous occurrence in a population of two or more alleles of a gene in which the frequency of the rarer of the alleles is greater than can be explained by recurrent mutation alone.

**Positional cloning:** cloning a gene simply on the basis of knowing its position in the genome without any idea of the function of that gene.

**Positive predictive value:** a measure of accuracy for a screening or diagnostic test; indicates what portion of those with an abnormal test result actually have the disease.

**Positron emission tomography:** use of radioactive tracers such as labeled glucose to identify regions in the body with altered metabolic activity.

**Premalignant:** changes in cells that may, but that do not always, become cancer. Also called "precancer."

**Prevalence:** a measure of the proportion of persons in the population with a particular disease at a given time.

**Prognosis:** prediction of the course and end of disease and the estimate of chance for recovery.

**Progression:** the growth or advancement of cancer, indicating a worsening of the disease.

**Prophylactic bilateral mastectomy:** surgical removal of both breasts with the intent of reducing the risk of developing breast cancer later in life.

**Proprietary rights:** exclusive rights held by a private individual or corporation under a trademark or patent.

**Proteome:** all of the proteins produced by a given species, just as the genome is the totality of the DNA possessed by that species.

**Protooncogene:** genes that promote cell growth and multiplication; normally found in all cells, but may undergo mutations that activate them, causing uncontrolled growth.

**Randomization:** a method that uses chance to assign participants to comparison groups in a trial by using a random-numbers table or a computer-generated random sequence. Random allocation implies that each individual being entered into a trial has the same chance of receiving each of the possible interventions.

**Relative risk:** a comparative measure of risk based on a comparison of disease incidence in two populations.

**Reverse transcriptase:** an RNA-dependent DNA polymerase, found in viruses, that catalyzes the synthesis of DNA from deoxyribonucleoside 5'-triphosphates, using RNA as a template.

**Risk:** a quantitative measure of the probability of developing or dying from a particular disease such as cancer.

**Scintimammography:** use of radioactive tracers to produce an image of the breast.

**Screen-film mammography:** conventional mammography in which the X rays are recorded on film.

**Screening:** systematic testing of an asymptomatic population to determine the presence of a particular disease or certain risk factors known to be associated with the disease.

**Screening mammography:** X-ray-based breast imaging in an asymptomatic population with the goal of detecting breast tumors at an early stage.

**Sensitivity:** a measure of how often a test correctly identifies women with breast cancer.

**Signal transduction:** the biochemical events that conduct the signal of a hormone growth factor from the cell exterior, through the cell membrane, and into the cytoplasm. This involves a number of molecules, including receptors, proteins, and messengers.

**Soft copy:** image display on a computer screen rather than on film.

**Somatic mutation:** uninherited mutation, acquired in cells during a person's lifetime.

**Specificity:** a measure of how often a test correctly identifies a woman as not having breast cancer.

**Specimen bank:** stored patient tissue samples that are used for biomedical research (also tumor or tissue banks).

**Spectroscopy:** analytical use of an instrument that separates radiant energy into its component frequencies or wavelengths by means of a prism or grating to form a spectrum for inspection.

**Stereotactic breast biopsy:** use of breast images (X ray or ultrasound) taken at various angles to generate a three-dimensional image for plotting the exact position of the suspicious lesion and for guiding the placement of a biopsy needle.

**Surrogate end points:** short-term, intermediate end points in a clinical study that are thought to be representative or predictive of longer-term outcomes.

**Systemic therapy:** treatment involving the whole body, usually using drugs.

**Telemammography:** the process of satellite or long-distance transmission of digital mammography for consultation.

**Thermography**: use of a device that detects and records the heat produced by tissues to generate an image.

**Thermotherapy**: use of lasers or high-intensity ultrasound to heat and destroy tumor cells.

**Tissue array**: small cylinders of tissue punched from 1,000 individual tumor biopsy specimens embedded in paraffin. These cylinders are then arrayed in a large paraffin block, from which 200 consecutive tissue sections can be cut, allowing rapid analysis of multiple arrayed samples by immunohistochemistry or in situ hybridization.

**Tomography**: any of several techniques for making X-ray pictures of a predetermined plane section of a solid object by blurring out the images of other planes.

**Tomosynthesis:** a variation of tomography in which several photographs of a patient are taken at different angles, and back-projection of the resulting radiographs produces a light distribution in a chosen three-dimensional volume of space that replicates the same volume in the patient.

**Transcription:** the first step of protein biosynthesis, in which DNA directs the production of RNA.

**Tumorigenesis:** the induction of the malignant growth of abnormal cells.

**Tumor marker:** any substance or characteristic that indicates the presence of a malignancy.

**Tumor suppressor genes:** genes that slow cell division or that cause cells to die at the appropriate time. Mutations in these genes can lead to uncontrolled cell growth and the development of cancer.

**Ultrasound**: use of inaudible, high-frequency sound waves to create an image of the body.

**Virtual reality imaging**: interactive computer graphic simulations that can be used to produce a three-dimensional visualization of an organ or tissue.

# References

Electronic Palpation Device Is Adjunct to Manual Breast Exam. *Oncology News International.* 1999(2).

FDA-cleared breast self-examination pad now available nationwide. *Primary Care and Cancer.* 1999;19:42.

Final Report of the Technology Transfer Workshop on Breast Cancer Detection, Diagnosis, and Treatment. Washington, D.C., USA. May 1-2, 1997. *Acad Radiol 1998 Nov;5 Suppl 3:S465-501.*

The Cancer Letter. 2000;15(2).

The Cancer Letter. 2000;15(3).

Using "Radar" to detect breast cancer. *Microwave News.* 2000;8.

Abbott R, Barber KR, Taylor DK, Pendel D. Utilization of early detection services: a recruitment and screening program for African American women [letter]. *J Health Care Poor Underserved.* 1999;10:269-80.

Alfano RR, Demos SG, Gayen SK. Advances in optical imaging of biomedical media. *Ann NY Acad Sci.* 1997;820:248-70; discussion 271.

Alizadeh AA, Eisen MB, Davis RE, et al. Distinct types of diffuse large B-cell lymphoma identified by gene expression profiling [see comments]. *Nature.* 2000;403:503-11.

Allen MW, Hendi P, Bassett L, Phelps ME, Gambhir SS. A study on the cost effectiveness of sestamibi scintimammography for screening women with dense breasts for breast cancer. *Breast Cancer Res Treat.* 1999;55:243-58.

Allred DC, Moshin SK; Biological features of human premalignant breast disease. In: Diseases of the Breast. Philadelphia: Lippincott Williams & Wilkins; 2000:355-366. Harris JR.

American Cancer Society. *Cancer Facts and Figures;* 2000.

American Society of Clinical Oncology. Statement on genetic testing for cancer susceptibility, Adopted on February 20, 1996. *J Clin Oncol.* 1996;14:1730-6; discussion 1737-40.

Amundadottir LT, Merlino G, Dickson RB. Transgenic mouse models of breast cancer. *Breast Cancer Res Treat.* 1996;39:119-35.

Anbar M. Mechanism of hyperthermia of the cancerous breast. *Biomedical Thermology.* 1995; 15:135-9.

Anbar M, Brown CA, Milescu L, Babalola JA. Clinical Applications of DAT using a QWIP FPA camera. Infrared Technology and Applications XXV: April 5, 1999-April 9, 1999; Orlando, FL. Part of the SPIE Conference on Infared Technology and Applications XXV.

Anbar M, Brown C, Milescu L. Objective identification of cancerous breasts by dynamic area telethermometry (DAT). *Thermology International*. 1999;127-33.

Anderson LF. Issues raised on availability of breast cancer materials for research [news]. *J Natl Cancer Inst*. 1994;86:1580-2.

Appleby JM, Barber JB, Levine E, et al. Absence of mutations in the ATM gene in breast cancer patients with severe responses to radiotherapy. *Br J Cancer*. 1997;76:1546-9.

Arfelli F, Assante M, Bonvicini V, et al. Low-dose phase contrast x-ray medical imaging. *Phys Med Biol*. 1998a;43:2845-52.

Arfelli F, Bonvicini V, Bravin A, et al. Mammography of a phantom and breast tissue with synchrotron radiation and a linear-array silicon detector. *Radiology*. 1998b;208:709-15.

Arfelli F, Bonvicini V, Bravin A, et al. Mammography with synchrotron radiation: phase-detection techniques. *Radiology*. 2000;215:286-93.

Aronowitz R. To screen or not to screen: What is the question? [editorial]. *J Gen Intern Med*. 1995;10:295-7.

Assurance Medical Inc. *The Clinical Assessment of Electronic Palpation Technology: A New Approach for the Early Detection and Monitoring of Breast Lesions*. 1999.

Aubry WM. Technology assessment and reimbursement for future new imaging technologies. *Acad Radiol*. 1998;5 Suppl 2:S389-91.

Baines CJ. The Canadian National Breast Screening Study: a perspective on criticisms. *Ann Intern Med*. 1994;120:326-34.

Baines CJ, To T, Wall C. Women's attitudes to screening after participation in the National Breast Screening Study. A questionnaire survey. *Cancer*. 1990;65:1663-9.

Banta HD, Thacker SB. The case for reassessment of health care technology. Once is not enough [see comments]. *JAMA*. 1990;264:235-40.

Barton MB, Harris R, Fletcher SW. Does this patient have breast cancer? The screening clinical breast examination: should it be done? How? *JAMA*. 1999;282:1270-80.

Baylin SB, Herman JG, Graff JR, Vertino PM, Issa JP. Alterations in DNA methylation: a fundamental aspect of neoplasia. *Adv Cancer Res*. 1998;72:141-96.

Beam CA, Layde PM, Sullivan DC. Variability in the interpretation of screening mammograms by US radiologists. Findings from a national sample. *Arch Intern Med*. 1996;156:209-13.

Beam CA, Sullivan DC, Layde PM. Effect of human variability on independent double reading in screening mammography. *Acad Radiol*. 1996;3:891-7.

Bergstraesser LM, Weitzman SA. Culture of normal and malignant primary human mammary epithelial cells in a physiological manner simulates in vivo growth patterns and allows discrimination of cell type. *Cancer Res*. 1993;53:2644-54.

Berlin L. The missed breast cancer: perceptions and realities [see comments]. *AJR Am J Roentgenol*. 1999;173:1161-7.

Berry DA. Benefits and risks of screening mammography for women in their forties: a statistical appraisal [see comments]. *J Natl Cancer Inst*. 1998;90:1431-9.

Berx G, Becker KF, Hofler H, van Roy F. Mutations of the human E-cadherin (CDH1) gene. *Hum Mutat*. 1998;12:226-37.

Blackman DK, Bennett EM, Miller DS. Trends in self-reported use of mammograms (1989-1997) and Papanicolaou tests (1991-1997)—Behavioral Risk Factor Surveillance System. *Mor Mortal Wkly Rep CDC Surveill Summ*. 1999;48:1-22.

Blanks RG, Moss SM, McGahan CE, Quinn MJ, Babb PJ. Effect of NHS breast screening programme on mortality from breast cancer in England and Wales, 1990-8: comparison of observed with predicted mortality. *BMJ*. 2000;321:665-669.

Blue Cross and Blue Shield Association Technology Evaluation Center AP. *Scintimammography*; 1997. Volume 12.

Bohorfoush AG. Tissue spectroscopy for gastrointestinal diseases. *Endoscopy.* 1996;28:372-80.

Bone B, Pentek Z, Perbeck L, Veress B. Diagnostic accuracy of mammography and contrast-enhanced MR imaging in 238 histologically verified breast lesions. *Acta Radiol.* 1997; 38:489-96.

Borresen AL. Role of genetic factors in breast cancer susceptibility. *Acta Oncol.* 1992;31: 151-5.

Bosanko CM, Baum JK, Clark K, Barth-Jones D, Levine AJ. Optical spectroscopy (INVOS) is unreliable in detecting breast cancer. *Am J Roentgenol.* 1990;155:43-7.

Bown SG, Bigio I, Briggs GM, Pickard CDO, Ripley P. Optical biopsy for the diagnosis of breast tumors. Era of Hope Department of Defense Breast Cancer Program Meeting: June, 2000.

Braslow NM, Shatin D, McCarthy DB, Newcomer LN. Role of technology assessment in health benefits coverage for medical devices. *Am J Manag Care.* 1998;4 Spec No:SP139-50.

Braun S, Pantel K, Muller P, et al. Cytokeratin-positive cells in the bone marrow and survival of patients with stage I, II, or III breast cancer [see comments] [published erratum appears in N Engl J Med 2000 Jul 27;343(4):308]. *N Engl J Med.* 2000;342:525-33.

Breast Cancer Progress Review Group. *Charting The Course: Priorities For Breast Cancer Research*: Breast Cancer Progress Review Group; 1998.

Brennan TA, Sox CM, Burstin HR. Relation between negligent adverse events and the outcomes of medical-malpractice litigation *N Engl J Med.* 1996;335:1963-7.

Brice J. Small change for big medicine: The crisis in breast imaging services. *Diagn Imaging (San Franc).* 2000;22.

Bridges JE, inventor; *Non-Invasive System for Breast Cancer Detection*5704355. 1998 Jan 6.

Broeks A, Urbanus JH, Floore AN, et al. ATM-heterozygous germline mutations contribute to breast cancer-susceptibility. *Am J Hum Genet.* 2000;66:494-500.

Brown AD, Garber AM. Cost-effectiveness of 3 methods to enhance the sensitivity of Papanicolaou testing. *JAMA.* 1999;281:347-53.

Brown ML, Fintor L. Cost-effectiveness of breast cancer screening: preliminary results of a systematic review of the literature. *Breast Cancer Res Treat.* 1993;25:113-8.

Brown ML, Houn F, Sickles EA, Kessler LG. Screening mammography in community practice: positive predictive value of abnormal findings and yield of follow-up diagnostic procedures. *AJR Am J Roentgenol.* 1995;165:1373-7.

Burattini E, Cossu E, Di Maggio C, et al. Mammography with synchrotron radiation. *Radiology.* 1995;195:239-44.

Burke HB, Henson DE. Specimen banks for cancer prognostic factor research. *Arch Pathol Lab Med.* 1998;122:871-4.

Burke W, Daly M, Garber J, et al. Recommendations for follow-up care of individuals with an inherited predisposition to cancer. II. BRCA1 and BRCA2. Cancer Genetics Studies Consortium [see comments]. *JAMA.* 1997;277:997-1003.

Burman ML, Taplin SH, Herta DF, Elmore JG. Effect of false-positive mammograms on interval breast cancer screening in a health maintenance organization. *Ann Intern Med.* 1999;131:1-6.

Byng JW, Yaffe MJ, Jong RA, et al. Analysis of mammographic density and breast cancer risk from digitized mammograms. *Radiographics.* 1998;18:1587-98.

Canadian Association of Radiation Oncologists. The palpable breast lump: information and recommendations to assist decision-making when a breast lump is detected. The Steering Committee on Clinical Practice Guidelines for the Care and Treatment of Breast Cancer. [see comments]. *CMAJ.* 1998;158 Suppl 3:S3-8.

Carson PL, Fowlkes JB, Roubidoux MA, et al. 3-D color Doppler image quantification of breast masses. *Ultrasound Med Biol.* 1998;24:945-52.

Center for Disease Control and Prevention. Use of cervical and breast cancer screening among women with and without functional limitations—United States, 1994-1995. *MMWR Morb Weekly Report.* 1998;47:853-6.

Chan HP, Sahiner B, Helvie MA, et al. Improvement of radiologists' characterization of mammographic masses by using computer-aided diagnosis: an ROC study. *Radiology.* 1999;212:817-27.

Chance B. Near-infrared images using continuous, phase-modulated, and pulsed light with quantitation of blood and blood oxygenation. *Ann N Y Acad Sci.* 1998;838:29-45.

Chang CH, Sibala JL, Fritz SL, Dwyer SJ 3d, Templeton AW. Specific value of computed tomographic breast scanner (CT/M) in diagnosis of breast diseases. *Radiology.* 1979;132:647-52.

Chang CH, Sibala JL, Fritz SL, et al. Computed tomography in detection and diagnosis of breast cancer. *Cancer.* 1980;46:939-46.

Chang CH, Sibala JL, Gallagher JH, et al. Computed tomography of the breast. A preliminary report. *Radiology.* 1977;124:827-9.

Chaudhary SS, Mishra RK, Swarup A, Thomas JM. Dielectric properties of normal & malignant human breast tissues at radiowave & microwave frequencies. *Indian J Biochem Biophys.* 1984;21:76-9.

Chen J, Birkholtz GG, Lindblom P, Rubio C, Lindblom A. The role of ataxia-telangiectasia heterozygotes in familial breast cancer. *Cancer Res.* 1998;58:1376-9.

Cheung KL, Graves CR, Robertson JF. Tumour marker measurements in the diagnosis and monitoring of breast cancer. *Cancer Treat Rev.* 2000;26:91-102.

Christiansen CL, Wang F, Barton MB, et al. Predicting the cumulative risk of false-positive mammograms. *J Natl Cancer Inst.* 2000;92:1657-66.

Clarke C, Titley J, Davies S, O'Hare MJ. An immunomagnetic separation method using superparamagnetic (MACS) beads for large-scale purification of human mammary luminal and myoepithelial cells. *Epithelial Cell Biol.* 1994;3:38-46.

Clarke J. SQUIDS. *Scientific American.* 1994;271:46-53.

Clemons M, Loijens L, Goss P. Breast cancer risk following irradiation for Hodgkin's disease. *Cancer Treat Rev.* 2000;26:291-302.

Clontech Laboratories Inc. *High Through Put Expression Profiling With Atlas;* 1999.

Cocconi G. The natural history of operable breast cancer after primary treatment. *Ann Oncol.* 1995;6 Suppl 2:11-21.

Coleman EA. Practice and effectiveness of breast self examination: a selective review of the literature (1977-1989). *J Cancer Educ.* 1991;6:83-92.

Concato J, Shah N, Horwitz RI. Randomized, controlled trials, observational studies, and the hierarchy of research design. *N Engl J Med.* 2000;342:1887-92.

Connor F, Bertwistle D, Mee PJ, et al. Tumorigenesis and a DNA repair defect in mice with a truncating BRCA2 mutation. *Nat Genet.* 1997;17:423-30.

Cooper TA, Mattox W. The regulation of splice-site selection, and its role in human disease. *Am J Hum Genet.* 1997;61:259-66.

Cortez D, Wang Y, Qin J, Elledge SJ. Requirement of ATM-dependent phosphorylation of brca1 in the DNA damage response to double-strand breaks. *Science.* 1999;286:1162-6.

Costello JF, Fruhwald MC, Smiraglia DJ, et al. Aberrant CpG-island methylation has nonrandom and tumour-type-specific patterns. *Nat Genet.* 2000;24:132-8.

Craft PS, Harris AL. Clinical prognostic significance of tumour angiogenesis. *Ann Oncol.* 1994;5:305-11.

Cutler M. Transillumination as an aid in the diagnosis of breast lesions. *Surg Gynecol Obstet.* 1929;48:721-9.

Cuzick J, Holland R, Barth V, et al. Electropotential measurements as a new diagnostic modality for breast cancer. *Lancet.* 1998;352:359-63.

Daly MB, Offit K, Li F, et al. Participation in the cooperative family registry for breast cancer studies: issues of informed consent. *J Natl Cancer Inst.* 2000;92:452-6.

Dawson PJ, Wolman SR, Tait L, Heppner GH, Miller FR. MCF10AT: a model for the evolution of cancer from proliferative breast disease. *Am J Pathol.* 1996;148:313-9.

DeBruhl ND, Bassett LW, Jessop NW, Mason AM. Mobile mammography: results of a national survey. *Radiology.* 1996;201:433-7.

Del Vecchio S, Ciarmiello A, Salvatore M. Clinical imaging of multidrug resistance in cancer. *Q J Nucl Med.* 1999;43:125-31.

Department of Labor et al., Genetic Information and the Workplace: (January 20, 1998).

Detsky AS, Naglie IG. A clinician's guide to cost-effectiveness analysis. *Ann Intern Med.* 1990;113:147-54.

Doi K, Giger ML, Nishikawa RM, Schmidt RA. Computer-Aided Diagnosis of Breast Cancer on Mammograms. *Breast Cancer.* 1997;4:228-233.

Doyle AJ, Murray KA, Nelson EW, Bragg DG. Selective use of image-guided large-core needle biopsy of the breast: accuracy and cost-effectiveness. *Am J Roentgenol.* 1995;165:281-4.

Duijm LE, Guit GL, Zaat JO, Koomen AR, Willebrand D. Sensitivity, specificity and predictive values of breast imaging in the detection of cancer. *Br J Cancer.* 1997;76:377-81.

Dunning AM, Healey CS, Pharoah PD, Teare MD, Ponder BA, Easton DF. A systematic review of genetic polymorphisms and breast cancer risk. *Cancer Epidemiol Biomarkers Prev.* 1999;8:843-54.

Eastern Research Group. *Cost and Benefit Analysis of Regulation Under the Mammograpgy Quality Standards Act of 1992 Preliminary Report;* 1996.

Easton DF, Bishop DT, Ford D, Crockford GP. Genetic linkage analysis in familial breast and ovarian cancer: results from 214 families. The Breast Cancer Linkage Consortium. *Am J Hum Genet.* 1993;52:678-701.

Edell SL, Eisen MD. Current imaging modalities for the diagnosis of breast cancer. *Del Med J.* 1999;71:377-82.

Eisen A, Rebbeck TR, Wood WC, Weber BL. Prophylactic surgery in women with a hereditary predisposition to breast and ovarian cancer. *J Clin Oncol.* 2000;18:1980-95.

Eisen MB, Spellman PT, Brown PO, Botstein D. Cluster analysis and display of genome-wide expression patterns. *Proc Natl Acad Sci U S A.* 1998;95:14863-8.

Eisenberg JM. Ten lessons for evidence-based technology assessment. *JAMA.* 1999;282:1865-9.

Eklund GW. Shortage of qualified breast imagers could lead to crisis. *Diagn Imaging (San Franc).* 2000;22(4):31-3,69.

Elmore JG, Barton MB, Moceri VM, Polk S, Arena PJ, Fletcher SW. Ten-year risk of false positive screening mammograms and clinical breast examinations. *N Engl J Med.* 1998a;338:1089-96.

Elmore JG, Wells CK, Howard DH. Does diagnostic accuracy in mammography depend on radiologists' experience? *J Womens Health.* 1998b;7:443-9.

Elmore JG, Wells CK, Lee CH, Howard DH, Feinstein AR. Variability in radiologists' interpretations of mammograms. *N Engl J Med.* 1994;331:1493-9.

Emmert-Buck MR, Bonner RF, Smith PD, et al. Laser capture microdissection. *Science.* 1996;274:998-1001.

Engel LW, Young NA. Human breast carcinoma cells in continuous culture: a review. *Cancer Res.* 1978;38:4327-39.

Ernster VL, Barclay J. Increases in ductal carcinoma in situ (DCIS) of the breast in relation to mammography: a dilemma. *J Natl Cancer Inst Monogr.* 1997:151-6.

Ernster VL, Barclay J, Kerlikowske K, Grady D, Henderson C. Incidence of and treatment for ductal carcinoma in situ of the breast. *JAMA*. 1996;275:913-8.

Fabian C., O'Shaughnessy J., Mayo M.S., et al. *Prevention Clinical Trial Models Utilizing Breast Intraepitheial Neoplasia as an Endpoint*. In press.

Fajardo LL, DeAngelis GA. The role of stereotactic biopsy in abnormal mammograms. *Surg Oncol Clin N Am*. 1997;6:285-99.

Farria DM, Debruhl N, Gorczyca D, Bassett LW. Magnetic Resonance Imaging of Breast Tumors. *Seminars In Breast Disease*. 1999;2:74-88.

Farria D, Feig SA. An introduction to economic issues in breast imaging. *Radiol Clin North Am*. 2000;38:825-42.

Faupel M, Vanel D, Barth V, et al. Electropotential evaluation as a new technique for diagnosing breast lesions. *Eur J Radiol*. 1997;24:33-8.

Fear EC, Stuchly MA. Microwave System for Breast Tumor Detection. *IEEE Microwave and Guided Wave Letters*. 1999;9:470-2.

Federal Register. *Medicare Program: Procedures for Making National Coverage Decisions*. 1999;64(80):22619-25.

Federal Register. *Medicare Program: Criteria for Making Coverage Decisions*. 2000;65(95):31124-29.

Feig. *SBI News, President's Message: Behind the Scenes of an SBI Epic Production*; 2000a.

Feig S. Principles and practice of breast imaging, Seminars in breast disease. 1999a;2:3-16.

Feig SA. Economic challenges in breast imaging. A survivor's guide to success. *Radiol Clin North Am*. 2000b;38:843-52.

Feig SA. *President's Message: SBI Residency Training Curriculum*; 1999b.

Feig SA. Role and evaluation of mammography and other imaging methods for breast cancer detection, diagnosis, and staging. *Semin Nucl Med*. 1999c;29:3-15.

Feig SA, Hendrick RE. Radiation risk from screening mammography of women aged 40-49 years. *J Natl Cancer Inst Monogr*. 1997:119-24.

Feig SA, Shaber GS, Schwartz GF, et al. Thermography, mammography, and clinical examination in breast cancer screening. Review of 16,000 studies. *Radiology*. 1977;122:123-7.

Fisher B, Costantino JP, Wickerham DL, et al. Tamoxifen for prevention of breast cancer: report of the National Surgical Adjuvant Breast and Bowel Project P-1 Study. *J Natl Cancer Inst*. 1998a;90:1371-88.

Fisher B, Dignam J, Wolmark N, et al. Lumpectomy and radiation therapy for the treatment of intraductal breast cancer: findings from National Surgical Adjuvant Breast and Bowel Project B-17. *J Clin Oncol*. 1998b;16:441-52.

FitzGerald MG, Bean JM, Hegde SR, et al. Heterozygous ATM mutations do not contribute to early onset of breast cancer. *Nat Genet*. 1997;15:307-10.

Fitzgibbons PL, Page DL, Weaver D, et al. Prognostic factors in breast cancer. College of American Pathologists Consensus Statement 1999. *Arch Pathol Lab Med*. 2000;124:966-78.

Fletcher RH., Fletcher SW, Wagner EH. *Clinical Epidemiology - the Essentials*. 3rd Ed. Baltimore, MD: Williams & Wilkins; 1996.

Fliss MS, Usadel H, Caballero OL, et al. Facile detection of mitochondrial DNA mutations in tumors and bodily fluids. *Science*. 2000;287:2017-9.

Foray N, Randrianarison V, Marot D, Perricaudet M, Lenoir G, Feunteun J. Gamma-rays-induced death of human cells carrying mutations of BRCA1 or BRCA2. *Oncogene*. 1999;18:7334-42.

Ford D, Easton DF, Bishop DT, Narod SA, Goldgar DE. Risks of cancer in BRCA1-mutation carriers. Breast Cancer Linkage Consortium. *Lancet*. 1994;343:692-5.

Foster KR. Thermographic detection of breast cancer [see comments]. *IEEE Eng Med Biol Mag*1998;17:10-4.

Fox SA, Stein JA. The effect of physician-patient communication on mammography utilization by different ethnic groups. *Med Care*. 1991;29:1065-82.

Fuchs VR. Health care for the elderly: how much? Who will pay for it? *Health Aff (Millwood)*. 1999;18:11-21.

Fukuda M, Shimizu K, Okamoto N, et al. Prospective evaluation of skin surface electropotentials in Japanese patients with suspicious breast lesions. *Jpn J Cancer Res*. 1996; 87:1092-6.

Fuller BP, Kahn MJ, Barr PA, et al. Privacy in genetics research. *Science*. 1999;285:1359-61.

Gail M, Rimer B. Risk-based recommendations for mammographic screening for women in their forties [see comments] [published erratum appears in J Clin Oncol 1999 Feb; 17(2):740]. *J Clin Oncol*. 1998;16:3105-14.

Gelijns and Rosenberg Diagnostic Devices. *The Sources of Industrial Leadership, Edited by David Mowery and Richard Nelson*. Cambridge; 1999.

Glasspool RM, Evans TR. Clinical imaging of cancer metastasis. *Eur J Cancer*. 2000;36: 1661-70.

Gold MR, Siegel JE, Russell LB, Weinstein MC. *Cost-Effectiveness in Health and Medicine*. New York: Oxford University Press; 1996.

Gold RH, Bassett LW, Widoff BE. Highlights from the history of mammography. *Radiographics*. 1990;10:1111-31.

Goldenberg DM, Nabi HA. Breast cancer imaging with radiolabeled antibodies. *Semin Nucl Med*. 1999;29:41-8.

Golub G. Heroic Myths and Probability: Confronting the Limits of Screening. From: Kramer, BS; Gohagan, JK; Prorok, PC *Cancer Screening: Theory and Practice*. New York: M. Dekker; 1999:13-26.

Goodman CJ, Lindsey JI, Whigham CJ, Robinson A. Diagnostic radiology residents in the classes of 1999 and 2000: fellowship and employment. *AJR Am J Roentgenol*. 2000;174: 1211-3.

Goodman CS. Healthcare technology assessment: methods, framework, and role in policy making. *Am J Manag Care*. 1998;4 Spec No:SP200-14; quiz SP215-6.

Gotzsche PC, Olsen O. Is screening for breast cancer with mammography justifiable? *Lancet*. 2000;355:129-34.

Grady KE, Lemkau JP, McVay JM, Reisine ST. The importance of physician encouragement in breast cancer screening of older women. *Prev Med*. 1992;21:766-80.

Graham-Rowe D. Closing in on cancer. *New Scientist*. 1999.

Gram IT, Lund E, Slenker SE. Quality of life following a false positive mammogram. *Br J Cancer*. 1990;62:1018-22.

Gribbestad IS, Singstad TE, Nilsen G, et al. In vivo 1H MRS of normal breast and breast tumors using a dedicated double breast coil. *J Magn Reson Imaging*. 1998;8:1191-7.

Gribbestad IS, Sitter B, Lundgren S, Krane J, Axelson D. Metabolite composition in breast tumors examined by proton nuclear magnetic resonance spectroscopy. *Anticancer Res*. 1999;19:1737-46.

Grizzle WE, Aamodt R, Clausen K, LiVolsi V, Pretlow TG, Qualman S. Providing human tissues for research: how to establish a program. *Arch Pathol Lab Med*. 1998;122:1065-76.

Hacia JG, Brody LC, Chee MS, Fodor SP, Collins FS. Detection of heterozygous mutations in BRCA1 using high density oligonucleotide arrays and two-colour fluorescence analysis [see comments]. *Nat Genet*. 1996;14:441-7.

Hacia JG, Collins FS. Mutational analysis using oligonucleotide microarrays. *J Med Genet*. 1999;36:730-6.

Hagness SC, Taflove A, Bridges JE. Two-dimensional FDTD analysis of a pulsed microwave confocal system for breast cancer detection: fixed-focus and antenna-array sensors [published erratum appears in IEEE Trans Biomed Eng 1999 Mar;46(3):364]. *IEEE Trans Biomed Eng*. 1998;45:1470-9.

Hakama M, Pukkala E, Heikkila M, Kallio M. Effectiveness of the public health policy for breast cancer screening in Finland: population based cohort study. *BMJ*. 1997;314: 864-7.

Haley S. Bill to create bioimaging, bioengineering institute at NIH clears House. Advocates hope for pre-recess vote on Lott-sponsored Senate companion bill. *Washington Fax*. 2000.

Hall HG, Farson DA, Bissell MJ. Lumen formation by epithelial cell lines in response to collagen overlay: a morphogenetic model in culture. *Proc Natl Acad Sci U S A*. 1982;79: 4672-6.

Hancock SL, Cox RS, McDougall IR. Thyroid diseases after treatment of Hodgkin's disease. *N Engl J Med*. 1991;325:599-605.

Hankinson SE, Willett WC, Colditz GA, et al. Circulating concentrations of insulin-like growth factor-I and risk of breast cancer. *Lancet*. 1998;351:1393-6.

Haran C. Services denied: why women with disabilities aren't screened for cancer. *MAMM*. 2000;3.

Harris EL. Genetic inheritance of cancer risk: applications to cancer screening. From: Kramer BS, Gohagan JK, Prorok PC, eds. *Cancer Screening: Theory and Practice*. New York: M. Dekker; 1999:595-609.

Harris R. Decision-making about screening: individual and policy levels. From: Kramer BS, Gohagan JK, Prorok PC, eds. *Cancer Screening: Theory and Practice*. New York: M. Dekker; 1999:55-75.

Hartmann LC, Schaid D, Sellers T, et al. Bilateral Prophylactic Mastectomy (PM) in BRCA1/2 Mutation Carriers. Proceedings of the Annual Meeting of the American Association for Cancer Research: 2000.

Harvey JA, Fajardo LL, Innis CA. Previous mammograms in patients with impalpable breast carcinoma: retrospective vs blinded interpretation. 1993 ARRS President's Award [see comments]. *AJR Am J Roentgenol*. 1993;161:1167-72.

Havighurst CC. Health care law and policy: readings, notes and questions. 1998. Edited by: Clark C. Havighurst, James F. Blumstein and Troyen A. Brennan. 2nd Edition. New York: Foundation Press, 1998.

Hayes DF, Bast RC, Desch CE, et al. Tumor marker utility grading system: a framework to evaluate clinical utility of tumor markers [see comments]. *J Natl Cancer Inst*. 1996;88: 1456-66.

Hayes DF, Trock B, Harris AL. Assessing the clinical impact of prognostic factors: when is "statistically significant" clinically useful? *Breast Cancer Res Treat*. 1998;52:305-19.

Head JF, Elliott RL. Thermography. Its relation to pathologic characteristics, vascularity, proliferation rate, and survival of patients with invasive ductal carcinoma of the breast [letter; comment]. *Cancer*. 1997;79:186-8.

Health and Human Services. *Investigational Device Exemptions Manual*; 1996. HHS Publication FDA 96-4159.

Health Care Financing Administration/Food and Drug Administration. Interagency Agreement Between the Food and Drug Administration and the Health Care Financing Administration Regarding Medicare Coverage of Certain Investigational Medical Devices (IDE Memorandum D95-2). 1995.

Hebden JC, Delpy DT. Diagnostic imaging with light. *Br J Radiol*. 1997;70 Spec No:S206-14.

Heimann R, Bradley J, Hellman S. The benefits of mammography are not limited to women of ages older than 50 years [see comments]. *Cancer*. 1998;82:2221-6.

Heimann R, Hellman S. Individual characterisation of the metastatic capacity of human breast carcinoma. *Eur J Cancer*. 2000;36:1631-9.

Henschke CI, McCauley DI, Yankelevitz DF, et al. Early Lung Cancer Action Project: overall design and findings from baseline screening [see comments]. *Lancet*. 1999;354:99-105.

Heppner GH, Wolman SR, Rosen J, Salomon D, Smith G, Mohla S. Research potential of a unique xenograft model of human proliferative breast disease. *Breast Cancer Res Treat.* 1999;58:183-6.

Hetelekidis S, Collins L, Silver B, et al. Predictors of local recurrence following excision alone for ductal carcinoma in situ. *Cancer.* 1999;85:427-31.

Hillner BE, Bear HD, Fajardo LL. Estimating the cost-effectiveness of stereotaxic biopsy for nonpalpable breast abnormalities: a decision analysis model. *Acad Radiol.* 1996;3: 351-60.

Hoffman C. *Uninsured in America: A Chart Book. The Kasier Commission on Medicaid and the Uninsured.* 1998.

Hoffman JM, Menkens AE. Molecular imaging in cancer: future directions and goals of the National Cancer Institute. *Acad Radiol.* 2000;7:905-7.

Holtzman NA. Are genetic tests adequately regulated? [editorial]. *Science.* 1999;286:409.

Houn F, Bright RA, Bushar HF, et al. Study design in the evaluation of breast cancer imaging technologies. *Acad Radiol.* 2000;7:684-92.

Hrung JM, Langlotz CP, Orel SG, Fox KR, Schnall MD, Schwartz JS. Cost-effectiveness of MR imaging and core-needle biopsy in the preoperative work-up of suspicious breast lesions. *Radiology.* 1999;213:39-49.

Hrung JM, Sonnad SS, Schwartz JS, Langlotz CP. Accuracy of MR imaging in the work-up of suspicious breast lesions: a diagnostic meta-analysis. *Acad Radiol.* 1999;6:387-97.

Hutchinson ML, Berger BM, Farber FL. Clinical and cost implications of new technologies for cervical cancer screening: the impact of test sensitivity. *Am J Managed Care.* 2000;6:766-80.

Inman M. The negative impact of MQSA (Mammography Quality Standards Act) on rural mammography programs. *Radiol Manage.* 1998;20:31-9.

Institute of Medicine. *Ensuring Quality Cancer Care.* M Hewitt and JV Simone, editors. Washington, D.C.: National Academy Press; 1999.

Institute of Medicine. *Extending Medicare Reimbursement in Clinical Trials.* Aaron HJ, Gelband H., editors. Washington, D.C.: National Academy Press; 2000.

Institute of Medicine. *Mathematics and Physics of Emerging Biomedical Imaging.* Washington, D.C.: National Academy Press; 1996.

Institute of Medicine. *A Review of the Department of Defense's Program for Breast Cancer Research.* Washington, D.C.: National Academy Press; 1997.

Institute of Medicine. *Strategies for Managing the Breast Cancer Research Program: A Report to the U.S. Army Medical Research and Development Command.* Washington, D.C.: National Academy Press; 1993.

Izatt L, Greenman J, Hodgson S, et al. Identification of germline missense mutations and rare allelic variants in the ATM gene in early-onset breast cancer. *Genes Chromosomes Cancer.* 1999;26:286-94.

Jatoi I. Breast cancer screening. *Am J Surg.* 1999;177:518-24.

Joines WT, Jirtle RL, Rafal MD, Schaefer DJ. Microwave power absorption differences between normal and malignant tissue. *Int J Radiat Oncol Biol Phys.* 1980;6:681-7.

Joines WT, Zhang Y, Li C, Jirtle RL. The measured electrical properties of normal and malignant human tissues from 50 to 900 MHz. *Med Phys.* 1994;21:547-50.

Jones BF. A reappraisal of the use of infrared thermal image analysis in medicine. *IEEE Trans Med Imaging.* 1998;17:1019-27.

Kahan J.S. The Framework for Regulation of Medical Devices. *Medical Devices, Obtaining FDA Market Clearence.* 1995. PARAXEL International Corporation, Waltham, MA.

Katz SJ, Hofer TP. Socioeconomic disparities in preventive care persist despite universal coverage. Breast and cervical cancer screening in Ontario and the United States. *JAMA.* 1994;272:530-4.

Kerlikowske K. Efficacy of screening mammography among women aged 40 to 49 years and 50 to 69 years: comparison of relative and absolute benefit. *J Natl Cancer Inst Monogr.* 1997:79-86.

Kerlikowske K, Grady D, Barclay J, Sickles EA, Eaton A, Ernster V. Positive predictive value of screening mammography by age and family history of breast cancer. *JAMA.* 1993;270:2444-50.

Kerlikowske K, Grady D, Barclay J, Sickles EA, Ernster V. Likelihood ratios for modern screening mammography. Risk of breast cancer based on age and mammographic interpretation. *JAMA.* 1996;276:39-43.

Kerlikowske K, Grady D, Rubin SM, Sandrock C, Ernster VL. Efficacy of screening mammography. A meta-analysis. *JAMA.* 1995;273:149-54.

Kerlikowske K, Salzmann P, Phillips KA, Cauley JA, Cummings SR. Continuing screening mammography in women aged 70 to 79 years: impact on life expectancy and cost-effectiveness. *JAMA.* 1999;282:2156-63.

Kevles B. *Naked to the Bone: Medical Imaging in the Twentieth Century.* New Brunswick, NJ: Rutgers University Press; 1997.

Khalkhali I, Mena I, Jouanne E, et al. Prone scintimammography in patients with suspicion of carcinoma of the breast. *J Am Coll Surg.* 1994;178:491-7.

Kinoshita J, Haga S, Shimizu T, Imamura H, Watanabe O, Kajiwara T. The expression of variant exon v7-v8 CD44 antigen in relation to lymphatic metastasis of human breast cancer. *Breast Cancer Res Treat.* 1999;53:177-83.

Kleiner K. More gain, less pain. *New Scientist.* 1999.

Knopp MV, Weiss E, Sinn HP, et al. Pathophysiologic basis of contrast enhancement in breast tumors. *J Magn Reson Imaging.* 1999;10:260-6.

Koenig BA, Greely HT, McConnell LM, Silverberg HL, Raffin TA. Genetic testing for BRCA1 and BRCA2: recommendations of the Stanford Program in Genomics, Ethics, and Society. Breast Cancer Working Group. *J Womens Health.* 1998;7:531-45.

Kolb GR. Multidisciplinary breast cancer survival, part I and II. ADVANCE for Administrators in Radiology and Radiation Oncology. 2000.

Kolb TM, Lichy J, Newhouse JH. Occult cancer in women with dense breasts: detection with screening US—diagnostic yield and tumor characteristics. *Radiology.* 1998;207: 191-9.

Kononen J, Bubendorf L, Kallioniemi A, et al. Tissue microarrays for high-throughput molecular profiling of tumor specimens. *Nat Med.* 1998;4:844-7.

Kopans DB. The positive predictive value of mammography. *Am J Roentgenol.* 1992;158: 521-6.

Kopans DB, Moore RH, McCarthy KA, et al. Positive predictive value of breast biopsy performed as a result of mammography: there is no abrupt change at age 50 years. *Radiology.* 1996;200:357-60.

Kruger DG, Abreu CC, Hendee EG, et al. Imaging characteristics of x-ray capillary optics in digital mammography. *Med Phys.* 1996;23:187-96.

Kruger RA, inventor; *Photoacoustic Breast Scanner* 5713356. 1998 Feb 3.

Kruger RA, Kiser Jr WL, Reinecke DR, Kruger GA. Application of thermoacoustic computed tomography to breast imaging. *SPIE.* 1999;3659:426-30.

Kruger RA, Kopecky KK, Aisen AM, Reinecke DR, Kruger GA, Kiser WL Jr. Thermoacoustic CT with radio waves: a medical imaging paradigm. *Radiology.* 1999;211:275-8.

Kuhl CK, Schmutzler RK, Leutner CC, et al. Breast MR imaging screening in 192 women proved or suspected to be carriers of a breast cancer susceptibility gene: preliminary results. *Radiology.* 2000;215:267-79.

Kvistad KA, Bakken IJ, Gribbestad IS, et al. Characterization of neoplastic and normal human breast tissues with in vivo (1)H MR spectroscopy. *J Magn Reson Imaging.* 1999;10: 159-64.

Lakin ND, Jackson SP. Regulation of p53 in response to DNA damage. *Oncogene*. 1999;18: 7644-55.

Land CE. Estimating cancer risks from low doses of ionizing radiation. *Science*. 1980;209: 1197-203.

Lane DS, Caplan LS, Grimson R. Trends in mammography use and their relation to physician and other factors. *Cancer Detect Prev*. 1996;20:332-41.

Larsen LE, Jacobi JH, Eds. *Medical Applications of Microwave Imaging*. Piscataway, NJ: IEEE Press; 1986.

Lawrence WF, Liang W, Mandelblatt JS, et al. Serendipity in diagnostic imaging: magnetic resonance imaging of the breast. *J Natl Cancer Inst*. 1998;90:1792-800.

Lawson RN. Implications of surface temperatures in the diagnosis of breast cancer. *Can. Med. Assoc. J*. 1956;75:309-10.

Laya MB, Larson EB, Taplin SH, White E. Effect of estrogen replacement therapy on the specificity and sensitivity of screening mammography. *J Natl Cancer Inst*. 1996;88: 643-9.

Lerman C, Trock B, Rimer BK, Jepson C, Brody D, Boyce A. Psychological side effects of breast cancer screening. *Health Psychol*. 1991;10:259-67.

Lerner B.H. *To See Today With the Eyes of Tomorrow: A History of Screening Mammography*. 2001. (see http://www4.nationalacademies.org/IOM/IOMHome.nsf/Pages/Breast+Cancer+Detection)

Lewin JM. Full-field digital mammography. A candid assessment. *Diagn Imaging (San Franc)*. 1999;21:40-5.

Lewin JM, Hendrick RE, D'Orsi CJ, Isaacs PK, Moss LJ, Karellas A, Sisney GA, Kuni CC, Cutter GR. Comparison of full-field digital mammography with screen-film mammography for cancer detection: results of 4945 paired examinations. Radiology 2001;218:873-80.

Lewin J, Hendrick RE, D'Orsi CJ, Moss LJ, Isaacs P. *Clinical Evaluation of Full-Field Digital Mammography in a Screening Population*. *2000 Annual Meeting of the Radiological Society of North America*.

Li S, Ting NS, Zheng L, et al. Functional link of BRCA1 and ataxia telangiectasia gene product in DNA damage response. *Nature*. 2000;406:210-5.

Liaw D, Marsh DJ, Li J, et al. Germline mutations of the PTEN gene in Cowden disease, an inherited breast and thyroid cancer syndrome. *Nat Genet*. 1997;16:64-7.

Lichtenstein P, Holm NV, Verkasalo PK, et al. Environmental and heritable factors in the causation of cancer—analyses of cohorts of twins from Sweden, Denmark, and Finland. *N Engl J Med*. 2000;343:78-85.

Lidbrink E, Elfving J, Frisell J, Jonsson E. Neglected aspects of false positive findings of mammography in breast cancer screening: analysis of false positive cases from the Stockholm trial. *BMJ*. 1996;312:273-6.

Lijmer JG, Mol BW, Heisterkamp S, et al. Empirical evidence of design-related bias in studies of diagnostic tests [published erratum appears in JAMA 2000 Apr 19;283(15):1963]. *JAMA*. 1999;282:1061-6.

Liotta LA, Petricoin EF. Beyond the genome to tissue proteomics. Breast Cancer Research . 2000;2:13-14.

Louie AY, Huber MM, Ahrens ET, et al. In vivo visualization of gene expression using magnetic resonance imaging. *Nat Biotechnol*. 2000;18:321-5.

Love SM, Barsky SH. Breast-duct endoscopy to study stages of cancerous breast disease. *Lancet*. 1996;348:997-9.

Love SM, Chou J, Offodile R, et al. Development of Intraductal Techniques for Breast Cancer Prevention, Diagnosis and Treatment. Proceedings, Era of Hope Dept. of Defense Breast Cancer Research Program Meeting. 2000 June.

Love SM, Lindsey K. *Dr. Susan Love's Breast Book*. Reading, PA: Addison-Wesley; 1995.

Lowe JB, Balanda KP, Del Mar C, Hawes E. Psychologic distress in women with abnormal findings in mass mammography screening. *Cancer.* 1999;85:1114-8.

Lu YJ, Osin P, Lakhani SR, Di Palma S, Gusterson BA, Shipley JM. Comparative genomic hybridization analysis of lobular carcinoma in situ and atypical lobular hyperplasia and potential roles for gains and losses of genetic material in breast neoplasia. *Cancer Res.* 1998;58:4721-7.

MacBeath G, Schreiber SL. Printing proteins as microarrays for high-throughput function determination. *Science.* 2000;289:1760-3.

Mackinnon WB, Barry PA, Malycha PL, et al. Fine-needle biopsy specimens of benign breast lesions distinguished from invasive cancer ex vivo with proton MR spectroscopy. *Radiology.* 1997;204:661-6.

Mahmood U, Tung CH, Bogdanov A Jr, Weissleder R. Near-infrared optical imaging of protease activity for tumor detection. *Radiology.* 1999;213:866-70.

Makuc DM, Breen N, Freid V. Low income, race, and the use of mammography. *Health Serv Res.* 1999;34:229-39.

Malkin D, Li FP, Strong LC, et al. Germ line p53 mutations in a familial syndrome of breast cancer, sarcomas, and other neoplasms. *Science.* 1990;250:1233-8.

Mandelblatt JS, Gold K, O'Malley AS, et al. Breast and cervix cancer screening among multiethnic women: role of age, health, and source of care. *Prev Med.* 1999;28:418-25.

Mandelblatt JS, Yabroff KR. Effectiveness of interventions designed to increase mammography use: a meta-analysis of provider-targeted strategies. *Cancer Epidemiol Biomarkers Prev.* 1999;8:759-67.

Mandelblatt J, Andrews H, Kao R, Wallace R, Kerner J. Impact of access and social context on breast cancer stage at diagnosis. *J Health Care Poor Underserved.* 1995;6:342-51.

Mandelson MT, Oestreicher N, Porter PL, et al. Breast density as a predictor of mammographic detection: comparison of interval- and screen-detected cancers. *J Natl Cancer Inst.* 2000;92:1081-7.

Mandelson MT, Wagner EH, Thompson RS. PSA screening: a public health dilemma. *Annu Rev Public Health.* 1995;16:283-306.

Mark HF, Jenkins R, Miller WA. Current applications of molecular cytogenetic technologies. *Ann Clin Lab Sci.* 1997;27:47-56.

Marshall E. The politics of breast cancer [news]. *Science.* 1993;259:616-7.

Martin S, Jansen F, Bokelmann J, Kolb H. Soluble CD44 splice variants in metastasizing human breast cancer. *Int J Cancer.* 1997;74:443-5.

Martinez B. Screening Crunch—As more women seek mammograms, many have to wait months. *Wall Street Journal.* 2000.

Matsumura Y, Tarin D. Significance of CD44 gene products for cancer diagnosis and disease evaluation. *Lancet.* 1992;340:1053-8.

May DS, Kiefe CI, Funkhouser E, Fouad MN. Compliance with mammography guidelines: physician recommendation and patient adherence. *Prev Med.* 1999;28:386-94.

Meaney PM, Paulsen KD, Chang JT, Fanning MW, Hartov A. Nonactive antenna compensation for fixed-array microwave imaging: Part II—Imaging results. *IEEE Trans Med Imaging.* 1999;18:508-18.

Medical Technology Leadership Forum. *MTLF Summit: Conditional Coverage of Investigational Technologies.* Bethesda, MD: Medical Technology Leadership Forum; 1999.

Mehta TS, Raza S, Baum JK. Use of Doppler ultrasound in the evaluation of breast carcinoma. *Semin Ultrasound CT MR.* 2000;21:297-307.

Merchant TE. MR spectroscopy of the breast. *Magn Reson Imaging Clin N Am.* 1994;2: 691-703.

Merritt CRB. Future directions in breast ultrasonography. *Seminars in Breast Disease.* 1999;2: 89-96.

Mettlin C. Global breast cancer mortality statistics. *CA Cancer J Clin.* 1999;49:138-44.

Meyer JE, Smith DN, DiPiro PJ, et al. Stereotactic breast biopsy of clustered microcalcifications with a directional, vacuum-assisted device. *Radiology*. 1997;204:575-6.

Miki Y, Swensen J, Shattuck-Eidens D, et al. A strong candidate for the breast and ovarian cancer susceptibility gene BRCA1. *Science*. 1994;266:66-71.

Milbank Memorial Fund. *Better Information, Better Outcomes? The Use of Health Technology Assessment and Clinical Effectiveness Data in the United Kingdom and the United States*; 2000.

Miller AB, Baines CJ, To T, Wall C. Canadian National Breast Screening Study: 2. Breast cancer detection and death rates among women aged 50 to 59 years [published erratum appears in Can Med Assoc J 1993 Mar 1;148(5):718]. *CMAJ*. 1992;147:1477-88.

Miller AB, To T, Baines CJ, Wall C. Canadian National Breast Screening Study-2: 13-Year Results of a Randomized Trial in Women Aged 50-59 Years. *J Natl Cancer Inst*. 2000;92: 1490-1499.

Mittra I, Baum M, Thornton H, Houghton J. Is clinical breast examination an acceptable alternative to mammographic screening? *BMJ*. 2000;321:1071-1073.

Monaghan P, Clarke CL, Perusinghe NP, Ormerod MG, O'Hare MJ. Epidermal growth factor receptor expression on human breast luminal and basal cells in vitro. *Epithelial Cell Biol*. 1995;4:52-62.

Morrow M. When can stereotactic core biopsy replace excisional biopsy?—A clinical perspective. *Breast Cancer Res Treat*. 1995;36:1-9.

Moskowitz M. Thermography as a risk indicator of breast cancer. Results of a study and a review of the recent literature. *J Reprod Med*. 1985;30:451-9.

Moskowitz M, D'Orsi CJ, Bartrum RJ, Swets J. *Breast Cancer Diagnosis by Lightscan (Revised) Final Report*: National Cancer Institute; 1989. Grant Number CA37970.

Moss MS. Breast cancer. In: Kramer BS, Gohagan JK, Prorok PC, eds. *Cancer Screening: Theory and Practice*. New York: M. Dekker; 1999:143-170.

Mountford C, Somorjai R, Gluch L, et al. Magnetic Resonance Spectroscopy Determines Pathology, Vascularisation and Node Status. Era of Hope. Department of Defense Breast Cancer Research Program Meeting: June, 2000; Atlanta, GA.

Mourant JR, Bigio IJ, Boyer J, Conn RL, Johnson T, Shimada T. Spectroscopic diagnosis of bladder cancer with elastic light scattering. *Lasers Surg Med*. 1995;17:350-7.

Mushlin AI, Kouides RW, Shapiro DE. Estimating the accuracy of screening mammography: a meta-analysis. *Am J Prev Med*. 1998;14:143-53.

Muthupillai R, Lomas DJ, Rossman PJ, Greenleaf JF, Manduca A, Ehman RL. Magnetic resonance elastography by direct visualization of propagating acoustic strain waves. *Science*. 1995;269:1854-7.

National Bioethics Advisory Commission. *Research Involving Human Biological Materials: Ethical Issues and Policy Guidance. Volume I, Report and Recommendations of the National Bioethics Advisory Commission*. Rockville, MD; 1999.

National Institutes of Health. National Institutes of Health Consensus Conference on Breast Cancer Screening for Women Ages 40-49. *J Natl Cancer Inst Monogr*. 1997:1-156. Proceedings. Bethesda, Maryland, USA.

National Research Council/ Board On Science Technology, and Economic Policy. *The Small Business Innovation Research Program: Challenges and Opportunities*. Washington, D.C.: National Academy Press; 1999.

Nayar R, Zhuang Z, Merino MJ, Silverberg SG. Loss of heterozygosity on chromosome 11q13 in lobular lesions of the breast using tissue microdissection and polymerase chain reaction. *Hum Pathol*. 1997;28:277-82.

Newman L. Larger debate underlies spiral CT screening for lung cancer [news]. *J Natl Cancer Inst*. 2000;92:592-4.

Nichols KE, Levitz S, Shannon KE, et al. Heterozygous germline ATM mutations do not contribute to radiation-associated malignancies after Hodgkin's disease. *J Clin Oncol.* 1999;17:1259.

Nields MW, Galaty RR Jr. Digital mammography: a model for assessing cost-effectiveness. *Acad Radiol.* 1998 Sep;5 Suppl 2:S310-3.

Nielsen M, Thomsen JL, Primdahl S, Dyreborg U, Andersen JA. Breast cancer and atypia among young and middle-aged women: a study of 110 medicolegal autopsies. *Br J Cancer.* 1987;56:814-9.

Niklason LT, Christian BT, Niklason LE, et al. Digital tomosynthesis in breast imaging. *Radiology.* 1997;205:399-406.

Nishikawa RM. Computer-aided diagnosis complements full-field digital mammography. *Diagn Imaging (San Franc).* 1999;21:47-51, 75.

Ntziachristos V, Yodh AG, Schnall M, Chance B. Concurrent MRI and diffuse optical tomography of breast after indocyanine green enhancement. *Proc Natl Acad Sci U S A.* 2000;97:2767-72.

Ophir J, Alam SK, Garra B, et al. Elastography: ultrasonic estimation and imaging of the elastic properties of tissues. *Proc Inst Mech Eng [H].* 1999;213:203-33.

Osin P, Shipley J, Lu YJ, Crook T, Gusterson BA. Experimental pathology and breast cancer genetics: new technologies. *Recent Results Cancer Res.* 1998;152:35-48.

Osterman KS, Kerner TE, Williams DB, Hartov A, Poplack SP, Paulsen KD. Multifrequency electrical impedance imaging: preliminary in vivo experience in breast. *Physiol Meas.* 2000;21:99-109.

Page MJ, Amess B, Townsend RR, et al. Proteomic definition of normal human luminal and myoepithelial breast cells purified from reduction mammoplasties. *Proc Natl Acad Sci U S A.* 1999;96:12589-94.

Pantel K, Cote RJ, Fodstad O. Detection and clinical importance of micrometastatic disease. *J Natl Cancer Inst.* 1999;91:1113-24.

Papanicolaou GN, Holmquist DG, Bader GM, Falk EA. Exfoliative cytology of the human mammary gland and its value in the diagnosis of cancer and other diseases of the breast. *Cancer (Phila.).* 1958;11:377-409.

Parmigiani G, Berry D, Aguilar O. Determining carrier probabilities for breast cancer-susceptibility genes BRCA1 and BRCA2. *Am J Hum Genet.* 1998;62:145-58.

Perou CM, Jeffrey SS, van de Rijn M, et al. Distinctive gene expression patterns in human mammary epithelial cells and breast cancers. *Proc Natl Acad Sci U S A.* 1999;96:9212-7.

Perou CM, Sorlie T, Eisen MB, et al. Molecular portraits of human breast tumours. *Nature.* 2000;406:747-52.

Perry S, Thamer M. Medical innovation and the critical role of health technology assessment. *JAMA.* 1999;282:1869-72.

Petersen OW, Ronnov-Jessen L, Howlett AR, Bissell MJ. Interaction with basement membrane serves to rapidly distinguish growth and differentiation pattern of normal and malignant human breast epithelial cells [published erratum appears in Proc Natl Acad Sci U S A 1993 Mar 15;90(6):2556]. *Proc Natl Acad Sci U S A.* 1992;89:9064-8.

Peto R, Boreham J, Clarke M, Davies C, Beral V. *UK and USA Breast Cancer Deaths Down 25% in Year 2000 at Ages 20-69 Years [Letter];* 2000.Lancet 355:9217-1822.

Phelps ME. PET: the merging of biology and imaging into molecular imaging. *J Nucl Med.* 2000;41:661-81.

Phillips KA, Kerlikowske K, Baker LC, Chang SW, Brown ML. Factors associated with women's adherence to mammography screening guidelines. *Health Serv Res.* 1998;33:29-53.

Physicians Insurers Association of America. *Breast Cancer Study.* Rockville, MD: Physicians Insurers Association of America; 1995.

Physicians Insurers Association of America. *Practice Standards Claims Survey*. Rockville, MD: Physicians Insurers Association of America; 1997.

Pisano ED, Earp J, Schell M, Vokaty K, Denham A. Screening behavior of women after a false-positive mammogram. *Radiology*. 1998a;208:245-9.

Pisano ED, Fajardo LL, Tsimikas J, et al. Rate of insufficient samples for fine-needle aspiration for nonpalpable breast lesions in a multicenter clinical trial: The Radiologic Diagnostic Oncology Group 5 Study. The RDOG5 investigators. *Cancer*. 1998b;82:679-88.

Pisano ED, Parham CA. Digital mammography, sestamibi breast scintigraphy, and positron emission tomography breast imaging. *Radiol Clin North Am*. 2000;38:861-9, x.

Pisano ED, Yaffe MJ, Hemminger BM, et al. Current status of full-field digital mammography. *Acad Radiol*. 2000;7:266-80.

Plevritis, SK. A framework for evaluating the cost-effectiveness of MRI screening for breast cancer. Eur. Radiology. 2000a;10 Suppl. 3:5430-2.

Plevritis SK. Simulation of breast cancer screening trials. Outcomes and Cost-effectiveness (Methology Development). *Lucas Annual 2000*. 2000b. Stanford, CA.

Plewes DB, Bishop J, Samani A, Sciarretta J. Visualization and quantification of breast cancer biomechanical properties with magnetic resonance elastography. *Phys Med Biol*. 2000;45:1591-610.

Pollack JR, Perou CM, Alizadeh AA, et al. Genome-wide analysis of DNA copy-number changes using cDNA microarrays. *Nat Genet*. 1999;23:41-6.

Pollak MN. Endocrine effects of IGF-I on normal and transformed breast epithelial cells: potential relevance to strategies for breast cancer treatment and prevention. *Breast Cancer Res Treat*. 1998;47:209-17.

Potosky AL, Breen N, Graubard BI, Parsons PE. The association between health care coverage and the use of cancer screening tests. Results from the 1992 National Health Interview Survey [published erratum appears in Med Care 1998 Oct;36(10):1470]. *Med Care*. 1998;36:257-70.

PricewaterhouseCoopers Money Tree ™ Survey, www.pwcmoneytree.com (accessed August 2000 and March 2001).

Prorok PC, Kramer BS, Gohagan JK. Screening theory and study design: the basics. From: Kramer BS, Gohagan JK, Prorok PC, eds. *Cancer Screening: Theory and Practice*. New York: M. Dekker; 1999:29-53.

Rao PN, Levine E, Myers MO, et al. Elevation of serum riboflavin carrier protein in breast cancer. *Cancer Epidemiol Biomarkers Prev*. 1999;8:985-90.

Rathore SS, McGreevey JD 3rd, Schulman KA, Atkins D. Mandated coverage for cancer-screening services: whose guidelines do states follow? *Am J Prev Med*. 2000;19:71-8.

Rettig RA. *Health Care in Transition: Technology Assessment in the Private Sector*. Santa Monica, CA: RAND; 1997.

Reynolds T. Gene patent race speeds ahead amid controversy, concern. *J Natl Cancer Inst*. 2000;92:184-6.

Ries LAG, Kosary CL, Hankey BFeale. *SEER Cancer Statistic Review, 1973-1996*. Bethesda, MD; 1999.

Rimer BK, Keintz MK, Kessler HB, Engstrom PF, Rosan JR. Why women resist screening mammography: patient-related barriers. *Radiology*. 1989;172:243-6.

Rodenko GN, Harms SE, Pruneda JM, et al. MR imaging in the management before surgery of lobular carcinoma of the breast: correlation with pathology. *Am J Roentgenol*. 1996;167:1415-9.

Roebuck JR, Cecil KM, Schnall MD, Lenkinski RE. Human breast lesions: characterization with proton MR spectroscopy. *Radiology*. 1998;209:269-75.

Rosen PP. Clinical implications of preinvasive and small invasive breast carcinomas. *Pathol Annu*. 1981;16:337-56.

Rosen PP, Braun DW Jr, Kinne DE. The clinical significance of pre-invasive breast carcinoma. *Cancer.* 1980;46:919-25.

Rosencwaig A. Photoacoustic spectroscopy. *Anal Chem.* 1975;47:592-602.

Rosenquist CJ, Lindfors KK. Screening mammography beginning at age 40 years: a reappraisal of cost-effectiveness. *Cancer.* 1998;82:2235-40.

Rothenberg K, Fuller B, Rothstein M, et al. Genetic information and the workplace: legislative approaches and policy changes. *Science.* 1997;275:1755-7.

Rubin M, Horiuchi K, Joy N, et al. Use of fine needle aspiration for solid breast lesions is accurate and cost-effective. *Am J Surg.* 1997;174:694-6; discussion 697-8.

Russo IH, Russo J. Mammary gland neoplasia in long-term rodent studies. *Environ Health Perspect.* 1996;104:938-67.

Russo J, Russo IHNMC, Daniel CWe. Development of human mammary gland. *The Mammary Gland.* 1987:67-105. Plenum: New York.

Sapirstein W. The conduct of clinical trials: a Food and Drug Agency perspective. *ASAIO J.* 2000;46:29-30.

Sauter ER, Ehya H, Babb J, et al. Biological markers of risk in nipple aspirate fluid are associated with residual cancer and tumour size. *Br J Cancer.* 1999;81:1222-7.

Sauter ER, Ross E, Daly M, et al. Nipple aspirate fluid: a promising non-invasive method to identify cellular markers of breast cancer risk. *Br J Cancer.* 1997;76:494-501.

Schubert EL, Lee MK, Newman B, King MC. Single nucleotide polymorphisms (SNPs) in the estrogen receptor gene and breast cancer susceptibility. *J Steroid Biochem Mol Biol.* 1999;71:21-7.

Scopinaro F, Pani R, De Vincentis G, Soluri A, Pellegrini R, Porfiri LM. High-resolution scintimammography improves the accuracy of technetium-99m methoxyisobutylisonitrile scintimammography: use of a new dedicated gamma camera. *Eur J Nucl Med.* 1999;26:1279-88.

Scott S, Morrow M. Breast cancer. Making the diagnosis. *Surg Clin North Am.* 1999;79:991-1005.

Semiglazov VF, Moiseenko VM, Manikhas AG, et al. Interim results of a prospective randomized study of self-examination for early detection of breast cancer (Russia/St. Petersburg/WHO). *Vopr Onkol.* 1999;45:265-71.

Semiglazov VF, Moiseyenko VM, Bavli JL, et al. The role of breast self-examination in early breast cancer detection (results of the 5-years USSR/WHO randomized study in Leningrad). *Eur J Epidemiol.* 1992;8:498-502.

Service RF. Biochemistry. Protein arrays step out of DNA's shadow. *Science.* 2000;289:1673.

Shafman TD, Levitz S, Nixon AJ, et al. Prevalence of germline truncating mutations in ATM in women with a second breast cancer after radiation therapy for a contralateral tumor. *Genes Chromosomes Cancer.* 2000;27:124-9.

Shalala D. "Report of the Secretary to the President: Health insurance in the age of genetics." (July 1997).

Shapiro S. Periodic screening for breast cancer: the HIP Randomized Controlled Trial. Health Insurance Plan. *J Natl Cancer Inst Monogr.* 1997:27-30.

Sharan SK, Morimatsu M, Albrecht U, et al. Embryonic lethality and radiation hypersensitivity mediated by Rad51 in mice lacking BRCA2. *Nature.* 1997;386:804-10.

Shayeghi M, Seal S, Regan J, et al. Heterozygosity for mutations in the ataxia telangiectasia gene is not a major cause of radiotherapy complications in breast cancer patients. *Br J Cancer.* 1998;78:922-7.

Sidransky D, Tokino T, Helzlsouer K, et al. Inherited p53 gene mutations in breast cancer. *Cancer Res.* 1992;52:2984-6.

Siegel JE, Weinstein MC, Russell LB, Gold MR. Recommendations for reporting cost-effectiveness analyses. Panel on Cost-Effectiveness in Health and Medicine. *JAMA.* 1996;276:1339-41.

Silverstein MJ, Lagios MD. Use of predictors of recurrence to plan therapy for DCIS of the breast. *Oncology (Huntingt)*. 1997;11:393-406, 409-10; discussion 413-5.

Sinkus R, Lorenzen J, Schrader D, Lorenzen M, Dargatz M, Holz D. High-resolution tensor MR elastography for breast tumour detection. *Phys Med Biol*. 2000;45:1649-64.

Sirovich BE, Sox HC Jr. Breast cancer screening. *Surg Clin North Am*. 1999;79:961-90.

Skoumal SM, Florell SR, Bydalek MK, Hunter WJ 3rd. Malpractice protection: communication of diagnostic uncertainty. *Diagn Cytopathol*. 1996;14:385-9.

Smith-Bindman R, Kerlikowske K, Gebretsadik T, Newman J. Is screening mammography effective in elderly women? *Am J Med*. 2000;108:112-9.

Smith HS, Lan S, Ceriani R, Hackett AJ, Stampfer MR. Clonal proliferation of cultured nonmalignant and malignant human breast epithelia. *Cancer Res*. 1981;41:4637-43.

Smith R.A. Risk-Based Screening For Breast Cancer: Is There a Practical Strategy? *Seminars in Breast Disease*. 1999;2:280-91.

Sneige N. A comparison of fine needle aspiration, core biopsy, and needle localization biopsy techniques in mammographically detectable nonpalpable breast lesions. *Pathol Case Rev*. 1991;1.

Softcheck J.T. President Clinton signs bill to create NIH Institute of Biomedical Imaging and Bioengineering: NIH effort to build Office of Bioengineering, Bioimaging and Bioinformatics effectively derailed. *Washington Fax*. 2001.

Stavros AT, Thickman D, Rapp CL, Dennis MA, Parker SH, Sisney GA. Solid breast nodules: use of sonography to distinguish between benign and malignant lesions. *Radiology*. 1995;196:123-34.

Straus E. Magnetic resonance imaging. Detecting enzyme activity in live animals [news]. *Science*. 2000;287:1575.

Strongin R. Medicare coverage and technology diffusion: past, present, and future. *Issue Brief Natl Health Policy Forum*. 1998:1-8.

Struewing JP, Hartge P, Wacholder S, et al. The risk of cancer associated with specific mutations of BRCA1 and BRCA2 among Ashkenazi Jews. *N Engl J Med*. 1997;336:1401-8.

Stuntz ME, Khalkhali I, Kakuda JT, Klein SR, Vargas HI. Scintimammography. *Seminars In Breast Disease*. 1999;2:97-106.

Suleiman OH, Spelic DC, McCrohan JL, Symonds GR, Houn F. Mammography in the 1990s: the United States and Canada. *Radiology*. 1999;210:345-51.

Swift M, Morrell D, Massey RB, Chase CL. Incidence of cancer in 161 families affected by ataxia-telangiectasia. *N Engl J Med*. 1991;325:1831-6.

Tabar L, Dean PB, Kaufman CS, Duffy SW, Chen HH. A new era in the diagnosis of breast cancer. *Surg Oncol Clin N Am*. 2000;9:233-77.

Tabar L, Duffy SW, Vitak B, Chen HH, Prevost TC. The natural history of breast carcinoma: what have we learned from screening? *Cancer*. 1999;86:449-62.

Tan JE, Orel SG, Schnall MD, Schultz DJ, Solin LJ. Role of magnetic resonance imaging and magnetic resonance imaging—guided surgery in the evaluation of patients with early-stage breast cancer for breast conservation treatment. *Am J Clin Oncol*. 1999;22:414-8.

Tavtigian SV, Simard J, Rommens J, et al. The complete BRCA2 gene and mutations in chromosome 13q-linked kindreds. *Nat Genet*. 1996;12:333-7.

Taylor-Papadimitriou J, Stampfer MR (Freshney RI, Editor); Culture of Human Mammary Epithelial Cells. *Culture of Epithelial Cells*. Wiley-Liss, USA; 1992:107-33.

The Lewin Group/AdvaMed. Outlook For Medical Technology Innovation. Will Patients Get The Care They Need? 1999;1.

The Lewin Group/AdvaMed. Outlook For Medical Technology Innovation. Will Patients Get The Care They Need? 2000;2.

Thomas DB, Gao DL, Self SG, et al. Randomized trial of breast self-examination in Shanghai: methodology and preliminary results. *J Natl Cancer Inst*. 1997;89:355-65.

Thomsen S, Tatman D. Physiological and pathological factors of human breast disease that can influence optical diagnosis. *Ann N Y Acad Sci 1998 Feb 9;838:171-93.*

Thurfjell EL, Lernevall KA, Taube AA. Benefit of independent double reading in a population-based mammography screening program. *Radiology.* 1994;191:241-4.

Thurfjell E, Thurfjell MG, Egge E, Bjurstam N. Sensitivity and specificity of computer-assisted breast cancer detection in mammography screening. *Acta Radiol.* 1998;39: 384-8.

Tonetti DA, Jordan VC. The role of estrogen receptor mutations in tamoxifen-stimulated breast cancer. *J Steroid Biochem Mol Biol.* 1997;62:119-28.

U.S. Congress, Office of Technology Assessment. "Identifying Health Technologies that Work: Searching for Evidence." OTA-H-608 (Washington, D.C., U.S. Government Printing Office, September, 1994).

U.S. Department of Health and Human Services. *Health, United States, 2000. With Adolescent Health Chartbook*: Department of Health and Human Services; 2000.

U.S. General Accounting Office. *Mammography Quality Standards Act: X-Ray Quality Improved, Access Unaffected, but Impact on Health Outcomes Unknown*; 1998a. GAO/HEHS-98-164.

U.S. General Accounting Office. *Mammography Services: Impact of Federal Legislation on Quality, Access, and Health Outcomes*; 1998b. GAO/HEHS-98-11.

U.S. Preventive Services Task Force, Screening for breast cancer. *In:. Guide to Clinical Preventive Services.* 2nd ed. Baltimore MD: Williams & Wilkins; 1996:73-88. HealthSTAR.

Van Dijck JA, Verbeek AL, Beex LVHJH, et al. Mammographic screening after the age of 65 years: evidence for a reduction in breast cancer mortality. *Int J Cancer.* 1996;66:727-31.

van Dijck JA, Verbeek AL, Hendriks JH, Holland R. The current detectability of breast cancer in a mammographic screening program. A review of the previous mammograms of interval and screen-detected cancers. *Cancer.* 1993;72:1933-8.

Velanovich V, Lewis FR Jr, Nathanson SD, et al. Comparison of mammographically guided breast biopsy techniques. *Ann Surg.* 1999;229:625-30; discussion 630-3.

Vernon SW, Laville EA, Jackson GL. Participation in breast screening programs: a review. *Soc Sci Med.* 1990;30:1107-18.

Vetto JT, Pommier RF, Schmidt WA, Eppich H, Alexander PW. Diagnosis of palpable breast lesions in younger women by the modified triple test is accurate and cost-effective. *Arch Surg.* 1996;131:967-72; discussion 972-4.

Wagner SK. Verdict on MQSA: quality up, but so is financial burden. *Diagn Imaging (San Franc).* 1999;21:33-4, 62.

Warren-Burhenne LJ, Wood SA, D'Orsi CJ, et al. Potential contribution of computer-aided detection to the sensitivity of screening mammography [published erratum appears in Radiology 2000 Jul;216(1):306]. *Radiology.* 2000;215:554-62.

Webber RL, Horton RA, Tyndall DA, Ludlow JB. Tuned-aperture computed tomography (TACT). Theory and application for three-dimensional dento-alveolar imaging. *Dentomaxillofac Radiol.* 1997;26:53-62.

Weidner N. Prognostic factors in breast carcinoma. *Curr Opin Obstet Gynecol.* 1995;7:4-9.

Weidner N, Folkman J, Pozza F, et al. Tumor angiogenesis: a new significant and independent prognostic indicator in early-stage breast carcinoma. *J Natl Cancer Inst.* 1992;84:1875-87.

Welch HG, Black WC. Using autopsy series to estimate the disease "reservoir" for ductal carcinoma in situ of the breast: how much more breast cancer can we find? *Ann Intern Med.* 1997;127:1023-8.

Welcsh PL, Owens KN, King MC. Insights into the functions of BRCA1 and BRCA2. *Trends Genet.* 2000;16:69-74.

Welsch CW, Medina D, Kidwell W, Heppner G, Anderson E. Rodent models to examine in vivo hormonal regulation of mammary gland tumorigenesis. *Cellular and Molecular Biology of Mammary Cancer.* 1987:163-79.

Wen H. Volumetric Hall effect tomography—a feasibility study. *Ultrason Imaging.* 1999;21: 186-200.

Wen H, Shah J, Balaban RS. Hall effect imaging. *IEEE Trans Biomed Eng.* 1998;45:119-24.

White E, Velentgas P, Mandelson MT, et al. Variation in mammographic breast density by time in menstrual cycle among women aged 40-49 years. *J Natl Cancer Inst.* 1998;90: 906-10.

Wilson JMG, Jungren G. Principles and practice of screening for disease. *Public Health Paper (No. 34). Geneva, World Health Organization.* 1968;26.

Wismar BA (Kramer EJ, Ivey SL, Ying Y-W, Editors); Breast and Cervical Cancer. *Immigrant Women's Health, Problems and Solutions.* San Francisco, CA: Jossey-Bass Publishers; 1999.

Wong AY, Salisbury E, Bilous M. Recent developments in stereotactic breast biopsy methodologies: an update for the surgical pathologist. *Adv Anat Pathol.* 2000;7:26-35.

Wooster R, Bignell G, Lancaster J, et al. Identification of the breast cancer susceptibility gene BRCA2 [published erratum appears in Nature 1996 Feb 22;379(6567):749]. *Nature.* 1995;378:789-92.

Wrensch MR, Petrakis NL, King EB, et al. Breast cancer incidence in women with abnormal cytology in nipple aspirates of breast fluid. *Am J Epidemiol.* 1992;135:130-41.

Wun LM, Merrill RM, Feuer EJ. Estimating lifetime and age-conditional probabilities of developing cancer. *Lifetime Data Anal.* 1998;4:169-86.

Yabroff KR, Mandelblatt JS. Interventions targeted toward patients to increase mammography use. *Cancer Epidemiol Biomarkers Prev.* 1999;8:749-57.

Yan H, Kinzler KW, Vogelstein B. Tech.sight. Genetic testing—present and future. *Science.* 2000;289:1890-2.

Yan PS, Perry MR, Laux DE, Asare AL, Caldwell CW, Huang TH. CpG island arrays: an application toward deciphering epigenetic signatures of breast cancer. *Clin Cancer Res.* 2000;6:1432-8.

Ziewacz JT, Neumann DP, Weiner RE. The difficult breast. *Surg Oncol Clin N Am.* 1999;8: 17-33.

# Appendix

# Workshop Speakers

## WORKSHOP 1, FEBRUARY 9–10, 2000

D. Craig Allred, M.D.
Professor of Pathology
Baylor College of Medicine

Ronald A. Castellino, M.D.
Medical Director
R2 Technology, Inc.
Professor Emeritus of Radiology
Stanford University and Cornell
    University

Britton Chance, Ph.D.
Professor Emeritus
Biophysics, Physical Chemistry,
    and Radiologic Physics
University of Pennsylvania

Carl D'Orsi, M.D.
Professor of Radiology
University of Massachusettes
    Medical School

Stefanie Jeffrey, M.D.
Chief of Breast Surgery
Stanford University School of
    Medicine

Michael Knopp, M.D.
German Cancer Research Center
Chief, Division of MRI and MRS
    (on leave)
Associate Professor of Radiology

Jean Latimer, Ph.D.
Investigator, Magee-Women's
    Research Institute
Pittsburgh, PA

Thomas Meade, Ph.D.
Beckman Institute
California Institute of Technology

Christopher Merritt, M.D.
Professor of Radiology
Thomas Jefferson University
    Hospital

Etta Pisano, M.D.
Professor of Radiology and Chief
  of Breast Imaging
University of North Carolina
  School of Medicine
UNC-Lineberger Comprehensive
  Cancer Center

David Piwnica-Worms, M.D.,
  Ph.D.
Departments of Radiology and
  Molecular Biology and
  Pharmacology
Washington University School of
  Medicine

Donald Plewes, Ph.D.
Department of Medical Biophysics
University of Toronto

Edward Sauter, M.D., Ph.D.
Department of Surgery
Thomas Jefferson University

Mitchell Schnall, M.D., Ph.D.
Chief, MRI
University of Pennsylvania
  Medical Center

## WORKSHOP 2, JUNE 19–20, 2000

Rachel Ballard-Barbash, M.D.
Associate Director
Applied Research Program
National Cancer Institute

Norman Boyd, M.D.
Princess Margaret Hospital

Carol Dahl, Ph.D.
Director, Office of Technologies
  and Industrial Relations
National Institutes of Health

Susan B. Foote, J.D.
Associate Professor & Division
  Head
University of Minnesota

Steven Gutman, M.D., MBA
Division Director
Food and Drug Administration
Clinical Laboratory Devices

Bruce J. Hillman, M.D.
Professor & Chairman, Medicine-
  Radiology
University of Virginia School of
  Medicine

Jon Kerner, Ph.D.
Assistant Deputy Director for
  Research, Dissemination, and
  Diffusion
National Cancer Institute

Diane Makuc, Ph.D.
Director, Division of Health and
  Utilization Analysis
National Center for Health
  Statistics

Bill McPhee
Mi3 Venture Capitol

John Neugebauer
Vice President of Marketing
Transcan Medical

Lee Newcomer, M.D.
EVP and Chief Medical Officer
Vivius, Inc.

Harold C. Sox, Jr., M.D.
Chairman, Dartmouth Hitchcock
   Medical Center

Alicia Toledano, Sc.D.,
Assistant Professor
Center for Statistical Sciences
Brown University

Charles Turkelson, Ph.D.
Chief Research Analyst
Health Technology Assessment
   Group
ECRI

## OTHER CONTRIBUTORS TO THE STUDY:

Karen Colbert
NCI Financial Management
   Branch

Rosemary Cuddy
NCI Division of Extramural
   Activities

Jeff Garwin
UltraTouch, Corporation

Marilyn Gaston
NCI Inquiry and Reporting
   Section

Constantine Gatsonis
Brown University

Richard Hartman
NIH Center for Information
   Technology

Hugh Hill
Health Care Financing
   Administration

Robert Kraus
Los Alamos National Laboratory

Robert Kruger
Optosonics, Inc

Herchel Lawson
Centers for Disease Control and
   Prevention

Anna Levy
NCI Office of Women's Health

Liz Lostumbo
National Breast Cancer Coalition

Morgan Nields
Fischer Imaging, Inc.

Daniel Schultz
Food and Drug Administration

Steven Seelig
Vysis, Inc.

Robert Smith
American Cancer Society

Earl Steinberg
Covance Health Economics and
   Outcomes Services Inc.

Celia Witten
Food and Drug Administration

Stacey Young-McCaughan
U.S. Army Medical Research and
    Material Command
Breast Cancer Research Program

# Index